Vertebral Manipulation

Fourth Edition

By the same author

Peripheral Manipulation

Vertebral Manipulation

Fourth Edition

G. D. Maitland
AUA, FCSP, MAPA

Part-time Senior Lecturer and Clinical Tutor for the 'Graduate Diploma in Advanced Manipulative Therapy' within the School of Physiotherapy of the South Australian Institute of Technology, Adelaide

with a contribution by

D. A. Brewerton
MD, FRCP

Consultant Physician, Rheumatology Department, Westminster Hospital, London

BUTTERWORTHS
LONDON - BOSTON
Sydney - Wellington - Durban - Toronto

The Butterworth Group

United Kingdom	Butterworth & Co (Publishers) Ltd
London	88 Kingsway, WC2B 6AB
Australia	Butterworths Pty Ltd
Sydney	586 Pacific Highway, Chatswood, NSW 2067 Also at Melbourne, Brisbane, Adelaide and Perth
South Africa	Butterworth & Co (South Africa) (Pty) Ltd
Durban	152–154 Gale Street
New Zealand	Butterworths of New Zealand Ltd
Wellington	77–85 Customhouse Quay, 1, CPO Box 472
Canada	Butterworth & Co (Canada) Ltd
Toronto	2265 Midland Avenue, Scarborough, Ontario, M1P 4S1
USA	Butterworth (Publishers) Inc
Boston	19 Cummings Park, Woburn, Mass. 01801

First published 1964
Second Edition 1968
Reprinted 1970
Third Edition 1973
Reprinted 1974
Reprinted 1975
Fourth Edition 1977
Reprinted 1978
Reprinted 1979

ISBN 0 407 43505 0

Library of Congress Cataloging in Publication Data
Maitland, Geoffrey Douglas.
Vertebral manipulation.

Includes bibliographical references and index.
1. Spine-Diseases. 2. Manipulation (Therapeutics)
1. Title. [DNLM: 1. Manipulation, Orthopedic.
RD768.M35 1977 615'.822 76–44222
ISBN 0 407 43505 0

Typeset by Butterworths Litho Preparation Department

Printed in Great Britain by Chapel River Press, Andover, Hants.

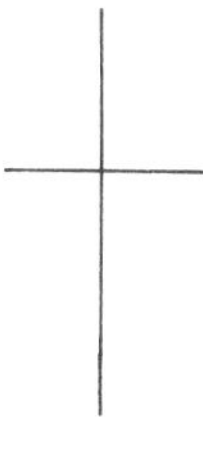

To my wife Anne
for her continuing patience and encouragement

Contents

Preface to the Fourth Edition

Education in the use of passive movement treatment has improved and grown rapidly in the last few years. However, some courses being conducted give cause for concern. Many types are conducted: one-week courses, two-week courses, weekend courses etc., none of them including supervised treatment of patients. Regrettably, some physiotherapists, having taken part in these short courses, then feel they are competent manipulators. Efforts should be directed to the time when such courses will be substituted by long-term courses with the necessary inclusion of adequate supervised treatment of patients.

Courses now exist which do include the vital sections of teaching supervised treatment of patients. These courses should be encouraged. Even with these courses it is necessary to emphasize to graduates that at least a further 1500 hours of clinical experience are required to reach the standard when they will be sufficiently critical of their own work to venture further, trying other techniques and combinations of techniques for different disorders.

It seems fitting to include in this edition a comprehensive chapter on 'Assessment' as it is assessment which makes up 90 per cent of the effective management of all patients treated by passive movement techniques. Assessment guides treatment throughout and provides constructive information to all: the doctor, the patient and the physiotherapist.

Two appendices explaining the depth of movement tests are included. They explain how movements can be effected and how they vary in their relationships to each other.

I am grateful to the people who have given considerable thought to their reviews of earlier editions. Many valuable points have helped to improve the text which follows. I would again like to thank my wife for her additional help, especially with the drawings.

Adelaide G. D. Maitland

Preface to the First Edition

Manipulation of the spine is associated so often with false diagnoses and 'hit or miss' methods of brute force. These associations have resulted in the exclusion of manipulative treatment from routine physical medicine. The cautious and apprehensive attitude towards this treatment would be largely eliminated if it were recognized that most patients can be relieved by the gentler procedures.

There are two ways of manipulating the conscious patient. The first, better thought of as mobilization, is the gentler coaxing of a movement by passive rhythmical oscillations performed within or at the limit of the range; the second is the forcing of a movement from the limit of the range by a sudden thrust. The difference between these two techniques may seem negligible when comparing a strongly applied mobilization with a gentle manipulative thrust, but there is an important difference. The patient can always resist the mobilization if it should become too painful, whereas the suddenness of the forceful manipulation prevents any control by the patient.

The practical approach to the use of manipulation is to relate treatment to the patient's symptoms and signs rather than to diagnoses. Such a plan avoids both the confusion caused by diagnostic titles calling to mind different symptoms to different people, and the controversy over pathology. Indeed, it is often impossible to know what the true pathology is. Also it will be agreed that under the umbrella of one diagnostic title, for example 'disc lesion', symptoms and signs may vary widely and require different treatments.

Only the spinal joints from the occiput to the sacrum are discussed in this book, and the text has been planned to lead the reader in logical sequence from the examination of the different intervertebral levels to the techniques of mobilization applicable in each case. The way is then prepared for further development into the more forceful manipulative procedures and their application. Guiding principles of treatment follow and are then applied to specific case histories in the final chapter. It should be understood that all treatment in this book when done by physiotherapists is only carried out on medical referral.

To the many people who have contributed so much towards the

final presentation of this book I am unable to express adequately my gratitude. Without the constructive help of those concerned with the typing and posing for the diagrams, my work would have been much more difficult.

Particular people were asked to undertake the task of reading and criticizing the manuscript in detail, so that it might meet as nearly as possible the needs for which it was undertaken and I am sure that they will be able to see how invaluable their guidance has been. In particular I wish to express my sincere thanks to Miss M. J. Hammond, A.U.A., M.C.S.P. (Teachers Cert.), Miss J-M. Ganne, M.C.S.P. (Teachers Cert.) Miss. M. Martin-Jones, M.C.S.P. (Teachers Cert.), Dr. A. W. Burnell, D.Phys.Med., Mrs. H. B. Culshaw, B.A., Dip.Ed., Mr. Lansell Bonnin, M.Ch.(Orth.), F.R.C.S. and Dr. Bryan Gandevia, M.D., B.S. (Melb.), M.R.A.C.P. (Consultant Editor, *Australian Journal of Physiotherapy*). These persons by their individual comments and criticisms gave considerable guidance concerning different aspects of the work, namely the teaching of physiotherapy students, medical acceptance and composition. My thanks are due also to my wife who so painstakingly produced all the drawings.

I am most grateful for the courtesy extended to me during a recent study tour in Great Britain, the United States of America and Canada.

Adelaide G. D. Maitland

1 The Doctor's Role in Diagnosis and Prescribing Vertebral Manipulation

By D. A. Brewerton, M.D., F.R.C.P.

Every patient who is to undergo spinal mobilization or manipulation by a physiotherapist should have consulted a doctor, who has the dual responsibility of determining the diagnosis and deciding the best treatment. Therefore the first purpose of this chapter is to indicate to doctors the types of patient who should or should not be referred to a physiotherapist for manipulation, mobilization or traction of the spine. The main emphasis is on the contraindications to such treatment. Unfortunately, any guide to doctors cannot yet be based on an analysis of proven facts. So far there have been few detailed studies of the results of treatment or controlled trials. These have begun and many more will follow, but several years will pass before they can act as a basis for a comprehensive scheme of treatment. At present it is essential to draw on the experience and impressions of many doctors and therapists.

The physiotherapist must assess and examine the patient before treatment is begun and repeatedly during a course of treatment. Without the ability to do this no physiotherapist should undertake the forms of treatment Mr. Maitland describes. This type of examination is detailed and expert, but largely confined to the musculoskeletal system. Consequently the second purpose of this chapter is to outline for physiotherapists some of the broader issues which a doctor must consider in his assessment.

Success depends largely on collaboration between doctor and physiotherapist. The doctor must explain to the therapist his clinical findings and general approach to treatment, and he must be prepared to discuss changes in the clinical situation which may develop during the course of treatment. The therapist does not require instructions in the details of treatment just in the broad aims.

ORGANIC DISORDERS NOT INVOLVING THE VERTEBRAE

The clinical history and examination by the doctor are essential in excluding a wide variety of disorders which may simulate spinal pain (Table 1.1). Special attention is always given to the patient who can move the relevant part of the spine freely without discomfort.

TABLE 1.1
Disorders which may Simulate Spinal Pain

Cervical pain	*Lumbar pain*
Malignant lymphadenopathy	Peptic ulcer
Pancoast tumour	Renal disease
Vertebral artery syndrome	Pancreatic carcinoma
Subarachnoid haemorrhage	Obstruction of aorta or iliac arteries
Coronary artery disease	Carcinoma of colon or rectum
Polymyalgia rheumatica	Other pelvic carcinoma
	Endometriosis
Thoracic pain	Pregnancy
Bronchogenic carcinoma	Disseminated sclerosis
Other lung disease	Spinal cord tumour
Coronary artery disease	Hip disease
Aortic aneurysm	Short leg
Massive cardiac enlargement	
Hiatus hernia	
Gall bladder disease	
Herpes zoster	

Most of the more serious diseases which are commonly quoted in textbooks seldom cause diagnostic difficulties. More problems are caused by gall disease, hiatus hernia or angina presenting with dorsal pain, or relatively minor peptic ulceration causing lumbar backache. Occlusion of the aorta or iliac arteries may present with lumbar pain on walking. No patient with dorsal pain should be treated without having had a chest radiograph.

There is no indication for manipulation if the cause of pain is not within the spine.

Pregnancy

Pregnancy in the last months is regarded by some authorities as a contraindication to manipulation. It is true that the pregnancy presents mechanical and technical problems, but, if marked pain is clearly originating within the spine, there is no absolute bar to manipulation provided sensible precautions are taken.

Disease of the spinal cord or cauda equina

Disease of the spinal cord or cauda equina or any evidence of pressure on them is an absolute contraindication to any form of mobilization or manipulation. This applies even to the slightest symptoms, such as mild bilateral paraesthesiae in the feet. The term 'spinal stenosis' describes a clinical syndrome which is usually produced by a massive disc protrusion compressing the cauda equina. This results in pain in both legs, with progressive pain, numbness and weakness on walking, and is easily mistaken for intermittent claudication due to peripheral arterial disease.

The vertebral arteries

The vertebral arteries may be occluded by atherosclerosis, or by disease or deformity of the spine. Some of the very rare tragedies following manipulation have been due to occlusion of the vertebral arteries, particularly on rotation of the neck. Before any mobilization or manipulation of the neck it is essential to ask specifically for any symptoms suggesting vertebral artery disease, particularly any giddiness or disturbance of vision related to neck posture. The physiotherapist should gently rotate the neck fully in both directions and hold each position for a few seconds to be certain that this does not produce symptoms before attempting even gentle mobilization.

VERTEBRAL DISEASE

A classification of the vertebral causes of spinal pain includes many well-known pathological disorders (Table 1.2). In practice most patients have changes which are difficult to classify and it is usually impossible to make a precise anatomical diagnosis. There is often a basis of underlying degenerative change and this is sometimes aggravated by strains and minor trauma.

General medical assessment and radiographs of the spine are essential before advising manipulation of the spine at any level.

Spondylolisthesis

Spondylolisthesis is a contraindication to forceful manipulation at that level but treatment is often successful when directed to the relief of a pain orginating higher in the spine.

Osteoporosis

Osteoporosis is an absolute contraindication to manipulation, and this restriction applies also to conditions likely to cause osteoporosis, including treatment with steroids. Age in itself is not a contraindication to manipulation and some of the most worthwhile results are obtained in older patients.

TABLE 1.2
Vertebral Causes of Spinal Pain

Developmental
- Spondylolisthesis
- Scoliosis
- Hypermobility
- Various uncommon disorders

Degenerative
- Disc lesions without root compression
- Disc lesions with root compression
- Disc lesions with compression of spinal cord or cauda equina
- Osteoarthrosis of apophyseal joints
- Hyperostosis
- Instability

Trauma
- Fracture
- Stress fracture
- Subluxation
- Ligamentous injury

Tumour
- Secondary carcinoma
- Myelomatosis

Infection
- Staphylococcal
- Tuberculous
- *E. coli*
- *Brucella melitensis*

Inflammatory arthropathy
- Ankylosing spondylitis
- Rheumatoid arthritis
- Reiter's disease
- Ulcerative colitis
- Crohn's disease
- Psoriasis

Metabolic
- Osteoporosis
- Osteomalacia

Unknown
- Paget's disease

Ankylosing spondylitis and rheumatoid arthritis

Ankylosing spondylitis and rheumatoid arthritis both commonly affect the spinal ligaments, which occasionally may lead to subluxation within the cervical spine and rarely to sudden death. Evidence of any inflammatory arthropathy of the spine is an absolute contra-indication to neck manipulation, even if there is no clinical or radiological evidence that the involvement includes the cervical spine.

Root pain

Root pain due to a disc protrusion or any local degenerative disorder may dominate the clinical picture, producing much more pain and more restriction of spinal movement than its underlying cause. It is one of the first essentials to decide whether or not there is an element of root pain before choosing the best treatment for a patient. This is easy if there is a full root distribution of pain accompanied by paraesthesiae, but very difficult when the involvement is partial. The extent of the radiation of pain may help: if it is beyond the elbow or the knee, root involvement is probable. It is also more likely if the pain includes paraesthesiae or other qualities suggesting nerve irritation. With root involvement, a gentle spinal movement may readily produce radiation of pain to a greater distance than would otherwise be expected; and maintenance of a spinal posture, such as rotation of the neck away from the pain, may reproduce the root symptoms if the position is held for 10–20 seconds.

Manipulation

Experts do not all agree whether patients with root symptoms should be subjected to forceful manipulation. Some claim that it is justified if there are no neurological signs; others advocate manipulation provided the symptoms do not extend beyond the elbow or the knee, using the argument that reference of pain that far need not imply root involvement. My own practice is to avoid forceful manipulation for all patients with any evidence of nerve root involvement, but this is a controversial issue which will not be settled until there have been detailed studies of patients with root symptoms to determine more accurately which do well and which do badly. While this knowledge is awaited, it is probably wise to exclude from forceful manipulation all patients whose symptoms appear to arise from root compression, however mild; but to permit manipulation of patients with pain of a similar distribution, provided that it is confidently diagnosed as being due to spinal derangement without root involvement. Nevertheless, it must be admitted that physiotherapists who are expert at passive mobilization and manipulation sometimes produce dramatic relief of symptoms from arm pain or sciatica, even when there are neurological signs. Also, it is probably right to make an exception when a patient has root symptoms of very long standing and then appears to get a stiff neck or back due to a mechanical derangement of the spine unrelated to the chronic nerve root pain.

Traction

Traction can be applied constantly to a patient confined to bed with severe root pain arising in the cervical or the lumbar spine, or intermittently on an out-patient basis. Traction in bed is used mostly for patients with particularly painful sciatica which has not settled after treatment by bed rest alone. The traction undoubtedly immobilizes the lumbar spine more effectively and probably the distraction aids in pain relief.

Intermittent traction

Intermittent traction on an out-patient basis is preferably given daily and can be applied to the cervical or lumbar spine. Cervical traction for patients with arm pain thought to be due to root compression has been the subject of a thorough study (Original Article, 1966). This showed that virtually every patient had marked relief of pain during the application of the traction, which was usually applied with the head in a flexed position. Often the pain relief lasted for a matter of hours, but the treatment did not influence the natural history of the condition or the long-term results. Three-quarters of the patients improved substantially within a month whether traction was used or not. This means that intermittent traction for out-patients should probably be reserved for patients with severe pain, who will be grateful for the temporary relief of pain even if the overall rate of recovery is not improved. Lumbar traction is commonly applied to patients with sciatic pain, although there has not yet been an adequate statistical evaluation of the results.

Impending root compression

Patients between the ages of 15 and 35 who develop acute lumbar or cervical pain are more likely to have true disc protrusions than older

Original Article (1966). 'Pain in the neck and arm: a multicentre trial of the effects of physiotherapy.' *Br. med. J.* **1**, 253 patients. Lumbar pain in the younger age group frequently presents in a way that suggests the likelihood of sciatica in the near future, and this is a contraindication to manipulation.

The remainder

Although the great majority of patients who complain of spinal pain cannot be classified or diagnosed accurately, this mixed and complicated group contains the patients who are most suitable for treatment by spinal mobilization or manipulation. The essence of selection is to choose patients whose pain originates in the spine and then exclude all those in whom there is any evidence of involvement of spinal cord, cauda equina, nerve roots or vertebral arteries, and those with any evidence of disease affecting their vertebrae or spinal ligaments.

In the management of this large remainder there are virtually no absolute contraindications to treatment, provided the correct techniques, as outlined by Mr. Maitland, are chosen. The main objects of treatment are to use the gentlest techniques that will produce the desired result and to modify the treatment on the basis of the patient's progress and repeated reassessments by the physiotherapist. Treatment starting with gentle mobilization and a small amplitude of movement should be perfectly safe for all patients in this mixed group. Everything depends on the techniques used: no-one would recommend the use of traction for a patient with acute lumbar back pain or forceful manipulation for a patient with sciatica or brachial neuropathy accompanied by neurological signs.

Some authorities advocate more clear-cut indications for treatment based on more accurate diagnosis, but it is doubtful whether such accuracy is really feasible. Although the origin of the pain may be located at the correct level within the spine, in the absence of root symptoms it is often only possible to make intelligent guesses as to whether the cause is a degenerative or protruded disc, vertebral instability, degenerative changes in an apophyseal joint, a torn interspinous ligament or some other precise diagnosis. Furthermore, it is impossible to give definite indications and contraindications for treatment within this ill-defined group of patients. Nor is it wise to say categorically which techniques are most likely to be effective: different manipulators get their best results with different techniques. At present all that can be said is that when these patients are treated by experienced physiotherapists many of them do well and they appear to recover more rapidly than with other methods. Regrettably we must await more detailed investigations and assessments before anything is more definite.

POSTURE AND WORK

Any physiotherapist treating a patient with spinal pain should automatically review with the patient the use of his spine for all everyday activities, emphasizing any posture or movement that aggravates the pain. It is wrong to concentrate on spinal mobilization while the patient is regularly making the pain worse by some unwise posture or by a repeated activity at work.

PSYCHOLOGICAL FACTORS

Pure psychogenic pain in the neck or back is not common, but virtually all chronic spinal pains are influenced by social and psychological circumstances, and the doctor's assessment is never complete if based on physical grounds alone. Given a chance to talk, many patients with these symptoms pour out their problems and make it obvious that they are suffering from depression, anxiety, marital or social problems or something else which demands help in its own right. Sometimes the patient has been told that he has 'arthritis of the spine' and he wishes to be protected from the ravages of a widespread, crippling disease.

While it is true that patients whose symptoms are predominantly psychological in origin may benefit considerably from manipulation and the general support given by the physiotherapist, this approach to treatment can never be an adequate substitute for psychological help, and better long-term results are usually obtained by doctor and patient facing up to the real problems. Furthermore, prolonged physical treatment with indifferent results may confirm the patient's suspicions that he has an organic disease which is too difficult to treat. This description applies to many patients who go from therapist to therapist receiving years of unsuccessful treatment.

Among patients with chronic spinal pain there are many with moderate or severe depression. They reject immediately any suggestion that their problems are psychological and usually they will not talk about their problems until they have received a course of anti-depressive drugs or other treatment. This is a much better approach for most of them than retreat into physical treatment.

A chronic anxiety state may be a form of depression, to be treated accordingly, or it may be based on a personality disorder. Obviously the personality cannot readily be changed, but these patients often have insight and recognize that they have had other symptoms due to tension. They may be surprisingly willing to discuss their pain in psychological terms. An explanation that 'some tense people get peptic ulcers, while others have tense neck muscles and a painful neck' may be understood and accepted, with obvious relief that the cause is nothing more serious.

Sometimes a double approach is required. When a patient cannot accept at once that his pain is psychological in origin he may tolerate the suggestion that psychological factors predominate provided he is also told that he has a minor organic condition which will probably respond to physical treatment.

2 Examination

Intelligent manipulative treatment is based on appreciation of the history of the patient's complaint and interpretation of the examination findings. It is taken for granted that all non-skeletal causes are excluded by the referring doctor. In mechanical problems of spinal joints the examination is concentrated on finding the intervertebral level responsible for the symptoms and assessing how movement of the joint has been affected.

A plan which encourages a clear and methodical examination progresses through the subjective section of the examination to the objective section, with a 'planning' stage interposed between them. The planning stage forces the inexperienced person to relate mentally the many facts of the patient's story to the parts which will require examination. These processes are carried out automatically by the experienced physiotherapist and do not require adherence to such a fixed plan. The inexperienced person, however, must have a starting point to encourage clarity and a systematic approach.

Although throughout this book the diagrams show both the patient and the operator as males, it would complicate the descriptive text if both patient and operator were referred to as 'he'. Some readers and reviewers have commented on this discrepancy though they all point out that it is of minor consequence. The word 'she' referring to the operator is deliberately chosen in an attempt to help emphasize the fact that passive movement treatment techniques can be very gentle procedures and that the additional strength a male manipulator may have is not necessary for the stronger manipulative techniques. One of the writer's aims is to present the subject of manipulation as one requiring skill rather than strength.

SUBJECTIVE EXAMINATION

The subjective examination relates to the patient's account of his complaint and past history. Methods of questioning will vary from patient to patient because although some patients are excellent witnesses, others frequently appear unable to understand some questions or to answer them simply. Skill in extracting the appropriate information requires care, patience and a critical attitude. If the technique is good much can be gained in addition to the answers to the questions. The patient gains confidence in the physiotherapist who in turn is able to understand the patient's plight. The influences of heredity and environment must be appreciated and it is necessary to remember that this colours the examiner's thinking as well as the patient's.

Communication is difficult and full of pitfalls. First the physiotherapist may not word the question in a way which clearly expresses what she has in mind to ask. Then the words used in the question may not mean the same to the patient as they do to the questioner, or the patient may misunderstand what is being asked. He may have problems which are important to him and he may incorrectly assume the question is directed at these. And so there are all manner of difficulties to spoil what is often assumed wrongly to be a simple process of discussion.

To make it easier for the patient, only one question should be asked at a time and it should be persisted with, within reason, until the answer is obtained. The question can be directed in different ways if it is not clearly understood by the patient and it should be carefully worded to avoid influencing the answer. It the patient gives what seems to be an incongruous answer to the question then the fault may lie in the way the question was put. It is kinder to rephrase or explain the question than to restate the question, even if it was so simply put that the error must have been the patient's. It is essential to approach each interview with a degree of humility and charity.

The first step in the subjective examination is to ascertain the area, depth, nature, behaviour and chronology of the patient's symptoms and to record those on a 'body chart'. Areas of sensory disturbance should also be included as should curt comments regarding areas of maximum intensity and type of pain. Reference to such a body chart gives a quick and clear reminder of the patient's symptoms.

The position of the pain in regard to area and depth may sometimes be related to dermatomes, myotomes and sclerotomes (*Figures 2.1–2.3*), and areas of paraesthesia or anaesthesia, particularly of distal distribution, can clearly indicate which nerve root may be involved.

The behaviour of the patient's pain with various activities will indicate how it affects him and give an idea of its severity. Questions should elicit facts against which subsequent progress can be evaluated. For example, a patient may say he can walk as far as the front gate

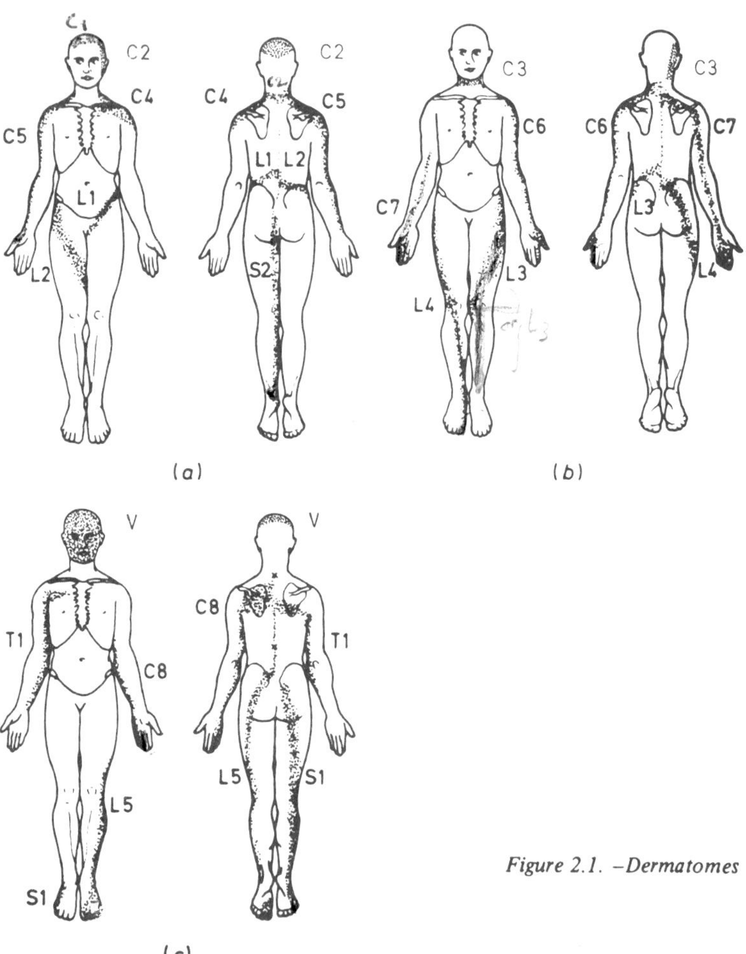

Figure 2.1. –Dermatomes

before his leg pain becomes severe. This fact is a basis for assessing progress if during treatment he reaches the stage of being able to walk further than the front gate. These subjective assessments then become objective facts.

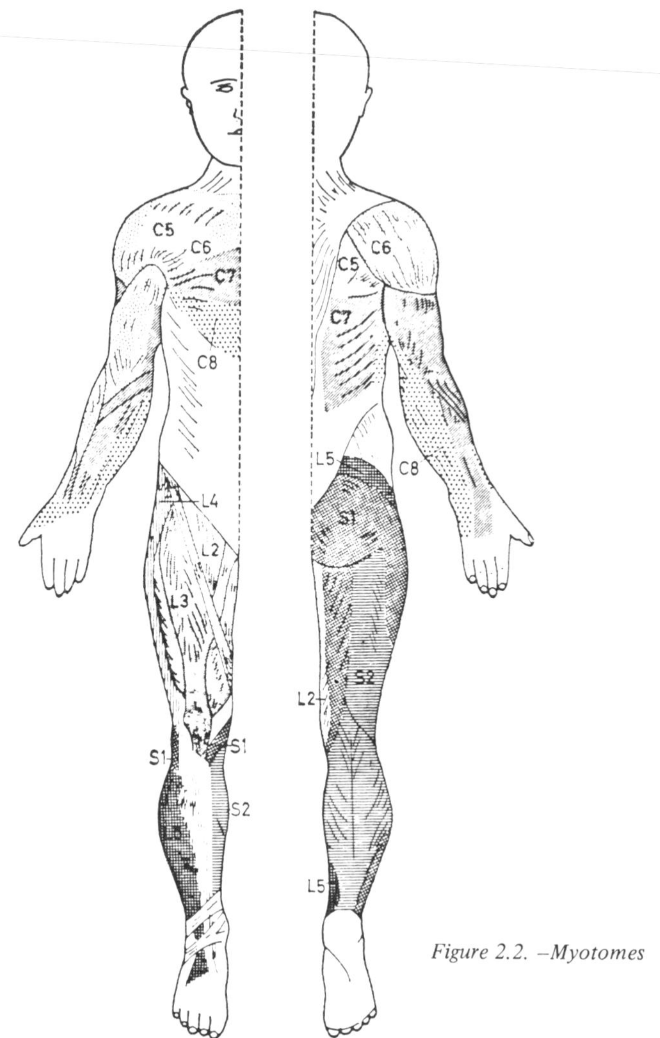

Figure 2.2. –Myotomes

Questions should be asked to determine how easily the patient's symptoms are aggravated by his activities and how readily the symptoms subside so that exacerbation of symptoms from excessive examination can be avoided. This is later referred to as 'irritability'.

No matter whether the patient's pain is constant or intermittent, present at rest or on activity, there will be movements, positions or

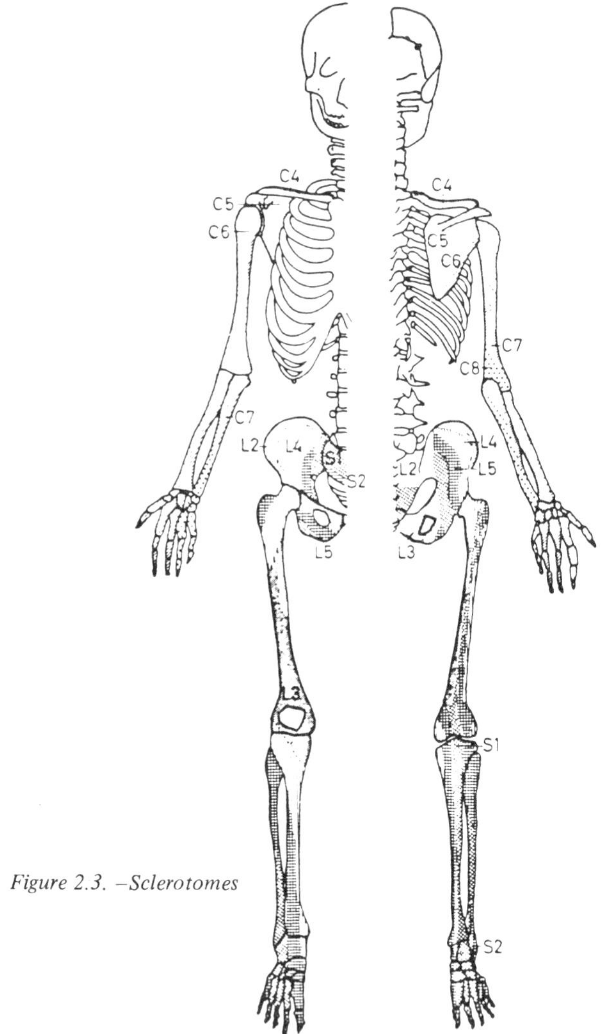

Figure 2.3. –Sclerotomes

activities which will aggravate or ease the pain. These positions or activities should be carefully noted as they may well guide the choice of positions to be adopted or avoided during treatment.

Care is required when assessing the effect of rest on pain. Frequently the patient will say the pain is worse when in bed, when in fact the symptoms may only be worse for the first hour or so as a result of the day's activities. On further questioning the pain is found to be considerably relieved by the following morning. However, pain which is worse at night and which is severe enough to make the patient get out of bed requires careful investigation because of the possibility of more serious pathology than the mechanical problems usually referred for physiotherapy.

Great difficulty can be encountered when endeavouring to assess the severity of the patient's pain. Different people have different pain thresholds (Keele, 1967) which have physiological and psychological bases. Assessment of pain may be assisted by applying stretch to one or two of the patient's normal joints while watching his reaction. Weighing this information against his history and his description of what he is unable to do because of his pain will all help in assessment.

The aim of the questioning is to know the patient's pain and problems so completely that the physiotherapist is able to 'live' them herself. It is then a natural step to ask about the onset and history of the present episode before asking about relevant previous history. Putting 'history' at the end of the sequence facilitates constructive questioning for the inexperienced physiotherapist.

PLANNING

Clinical evidence and experimental work have shown that pain from a muscle lesion is localized to the site of the lesion, although it spreads in area as the intensity increases. Lesions of synovial joints and the supporting inert structures on the other hand, although usually causing pain localized to the joint, can also cause pain referred for some distance from the joint. Synovial joint lesions can sometimes be responsible for referred pain without any pain in the region of the joint. For example the osteroarthritic hip causing knee pain is well known and lesions of the vertebral column frequently refer pain to the abdomen and thorax. Clinical investigation has shown that the intervertebral disc is capable of causing local and referred pain without any sign of herniation or nerve root compression (Cloward, 1959). It would seem that this pain is never more pronounced in the distal segment of a dermatome. However, when herniation of disc material compresses a nerve root the pain is commonly felt more severely in a distal area such as the

Keele, K. E. (1967). 'Discussion on research into pain.' *Practitioner,* **198,** 287
Cloward, R. B. (1959). 'Cervical diskography. A contribution to the etiology of neck shoulder and arm pain.' *Ann. Surg.* **150,** 1052

calf or forearm. Symptoms can be referred into superficial areas which may become hyperaesthetic (Glover, 1960), or into the muscles, making them tender, or they may be referred to joints which may then become painful on movement (Brain, 1957).

Following the subjective examination the inexperienced person should plan the objective examination of the patient. The plan can be considered in four sections:

(A) With a thorough knowledge of the patterns of pain from disorders affecting muscles, discs, synovial joints and nerve roots, it is possible to list the names of the joints and muscles which must be examined as a possible cause of pain.

1. The joints which lie under the area of pain.
2. The joints which do not lie under the area of pain but can refer pain into the area.
3. The muscles which lie under the area of pain.

(B) The second part to consider is the effect of the pain on the patient.

(C) The third indicates the kind of examination (for example the extent and strength of test movements) required.

(D) The last aspect deals with examination of the underlying abnormalities to ascertain the reasons which may have predisposed to the onset of the patient's pain, or which may, if uncorrected, lead to recurrences.

An example of such a 'Planning the Examination' sheet is shown in Table 2.2 on Page 74.

In the discussion which follows in this text, aspects of examination relating to general health, posture, muscle balance and other allied factors are omitted. They have been omitted deliberately for the purpose of emphasizing the aspects which are so vital to the choice of the mobilizing and manipulating techniques to be used during treatment and to the assessment of their effect.

An example will make the point of 'planning' clearer, and in this example the word 'joint' refers to the inert structures affected by passive movement.

A patient has pain spreading from C6 to T6 centrally and laterally across the left posterior thoracic wall from the top of the shoulder to the inferior angle of the scapula. The pain spreads into the left

Glover, J. R. (1960). 'Back pain and hyperaesthesia.' *Lancet* **1**, 1165
Brain, Sir Russell (1957). 'The treatment of pain.' *S. Afr. med. J.* **31**, 973

triceps area and down the posterior aspects of the forearm to the wrist. If the spread of pain from joints, muscles or nerve root lesions is borne in mind, it will be necessary to examine the following structures as being the possible cause, in part or in full, of these symptoms.

The joints which lie under the area of pain

C6 to T6
Left costovertebral joints T1 to T6
Intercostal movement between ribs 1 to 6 on the left
Scapulothoracic movement on the left
Left glenohumeral joint and rotator cuff
Left elbow
Left wrist

The joints which do not lie under the area of pain but can refer pain into the area

(Other joints need to be included to allow for a pre- or post-fixed plexus and for errors of interpretation of pain areas)
C4 to C6
T6 to T8 including the costovertebral joints and intercostal movement

The muscles which lie under the area of pain

Elevators and retractors of scapula
Extensors of elbow
Extensors of wrist and fingers

Experienced physiotherapists will only briefly examine some of the structures listed because the history and behaviour of the pain make it clear that these structures are unlikely to be causing pain. However, such examination should never be completely omitted on the *assumption* that they are *not* contributing to the pain.

OBJECTIVE EXAMINATION

The purpose of the physiotherapist's objective examination is to (*a*) interpret the patient's concept of his disability in terms of muscles, joints and nerves causing pain, and (*b*) to determine physical factors which may have predisposed to the onset of pain. It is possible by tests using isometric resisted contraction and passive movements to differentiate between pain from muscles and pain from joints. It is also necessary to make assessment of active movements to indicate the functional limits caused by the condition and to show the patient's willingness to move.

When the inert structures of a joint are painful passive movement of that joint will be painful at some point in the range. To elicit the pain it may be necessary to move the joint while holding the joint surfaces compressed or to test accessory movements. When a lesion occurs in a muscle, passive joint movement will not be painful unless it is a movement which stretches or pinches the muscle. However, pain will always be reproduced when fibres involved in the lesion are made to contract strongly. Joint problems are therefore determined by passive movement tests and muscular lesions by isometric muscle contraction tests which exclude joint movement.

The passive and isometric tests do not always provide clear answers, because an isometric test necessarily results in compression of the joint surface. Similarly, isometric tests in the lumbar and cervical areas always produce considerable intervertebral movement. Under these circumstances the isometric test may cause pain because the joint is moving. Therefore it may be necessary to test the muscle isometrically in different positions of the joint range and to compare the degree of pain produced by an active resisted movement with that of a passive movement.

The examination of a joint does not differentiate between pain caused by the intervertebral disc, the apophyseal joints or their ligaments. It does however reveal a disturbance of movement. It should be remembered that consideration of movement must not be limited to that of the disc and apophyseal joints. The spinal cord and its investments and the nerve roots with their sleeves must be able to move freely in the vertebral canal and intervertebral foramen. Tests for movement of these structures must also be part of the physiotherapist's objective examination.

The examination of the intervertebral segment can be divided into the following sequence.

1. Active tests
   - (*a*) Active movements.
   - (*b*) Auxiliary tests associated with active movements tests, for example joint compression tests and tests for vertebral artery insufficiency.
2. Passive tests
   - (*c*) Movement of the pain-sensitive structures in the vertebral canal and intervertebral foramen. Neurological examination forms an essential part of the examination of the neural elements.
   - (*d*) Palpation.
   - (*e*) Passive range of intervertebral movement.

Active tests

When a joint is found to cause pain a careful assessment of active and passive movements should be made. The active movements should be tested first because the patient will perform these within his own limits of pain, and therefore in safety; the assessment of these movements will indicate the severity of the disability and guide the examiner in how much passive handling the joint will tolerate. Active movements of the thoracic and lumbar spine are tested in standing, except for rotation which is best tested in sitting. Sitting is also the position most suitable for testing cervical movements because the trunk is more stable.

Before testing movement, the patient's present symptoms should be assessed. If he has no pain before moving he should be asked to bend in the direction being tested until pain is felt; if he has some pain present before moving, he should be asked to bend until the pain begins to increase. Measurement of this range should be made noting the area in which pain is caused by the movement. If the pain is not severe nor of a kind which must not be aggravated, the patient should be asked to move further into the range reporting any increase in severity of pain or alteration in its distribution so that the severity and behaviour of the pain with the further movement can be determined.

When no restrictions need to be placed on the examination of movements the patient should be encouraged to move to the limit of the range and the physiotherapist should then apply controlled over-pressure to determine the 'end-feel' of the movement.

This over-pressure is essential if, on examination, a movement appears to be full range and painless. It is incorrect to record the movement as normal unless pressure producing small oscillatory movements can be applied painlessly at the limit of the range. Care is required when applying this over-pressure to certain movements. With cervical extension, whether the pressure is applied by lifting under the chin or pressing against the forehead, care should be exercised to prevent it being merely one of traction or compression. Cervical lateral flexion should be tested with the physiotherapist's hands placed on either side of the patient's head and neck. She places the hand, on the side to which the patient bends, against the articular pillar, localizing the movement with the ulnar border of her hand, and the other hand she places against the side of the patient's head.

When pain is produced on either flexion or extension of the neck it is possible to differentiate between an upper and lower cervical disorder by extending the upper cervical spine while flexing the lower cervical spine. This movement is achieved by asking the patient to poke his chin forward. Similarly, by retracting the head the upper cervical spine can be flexed while the lower spine is extended. Comparison of pain caused by these two movements with that produced by the normal flexion and extension tests can indicate whether it is the upper or lower joints causing pain.

There are three points to be mentioned in relation to testing active movements which apply when a movement reveals little in the way of pain.

1. Occasionally it is necessary for a patient to perform a test movement quickly if pain is not provoked by the full range movement performed at the usual speed. For example a patient may say that turning his head is painful yet on examination of movements at the usual speed the movement is normal and over-pressure can be applied at the limit of the range without pain. However, if he is asked to turn his head sharply the pain is frequently reproduced.
2. If a patient says forward flexion of the lumbar spine is not very painful, yet the movement is limited, it is as well to find out how far he was able to bend before his symptoms began. There are some people who cannot reach their toes normally, including some who are unable to reach beyond their knees. Cervical rotation, in the presence of marked spondylitic change, is another movement of which prior knowledge of range is helpful. Stiffness under these circumstances may not be a primary objective sign in the patient's present condition.
3. When flexion of the thoracic and lumbar spines appears to be normal it is useful, particularly if on continued examination little is found, to tap each spinous process sharply in turn either with a reflex hammer or with the finger tips. A joint causing pain is found to respond painfully to this tap-test.

Following the test for range and pain the patient should, provided pain permits, move back and forth from the starting position while the physiotherapist watches for disturbances of the normal rhythm of intervertebral movement. Repeated movements should be avoided if a movement is very painful as they unjustifiably provoke and increase the patient's discomfort. The experienced physiotherapist is able to assess the rhythm of movement during the assessment of movement for range and pain described in the preceding paragraphs. Initially however, the physiotherapist may require the patient to make many movements.

Disturbances of the normal rhythm of intervertebral movement during flexion and lateral flexion of the lumbar and thoracic spines are readily seen from behind (*Figures 2.4* and *2.5*). Abnormalities in trunk

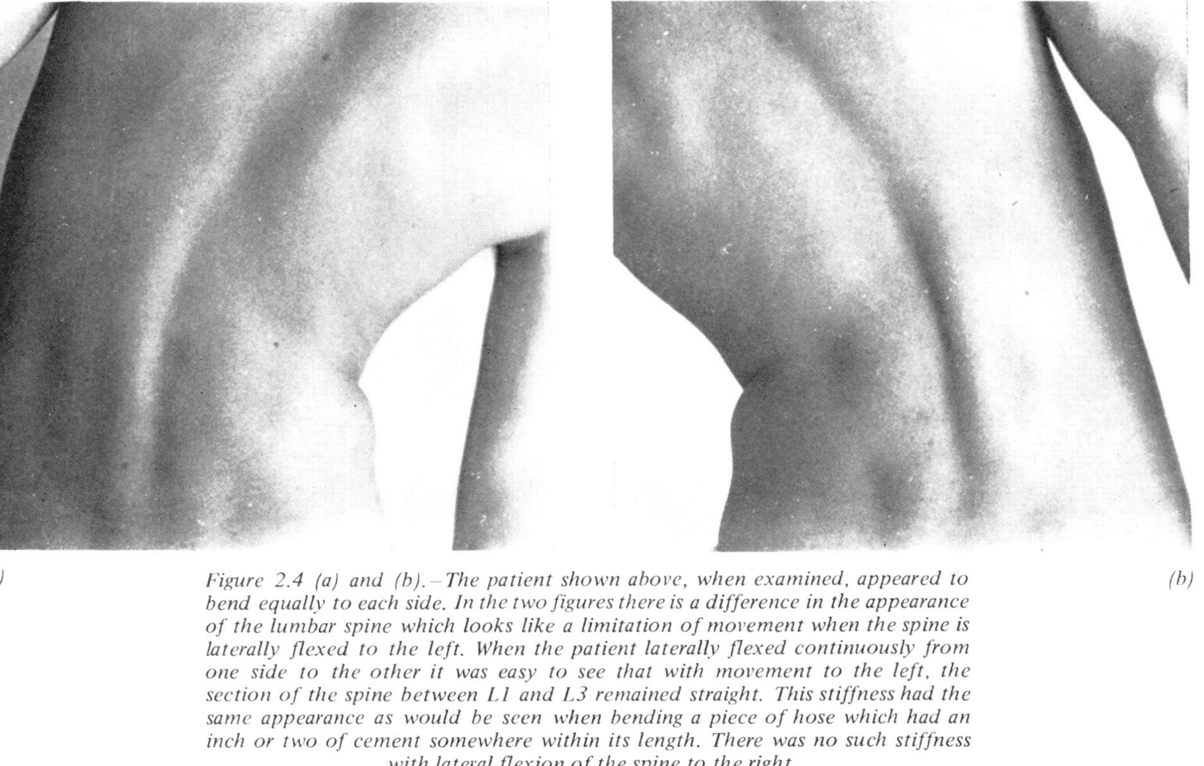

(a) (b)

Figure 2.4 (a) and (b).–The patient shown above, when examined, appeared to bend equally to each side. In the two figures there is a difference in the appearance of the lumbar spine which looks like a limitation of movement when the spine is laterally flexed to the left. When the patient laterally flexed continuously from one side to the other it was easy to see that with movement to the left, the section of the spine between L1 and L3 remained straight. This stiffness had the same appearance as would be seen when bending a piece of hose which had an inch or two of cement somewhere within its length. There was no such stiffness with lateral flexion of the spine to the right

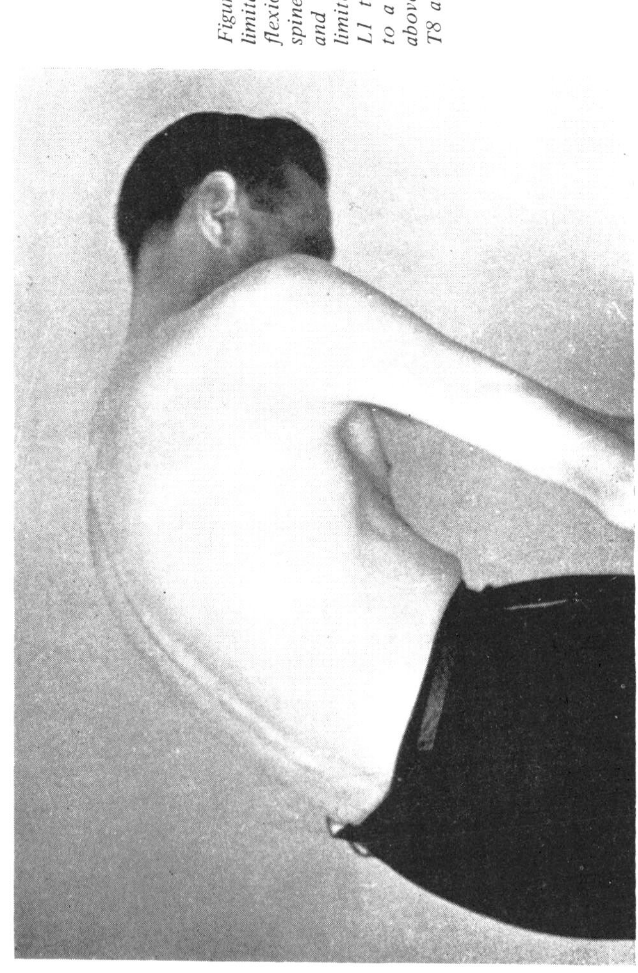

Figure 2.5. – This figure shows a limitation in the range of forward flexion at two levels of the thoracic spine. Between approximately T5 and T8 forward flexion is very limited, whereas between T10 and L1 the movement appears limited to a lesser degree. The movement above T5, below L1 and between T8 and T10 appears to be normal

rotation are much more difficult to notice. To watch intervertebral movement during lumbar extension the physiotherapist may need to kneel behind the patient while supporting his shoulders to prevent overbalancing (*Figure 2.6*).

A patient with low lumbar pain may appear to have a full painless range of extension in standing. If it is thought that the pain may be

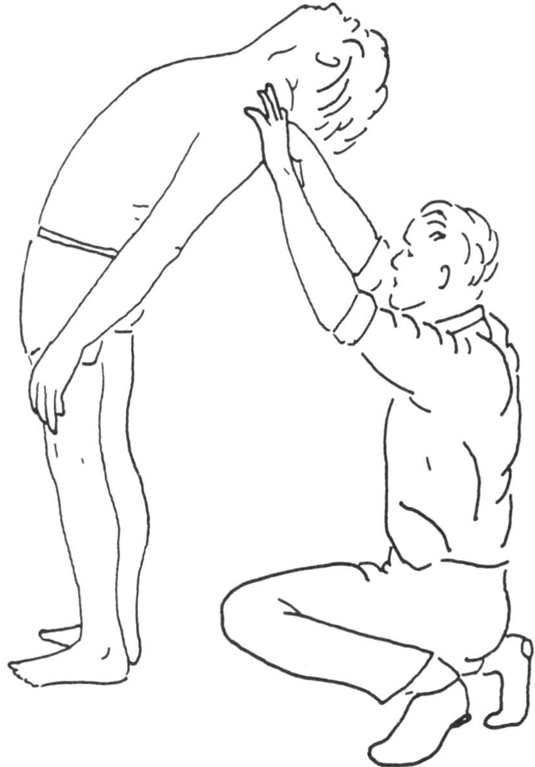

Figure 2.6.– Viewing lumbar extension

coming from the lumbosacral level it is advisable to include the following test: the standing patient should be asked to flex his pelvis (i.e. tuck his tail between his legs as a cat or dog can) and then extend his pelvis. This movement, particularly extension, may reproduce back pain in comparison with a pain-free arching backwards of his trunk. When arching backwards, the movement starts from the top and gradually the lower joints take part in the movement and it is possible that the low lumbar area is so protected by muscle spasm that the movement is pain free. If the extension movement is done in reverse by moving the pelvis, the intervertebral movement starts from the lowest moving joint and then it extends upwards. If pelvic movement reproduces the patient's back pain, the cause will almost certainly lie in the lumbosacral joint.

All cervical movements should be watched carefully from the front as each can reveal useful information (*Figure 2.7*) but the contour of the neck when fully flexed is best seen from behind or above. The patient may rotate his neck with more flexion when turning to one side than the other, indicating perhaps a painful lesion in the middle or upper cervical area. Any abnormal movement found on examination must be present each time the movement is repeated for it to be judged significant.

The importance of watching the repeated movement lies in the fact that if movement is tested only to note the range at which pain begins, only the gross movement of the vertebral column is assessed and insufficient account is taken of what is happening at an individual segment.

An abnormal movement may be present because of a painful lesion or it may be due to an abnormality such as joint stiffness which is painless. If it is caused by a painful lesion, pain will be provoked by preventing the abnormality occurring during the movement; if it is caused by joint stiffness there will be no pain response. For example, if a patient who has a painful neck flexes his neck more when turning his head to the left than to the right, the physiotherapist should support his head and neck to prevent the flexion occurring during rotation to the left. If there is no pain response during this test the abnormality is unrelated to the lesion causing the patient's pain. If the patient's pain were reproduced by this test it would be an example of 'protective deformity'.

Two common examples of static protective deformity are 'sciatic scoliosis' and 'wry neck'. Attempted passive correction of these deformities will also cause pain. Most of the descriptive titles for these abnormalities are open to misinterpretation, and the clearest method is to name them 'ipsilateral list' or 'contralateral list' depending on the relationship of the 'list' of the patient's thorax to the side of the pain. An ipsilateral list is a lateral displacement of the patient's thorax towards the painful side and a contralateral list is when his thorax is displaced away from the side of pain. The relationship of the list to the side of pain is important, but even more important is what happens to the list during movement. Sometimes it will straighten out and at other times

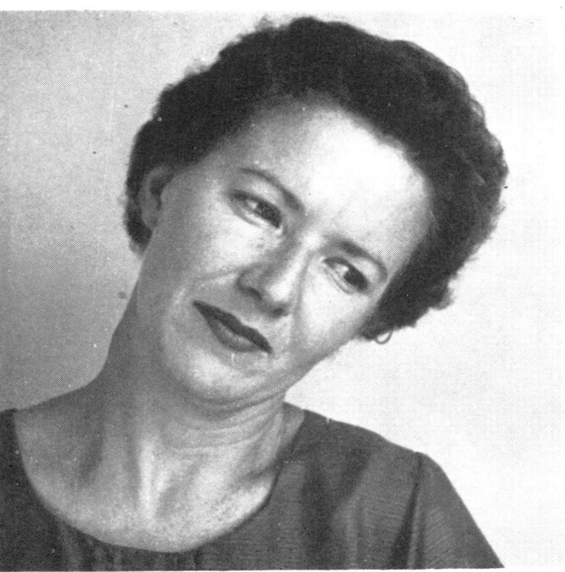

(a)

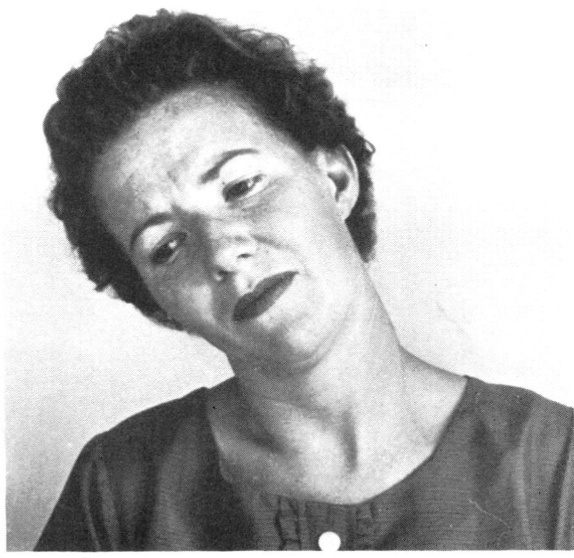

(b)

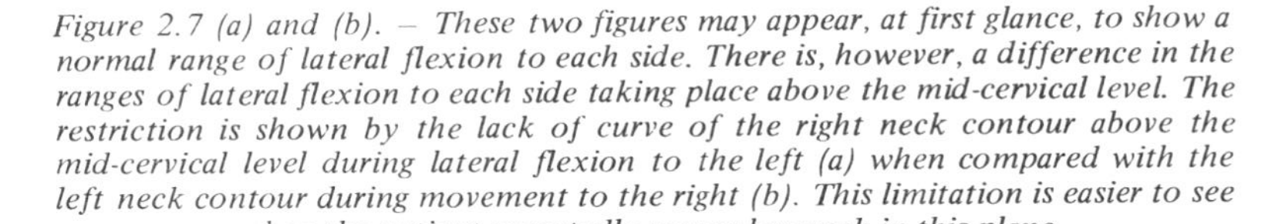

Figure 2.7 (a) and (b). – These two figures may appear, at first glance, to show a normal range of lateral flexion to each side. There is, however, a difference in the ranges of lateral flexion to each side taking place above the mid-cervical level. The restriction is shown by the lack of curve of the right neck contour above the mid-cervical level during lateral flexion to the left (a) when compared with the left neck contour during movement to the right (b). This limitation is easier to see when the patient repeatedly moves her neck in this plane

it will increase and further movement will be impossible. A patient whose list increases with further movement will respond less easily to conservative treatment than will the patient whose list decreases or disappears.

De Sèze (1955) describes and illustrates the common varieties of protective deformity very clearly. He states that the L5 sciaticas caused by the L 4/5 disc are accompanied most commonly by a contralateral list while the ipsilateral list occurs more frequently with S1 sciaticas caused by the lumbosacral disc. Lumbar kyphosis occurs with equal frequency at the L 4/5 and lumbosacral levels. Sometimes the patient's inability to extend his lumbar spine or laterally flex it towards the painful side is expressed in a one-legged stance with the leg on the painful side resting on the ball of the foot with hip and knee slightly flexed. Although De Sèze discusses the alternating list he does not mention the arc of list which can occur during forward flexion. This may be seen as a deviation of the patient's thorax to one side during the middle third of the flexion movement, or alternatively the patient's pelvis may displace backwards on the opposite side. Nor does he mention that these lists can be present only on extension. In addition they can be present in conjunction with a protective spasm of either the flexor or extensor muscles. The flexor or extensor spasm can also be present without any list. When spasm is present in the extensor muscles response to treatment is slow whether this spasm is bilateral, causing a marked lordosis localized to two vertebrae, or unilateral.

Whenever a deformity of the section of spine under examination is evident, whether as a static protective type of deformity or as an abnormal movement, it must be tested by countering the abnormality so that its significance in relation to the patient's complaint can be determined. The degree of reproduction of the patient's pain caused by countering the deformity is the important assessment but an attempt should be made to relate the deformity to previous history. It is possible that the same protective deformity may have been present during previous bouts and may not have completely recovered. In such an event the significance of a current protective deformity would be less. For example, if a patient on standing is seen to have a lumbar kyphosis it is possible that some of his deformity is of a long-standing nature particularly if previous episodes of back pain have been of similar severity. As such deformity does not usually completely disappear it is likely that at least 50 per cent of his present lumbar kyphosis is unrelated to his present pain.

De Sèze, S. (1955). 'Les attitudes antalgiques dans la sciatique discoradiculaire commune.' *Sem. Hôp. Paris* **31**, 2291

When the origin of a patient's arm pain is in doubt it may be necessary to try to reproduce the pain by cervical movements. It is unwise, and unnecessary to do this with severe nerve root pain. If the normal tests of cervical movement do not reproduce the pain, rotation and lateral flexion towards the painful side and extension are three movements which should be tested in a special way. The head should be moved to the limit of the range or to the point where pain begins. If there is no pain or the pain is felt only in the neck, gentle pressure should be applied, increasing the movement and holding it for 10 seconds to see if pain spreads into the referred area. Occasionally referred pain may not be felt while the position is being held but may occur when the movement is released. A similar test can be performed in the lumbar spine using the movements of lateral flexion towards the side of the pain and extension. There is one further test which can be applied to the cervical spine to determine whether a referred pain is intervertebral in origin. It involves applying compression to the crown of the head while the cervical spine is slightly flexed towards the painful side and minimally extended. The compression should be applied slowly and only increased to stronger pressure if the lesser pressure is not painful. Reproduction of the referred pain indicates that it is of cervical origin.

An auxiliary test which may elicit joint signs when active movement tests followed by passive over-pressure are painless is the movement of combined extension lateral flexion and rotation towards the side of pain. The technique for testing the lower cervical spine by this 'quadrant' movement varies appreciably from that used for the upper cervical spine. To test the lower cervical spine for left-sided pain the neck is tilted back into the left corner until the lower cervical spine is fully extended and laterally flexed to the left (*Figure 2.8*). With extension and left lateral flexion held in this combined position, rotation to the left side is added. To test the left quadrant for the left side of the upper cervical spine the physiotherapist stands by the left side of the patient and guides his head into extension and applies pressure to localize the movement to the upper cervical joints. This is done by grasping the patient's chin from underneath in the left hand and his forehead in the right. At the same time his trunk should be stabilized by the physiotherapist's arm from behind and her side from in front while applying pressure through her hands to flex the lower cervical spine with the head held in extension. While head extension is maintained rotation to the left is added. The axis of rotation has changed from the vertical when the head is in the upright position to almost horizontal when the head is in full extension. It is the head which is turned and the technique is to produce oscillatory movements so that the limit of the rotatory range can be felt. When the head is fully turned towards the physiotherapist she then adds the lateral flexion component. The lateral flexion movement involves tilting the crown of the patient's head towards her and his chin away from her. This movement is also performed in an oscillatory fashion until the limit of the range is reached (*Figure 2.9*). This is a very difficult test movement to carry out accurately and much practice is necessary to perform it well.

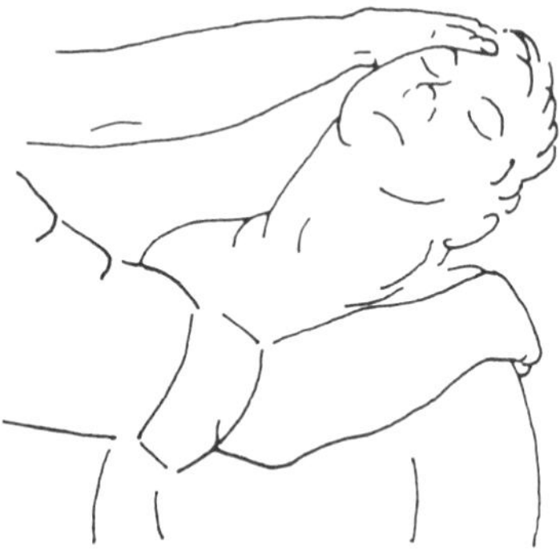

Figure 2.8. – Lower cervical quadrant position

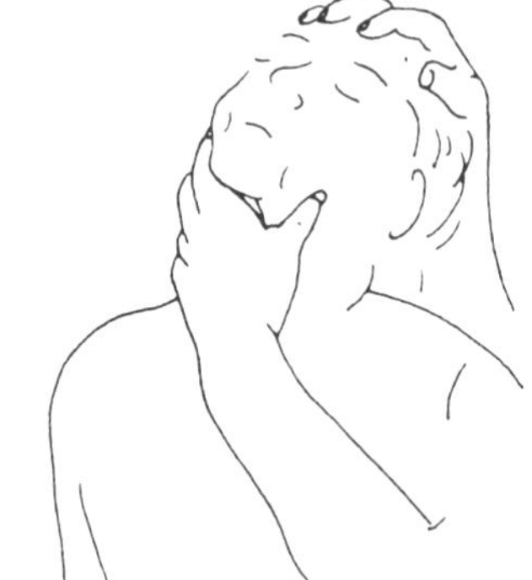

Figure 2.9. – Upper cervical quadrant position

When using the quadrant test for the lumbar spine the physiotherapist should stand behind the patient on the side away from which she intends turning the patient. She encourages him to extend to the limit of his range and then places her hands over his shoulders for control. Then, and only then, should she apply through her hands some pressure to the extension while ensuring that her near-side shoulder is near his occiput to take the weight of his head if he so chooses to use it. By using her hands on his shoulders she then guides his trunk into the corner by laterally flexing and rotating his trunk away from her. Movement is continued until the limit of the range is reached (*Figure 2.10*).

Tests for vertebral artery insufficiency can be introduced at this point in examination of the cervical spine. Vertebral artery insufficiency is one of the contraindications to cervical manipulation and questioning regarding dizziness associated with neck movements or positions should be a routine part of the initial interrogation. Ryan and Cope (1955) have discussed the tests for cervical vertigo. The objective examination to determine the extent to which positions of the neck provoke vertigo

Ryan, G. M. S. and Cope, S. (1955). 'Cervical vertigo.' *Lancet* **2**, 1355

consists mainly of sustaining three positions, head and neck extension and rotation to each side. To assess the relationship of neck movements to vertigo requires testing repeated neck rotation without turning the head. This is the only way of eliminating the effect of the middle ear.

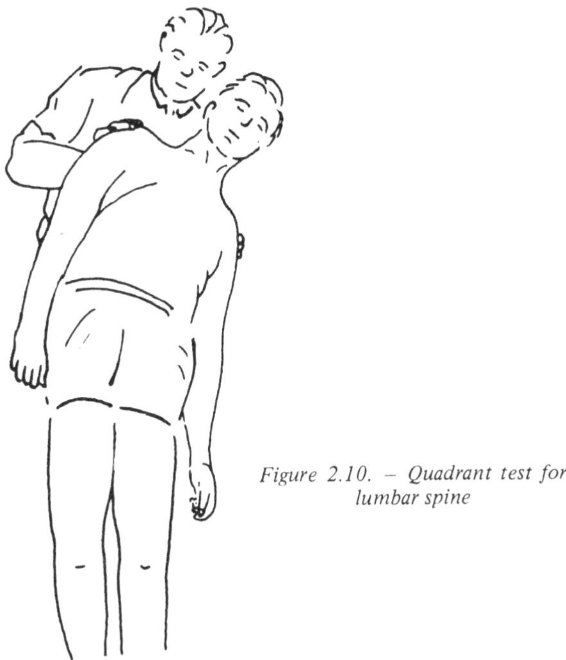

Figure 2.10. – Quadrant test for lumbar spine

To achieve this movement the patient stands while the physiotherapist, standing in front of the patient, holds his head in her hands. The patient then twists his trunk fully from side to side while his feet remain stationary. Thus his trunk rotates under his head and in this way repeated rapid neck rotation can be achieved without movement of his head. Dizziness provoked by this test is not caused by middle ear disturbance.

Passive tests

There are many passive movement tests which form part of examination.

1. The movement of the pain-sensitive structures in the vertebral canal and intervertebral foramen.

2. The tension in soft tissue and the quality of movement of the intervertebral joint by palpation with special emphasis on accessory movements.
3. The passive range of movement of the intervertebral joint.

MOVEMENT IN THE VERTEBRAL CANAL AND INTERVERTEBRAL FORAMEN

To be able to flex the spine fully and touch the toes requires free movement of the spinal cord, lumbosacral nerve roots and their investments. If forward flexion is restricted it may be that the intervertebral joint is stiff or it may be that there is loss of movement of the structures in the canal or foramen. The tests which can be applied to move the structures in the vertebral canal without also moving the intervertebral joints are few in number.

Straight leg raising tests the free movement of the low lumbar and sacral nerve roots and their sleeves within the vertebral canal and intervertebral foramen. Although straight leg raising restricted to 40 degrees can be indicative of nerve root restriction from herniated disc material (Charnley, 1951), pain at full range can indicate some interference with the painless movement of the structures in the canal or foramen. Gross limitation of passive knee flexion while the patient lies prone is similarly a sign of restriction of movement of one of the nerve roots of the lumbar plexus, while any reproduction of pain with an almost full range of movement may indicate mild interference and should be noted.

Care is required when testing straight leg raising because minimal restriction may be missed if the test is not done correctly or repeated two or three times in quick succession while watching carefully for any abnormality of pelvic movement or difference in tension when compared with movement of the other leg. When raising the leg the knee must not be allowed to bend and the pelvis must not be allowed to rise or hitch on the side being tested. The leg being tested should be held in a slight degree of adduction, while lateral rotation at the hip must be prevented. It is possible to increase the tension on the lower lumbar and sacral nerve roots and their sleeves when testing straight leg raising by passively dorsiflexing the patient's foot while holding his leg at the limit of straight leg raising and fully flexing his head and neck.

Charnley, J. (1951). 'Orthopaedic signs in the diagnosis of disc protrusion.' *Lancet* **1**, 186

Another aspect relevant to the straight leg raising test is that, as there is an increase in intradiscal pressure when the patient sits or stands compared with when lying (Nachemson and Morris, 1964), this may effect a discrepancy in the degree of limitation of straight leg raising performed in the standing and lying positions. Testing in both positions, therefore, can be of value.

Movement of the dural investments of the spinal cord can also be effected in the supine patient by passively flexing his head and neck. As an example, a patient may have gluteal pain for which examination findings do not clearly identify the lumbar spine or the hip as being the cause. If passive flexion of the head and neck while the patient lies supine reproduces the gluteal pain, and particularly if the range of movement is limited by the pain, restriction of movement of pain-sensitive structures in the vertebral canal is identified as the cause of the pain. This test is used for the thoracic and lumbar spines. Maximum tension can be exerted on the canal structures if the patient sits slumped with his chin on his chest.

It is not possible to test the movements of the cervical or thoracic nerve roots or their sleeves by applying tension. However information of a similar nature may be gleaned when the patient is afforded relief of symptoms by placing his hand on his head thus relieving tension on the fifth cervical nerve root, or by supporting his elbow in his other hand in a sling-like fashion to relieve tension on the seventh cervical nerve root. Conversely tension can sometimes be increased by protracting the shoulder and stretching the arm across in front of the body.

In summary the main tests used, either singly or in combination, are (1) straight leg raising; (2) prone lying knee flexion; and (3) supine neck flexion.

INTERVERTEBRAL TESTS BY PALPATION

In relation to examining the normality or otherwise of intervertebral movements, the most important techniques are those which follow. It is possible for a patient's physiological movements to appear normal yet the palpation tests for intervertebral movement will reveal positive appropriate joint signs. If a patient has nerve root pain and when this pain is only felt in the distal extent of the dermatome then the patient's symptoms can frequently be reproduced by the specific physiological movements described on page 27. These tests are the sustained positional

Nachemson, A. and Morris, J. M. (1964). '*In vivo* measurements of intradiscal pressure.' *J. Bone Jt Surg.* **46A,** 1077 tests and the quadrant tests. The method by which these test movements reproduce the symptoms is that they alter the relationships of pain-sensitive structures in the intervertebral canal. Under these circumstances passive tests of movement of the intervertebral segments can be negative. In contrast to this if the patient has symptoms arising from the intervertebral joint, in the absence of any abnormality of movement of the pain-sensitive structures in the vertebral canal, then the tests by palpation will always, without exception, be positive. They may be difficult to ascertain but if the directions of movement are tested properly as described in the following section, positive signs of pain, restriction or muscle spasm will be found in one or more directions of the palpation movement. It is also necessary to point out that testing physiological movements either actively or passively does not involve the accessory movements of the intervertebral joints, whereas the palpation movement tests can be directly related to the accessory movements.

Under the above heading the examination includes the following tests.

1. Skin temperature and sweating
2. Soft tissue tension
3. Position of vertebrae
4. Movement of vertebrae

When the spine is being examined the patient lies prone and the skin is checked for sweating and temperature. Palpation for muscle spasm and general tissue tension then follows. Finally, before testing inter-vertebral movement, the positions of the vertebrae should be assessed in relation to adjacent vertebrae. Not too much importance should be placed on abnormalities found on this assessment as they are only relevant if they can be verified by radiography. As there are some differences in procedure for testing some levels of the spine, each will be described separately. Description of the tests for movement will then follow.

Position tests

C1

The patient lies prone and rests his forehead on his hands while the physiotherapist palpates between the spinous process of C2 and the occiput to ascertain whether the posterior tubercle of C1 is palpable. From this point she palpates bilaterally through the relaxed suboccipital muscles, moving laterally until the tip of the transverse process is reached. The relationship which each side of C1 bears to the occiput and to C2 should be assessed. This finding is assisted by also palpating the tip of C1 laterally to assess its relationship to the anterior border of the mastoid process.

C2–C7

The spinous processes are unreliable as the sole source of information regarding position of the vertebrae. They frequently veer to one side without there being any deviation of the body of the vertebra, and absence of one or other terminal tubercle is common. However as they are accessible they are palpated first. If a spinous process is not central, the articular pillar and interlaminar space are then palpated to see if their position indicates any rotation or lateral flexion. The articular pillar is also palpated laterally, and the transverse processes antero-laterally. Apophyseal joint exostoses can be clearly felt. With practice it is possible to appreciate even a small loss of the normal cervical lordosis.

T1–T11

As in the cervical spine, when the thoracic spinous processes which are readily accessible do not lie centrally, rotation or lateral flexion of the vertebra is not necessarily indicated. The spinous process should be palpated at the terminal tubercle and on its lateral surfaces. The interspinous and supraspinous ligaments can also be palpated in this position for undue thickening. If, following such examination, rotation or lateral flexion is indicated, the transverse processes should be palpated. Although these bony points are deeply set they can be found and a reasonable assessment made by comparing one transverse process with that on the other side and also with the adjacent transverse processes above and below. The position of one rib in relation to its neighbours, particularly that part of the rib immediately lateral to its angle, may assist in the vertebral assessment. The closeness of one spinous process to one of its neighbours, or the prominence of one spinous process compared to the adjacent processes are common findings which are easy to appreciate but cannot be radiologically confirmed as easily as positional abnormalities in the cervical spine.

T12–S1

The spinous processes are more reliable indicators of vertebral position in this section of the spine, but the transverse processes are so padded that palpation is less than useful except in the case of L3 where the processes are longer. Palpation of the spinous process posteriorly and laterally is useful both in regard to the position of the vertebra and to the state of the interspinous and supraspinous ligaments.

The sacro-iliac joints, particularly adjacent to the posterior superior iliac spine, can be palpated as can the sacrococcygeal joint and the coccyx. For the sacro-iliac joints, pressure, through the physiotherapist's pisiform (*see Figure 3.27*), should be exerted on the sacrum centrally from the proximal end to the distal end, as well as at different angles on each posterosuperior iliac spine.

Movement tests

Testing movement by palpation involves techniques which are used for treatment as well as examination. The test seeks information not only of range but also of the 'end-feel' of the range, the behaviour of pain throughout the range, and the quality of any resistance or muscle spasm which may be present. Such information is determined for both the physiological movements and the accessory movement of gapping, rocking and shearing or gliding. Detailed description of the techniques is given in Chapter 3 and these will be referred to when the test movements for the different sections of the spine are described.

The passive intervertebral movements are produced by pressure against palpable parts of the vertebra and these pressures should be applied at the right speed to appreciate the movement of the vertebra in relation to adjacent vertebrae. If the pressure is applied as a single slow pressure, the vertebral movement will not be appreciated at all; if it is applied too quickly it can only be interpreted as shaking. However, if the pressure is applied then relaxed and reapplied and repeated two or three times a second, the amount of movement which can take place will be readily appreciated.

When examining movement the first pressures should be applied extremely gently. When a section of the spine is being treated in this way no more than two or three gentle pressures are applied to each vertebra in turn. If there is no pain response to the gentle movements the amplitude and depth of the movement is increased, still only two or three pressures per vertebra. The testing should be repeated more deeply until pain or abnormality is detected or until the movement achieved indicates that the joint has painless range in this direction. If pain is produced during movement, or if physical resistance or protective muscle contraction are encountered during the movement, their extent should be assessed. Occasionally a full assessment may not be possible until the second examination because pain with movement may not be evident until the joint has reacted to the first examination.

The costovertebral joints are tested in the same manner as described for the intervertebral joints except that the pressure is directed through the angle of each rib in turn.

The three primary directions in which the pressures are applied to the vertebrae are as follows.

1. Postero-anteriorly on the spinous process (*Figure 2.11a*).
2. Postero-anteriorly on the articular pillar (*Figure 2.11b*).
3. Transversely on the lateral surface of the spinous process (*Figure 2.11c*).

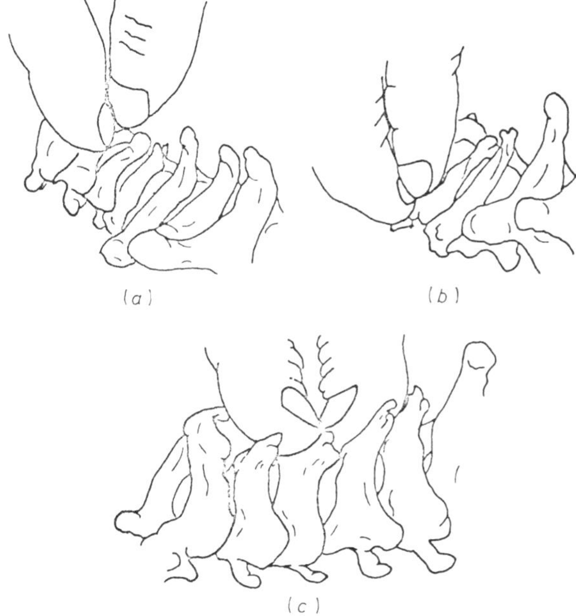

Figure 2.11. – (a) Postero-anterior pressure on the spinous process; (b) postero-anterior pressure on the articular pillar; (c) transverse pressure on the lateral surface of the spinous process

The test can then be further defined to determine the joint disturbance in greater detail by varying the direction of the above three pressures as follows.

Postero-anteriorly on the spinous process

The direction of these pressures can be varied between:

1. an inclination towards the patient's head (*Figure 2.12a*); and
2. an inclination towards his feet (*Figure 2.12b*).

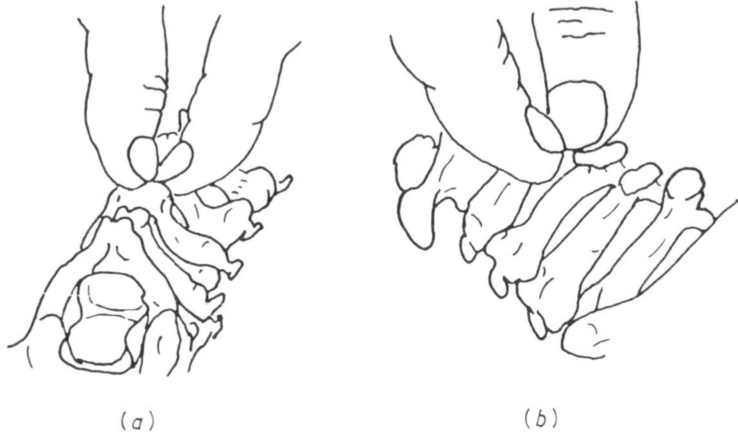

Figure 2.12. – Postero-anterior pressure on the spinous process (a) inclined towards the patient's head; (b) inclined towards the patient's feet

Postero-anteriorly over the articular pillar

This test can be varied in two ways. Firstly it can be inclined:

1. towards the patients head; or
2. towards his feet, as stated above.

The second variation is to incline the postero-anterior pressure:

3. laterally, away from the spinous process (*Figure 2.13a*); or
4. medially towards the spinous process (*Figure 2.13b*).

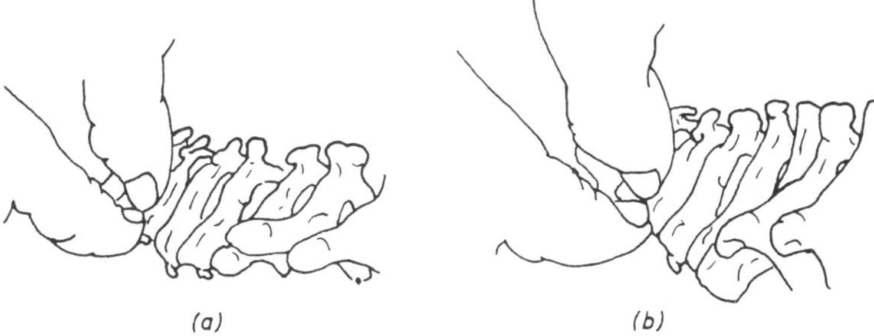

Figure 2.13. – Postero-anterior pressure on the articular pillar (a) inclined laterally away from the spinous process; (b) inclined medially towards the spinous process

Transverse pressure against the spinous process

This can be varied by inclining the direction of the pressure:

1. towards the patient's feet; or
2. towards his head.
3. It is even more important to vary the pressure from being applied transversely against the lateral surface of the spinous process, through an arc which ends as a postero-anterior pressure against the lamina or articular pillar of the same side of the vertebra (*Figure 2.14*).

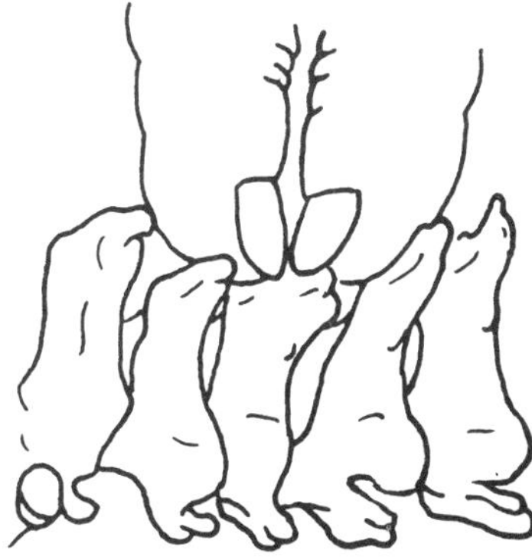

Figure 2.14. – Transverse pressure against the spinous process inclined postero-anteriorly

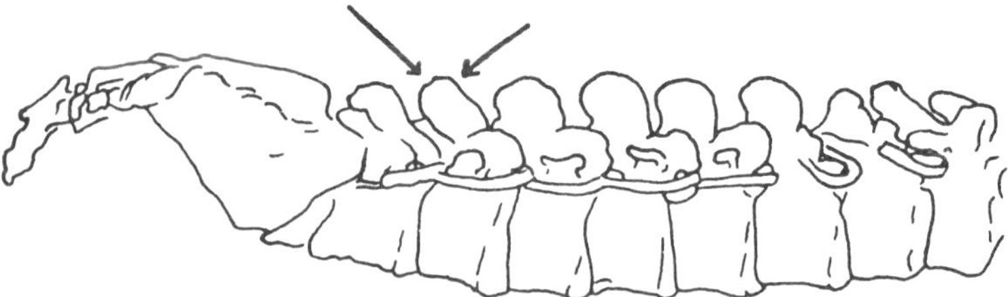

Figure 2.15. – Postero-anterior central pressure inclined cephalad and caudad

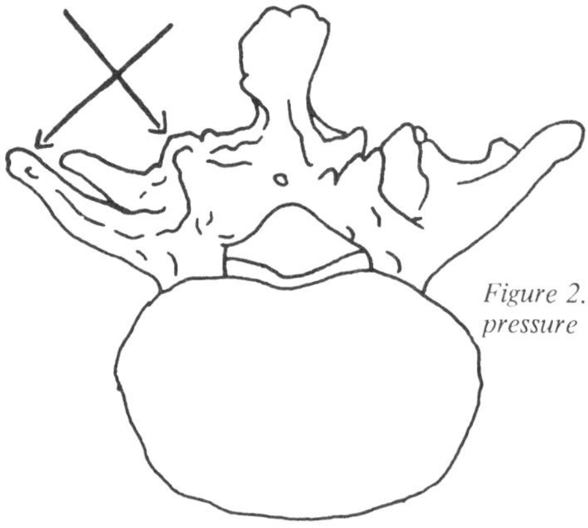

Figure 2.16. – Postero-anterior unilateral pressure inclined medially and laterally

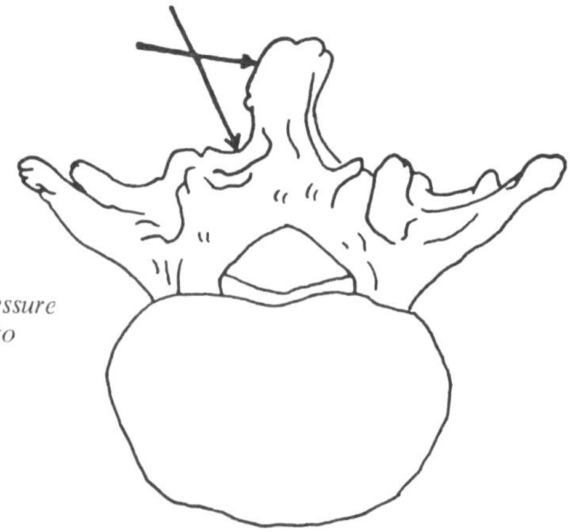

Figure 2.17. – Transverse pressure inclined from transverse to postero-anterior

Figures 2.15–2.17 show the direction of the pressure applied to the processes illustrated in *Figures 2.12–2.14.*

As well as varying the angles of pressures applied to the vertebrae, the point of contact at the intervertebral joint should also be varied. For example, if the C2/3 joint is being examined by postero-anterior unilateral vertebral pressure on the left, the point of contact should be varied by pressure on C2, then on C3 and lastly on the C2/3 joint line.

These tests, carried out effectively, will reveal not only the particular intervertebral joint at fault and the movements of the joint which are affected but also the manner in which each movement is affected.

There are three variables to be considered when determining the manner in which joint movement is affected. They are pain, muscle spasm and physical resistance. It is important to realize that each of these factors, when present, may follow one of many different patterns. Pain, for example, may be present only when joint movement is stretched to the limit of the range; or the opposite may be the case, the joint being painful even when it is at rest. It may vary in other ways too; if pain starts early in a range of movement, it does not always worsen in the same pattern when the joint is moved further. For example, the pain felt during movement may be quite moderate until nearing the limit of the range, when it suddenly increases to become severe. On the other hand, the pain may increase in intensity considerably in the first part of the movement and then maintain a steady degree of pain until the limit of the range is reached (*see* Appendix 1). Different patterns of behaviour of pain require different treatment techniques.

Physical resistance of the type offered by contracted fibrous tissue can also vary considerably in its presentation. Movement before the limit of the range may be perfectly free, with resistance being felt at the limit of the range. The more common presentation, however, is for the slight resistance to be felt some distance before reaching the limit of the range. The amplitude and strength of this slight resistance also vary widely (*see* Appendix 1, p. 322). These variations also influence the type of treatment technique used.

Muscle spasm is the third variable in normal joint movement. The range of movement may be limited by very strong muscle spasm, or the spasm may be of a type which is only evident if a joint movement is performed in a particular way. For example, if the joint is moved slowly and carefully no muscle spasm is felt, but if the movement is quick and jerky, spasm protects the joint from movement which would be painful. Movements used in treatments, therefore, must be modified to suit the particular combination and behaviour of pain, resistance and spasm (*see* Appendix 1, p. 323).

When any of the passive movements are found to be painful the physiotherapist should endeavour to assess at what stage in the range the movement becomes painful. She should then determine how the intensity or area of pain varies if the movement is carried further into the range. If pain is not too great and the movement can be carried further, an assessment of the possible range should be made. When physical resistance prevents a full range being achieved, the type of resistance, that is whether it is a protective muscle spasm or just tightness of inert structures, should be noted.

These tests will provide information about joint disorders which is more valuable than that determined by testing in any other way. Details regarding learning to feel these factors found on joint movement, and a method of recording them diagrammatically for purposes of communication and teaching, are explained at length in Appendices 1 and 2. It is sufficient to say that an extremely valuable and detailed assessment of intervertebral joint movement can be made by this examination.

When testing these movements it is necessary, when an abnormality is found, to test the same movement in the intervertebral joints above and below, and in the same joints on the opposite side. The physiotherapist should also make use of her experience to compare what is found on examination against that which she feels should be normal.

As tests vary for different levels of the spine each level will be described separately.

Upper cervical spine

Movement of C1 produced by postero-anterior pressure against the arch of the atlas is tested first with the patient prone resting his forehead on his hands (*see Figure 3.6*). The physiotherapist applies pressure to three main points: centrally over the posterior tubercle, laterally behind the occipito-atlantal joint and more laterally where the bony arch of the atlas is freely accessible. Occipito-atlantal movement can also be tested by pressure against the anterior surface of C1 at its lateral limits (*see Figure 3.9a*).

The main testing pressures for the second cervical vertebra with the patient's head still in the same position are directed postero-anteriorly first against the spinous process (*see Figure 3.6*) and then transversely against the tip of the spinous process (*see Figure 3.10*).

The patient is then asked to turn his head to one side (say to the right) placing his right arm at the level of his head and his left arm by his side. This position allows the right shoulder to lift slightly taking all strain off the cervical rotation. In this position two tests are carried out. The first is transverse pressure on the tip of the lateral mass of the first cervical vertebra (*see Figure 3.12*); the second is a postero-anterior pressure on the articular pillar of the second cervical vertebra (*see Figure 3.8*). It must be understood that when the patient lies in this position the head, and with it the first cervical vertebra, has rotated to the right; C2 has not moved. Therefore the position of the spinous process of C2 will be the same as it would have been had the head not been rotated. The postero-anterior pressure on the articular pillar of C2 on the right will test the rotation between C1 and C2.

Middle and lower cervical spine

The routine tests in this area include postero-anterior pressures against the spinous process and articular pillar (*see Figures 3.6* and *3.7*). When testing below C2 the medially directed pressure should routinely be tested (*see Figure 2.13b*). The spinous processes of the mid-cervical vertebra are not sufficiently accessible to test with transverse pressure but a similar test can be achieved by pressure against the articular pillar laterally (*see Figure 3.11*). In the lower cervical spine transverse pressure against the spinous process can be effected easily. All variations of the directions of the pressures should be assessed if required (*see* text and figures on pages 34–39).

Thoracic and lumbar spine

The tests here are by postero-anterior and transverse pressures against the spinous processes and varying these pressures cephalad and caudad is especially helpful. Also in the thoracic spine postero-anterior pressure against the transverse process forms part of routine examination. Although it is used in the lumbar spine, the paravertebral musculature makes assessment of movement more difficult. However, if the postero-anterior pressure contacts the vertebra where the spinous process meets the lamina, and its direction is angled midway between a transverse pressure and a postero-anterior pressure, the test becomes very useful (*see Figure 2.15*).

Many of the procedures which constitute intervertebral joint movement tests have been outlined on pages 31–41. Other tests (Passive Physiological Intervertebral Movement) only assess range. No one aspect of examination technique can be considered in isolation. In fact it is the combined findings with different tests which give the final information about movement. However, the preceding tests by palpation techniques are the most important, as they reveal range, pain, resistance and muscle spasm of each intervertebral joint tested. They also test accessory movements as well as the physiological movements. These tests can also be used as very effective treatment techniques. Under these circumstances the tests become highly informative. C. P. Snow (1965) summed up the above situation relating to the interplay between range, pain, stiffness and spasm when he wrote,

> Geography would be incomprehensible without maps. They've reduced a tremendous muddle of facts into something you can read at a glance. Now I suspect (passive movement) is fundamentally no more difficult than geography except that it's about things in motion. If only somebody would invent a dynamic map.

Diagrammatic representation of the available range and the three factors (pain, resistance and spasm) and their behaviour through range, in graphic form, could well be the 'dynamic map' suggested by C. P. Snow in the quotation above. Appendix 1 describes the theoretical background of the Movement Diagram, while Appendix 2 describes the details as to how the Movement Diagram can be compiled for any test movement, whether it be cervical extension or postero-anterior pressure on the spinous process of C4, etc.

In relation to these appendices it is essential to appreciate that the movement diagram is intended to serve only two purposes: to enable the novice to analyse what her hands are feeling when moving a joint passively and for use as a means of communication.

PASSIVE PHYSIOLOGICAL INTERVERTEBRAL MOVEMENT

Before describing specialized tests for testing the passive range of movement between each pair of vertebrae it is necessary to describe the less specific passive movement tests for sections of the spine.

The physiological movements of flexion, extension, lateral flexion and rotation in sitting and standing can be repeated passively in the non-weight-bearing position. This very general test of movement is only required when it is necessary to determine whether load through the joint makes any difference to the pain felt on movement.

The physiological movements of the spine are tested passively in the lying position. The techniques, except for lumbar lateral flexion and

C. P. Snow (1965). *Strangers and Brothers*, p. 67. London; Penguin Books lumbar rotation, are obvious and do not require description. Lateral flexion in the lumbar spine however is performed by the physiotherapist supporting the patient's flexed knees and hips at a right angle and pivoting his feet away from her. When hip rotation reaches the limit of the range the pelvis tilts laterally and lateral flexion then takes

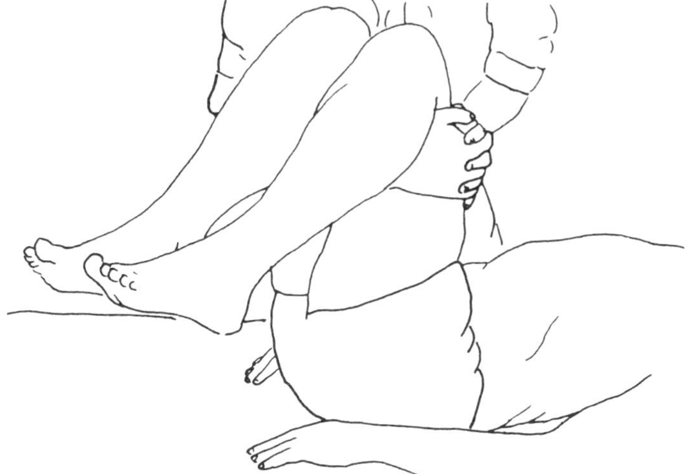

Figure 2.18. – Passive lumbar lateral flexion

place in the lumbar spine. Lateral flexion in the opposite direction is tested by pivoting the patient's feet in the opposite direction (*Figure 2.18*). Rotation is produced by flexing one of the patient's hips and knees to a right angle and carrying the knee across the patient to rotate his pelvis and lumbar spine with his leg.

Description of the specialized tests is different for each individual spinal joint. There are two important occasions when examination requires an assessment of flexion, extension lateral flexion and rotation as they exist at a single intervertebral joint.

1. When preceding examination shows that the faulty joint is stiff but not painful.
2. When a joint has suddenly become fixed in an abnormal position.

The information found on examination is also used in assessing improvement in the range of movement which may result from treatment. To estimate the range, the examiner moves the intervertebral joint through a full range of movement between palpable parts of the two adjacent vertebrae. This movement is compared with the following movements.

1. Movement found at the joint above and below.
2. Movement found on the opposite side.
3. Movement which can be expected to be normal for that particular joint in that particular patient.

Description of the method for testing each spinal joint from the occiput to the sacrum follows. These movements are tested:

1. through the range which is available; and
2. by stronger pressure at the end of the range to discern the fullest range possible and to determine the 'end-of-range feel'. The oscillatory test movement is performed somewhat more slowly than the oscillatory mobilization technique.

Occipito-atlantal joint (lateral flexion)

Starting position

In this examination, the patient lies supine with the crown of his head projecting beyond the end of the couch. Standing at the head of the couch the physiotherapist cradles the patient's occiput in her left hand and grasps the forehead in her right hand with the fingers pointing towards the right and the thumb towards the left. While the tip of the left thumb is in a position to palpate deeply between the left transverse process of the first cervical vertebra and the adjacent mastoid process, the fingers reach beyond the midline to the right occipital area. Pressure is then applied to the crown of the patient's head by the physiotherapist's abdomen to assist in steadying head movement during examination (*Figure 2.19*).

Method

Although the patient's head must be laterally flexed to the right, the crown of the head remains near the midline. To do this the physiotherapist's hands combine to tilt the head by displacing the upper cervical area to the left. This movement is aided by pressure against the crown of the head. When the neck is fully stretched in lateral flexion, the position of the physiotherapist's left thumb, between the transverse process and the mastoid process, must be checked. Care must be taken when producing the lateral flexion movement to

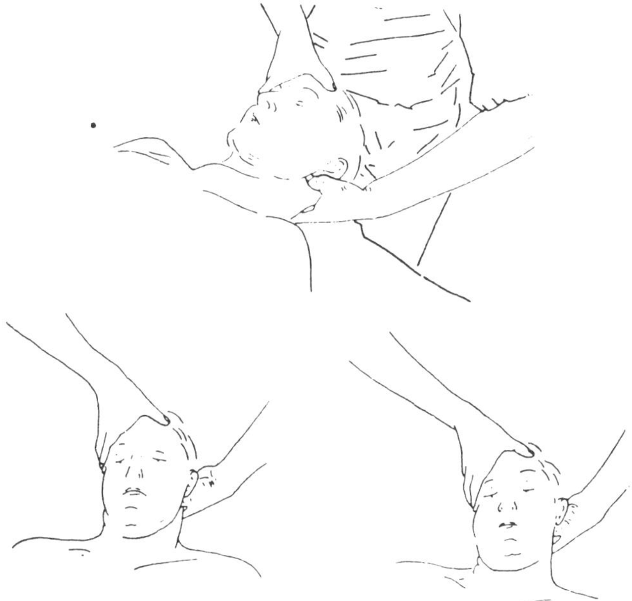

Figure 2.19. — *Occipito-atlantal movement (lateral flexion)*

ensure that it is a 'head on neck' movement. It is so easy to be misled into performing lower cervical movement without any occipito-atlantal movement.

As the head and neck are moved back and forth in the inner third (approximately 15 degrees) of the lateral flexion range the thumb can feel the opening and closing of the gap between the two bony points and the resulting changes in tension of the tissues.

Occipito-atlantal joint (rotation)

The starting position is identical with that described for testing lateral flexion (*Figure 2.20*).

Method

When the patient's head has been turned fully to the right the position of the tip of the left thumb between the left mastoid process and the left transverse process of C1 must be checked. The patient's head is

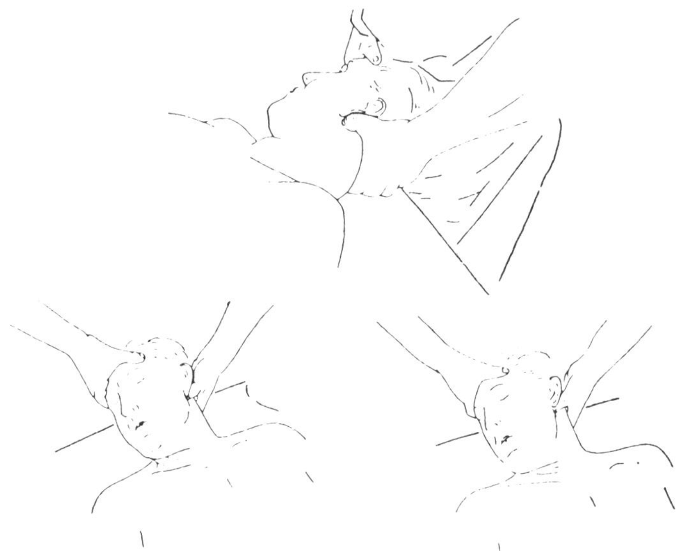

Figure 2.20. – Occipito-atlantal movement (rotation)

then rotated back and forth in the inner third of the range (approximately 20 degrees). As maximum rotation is approached the transverse process is felt to draw nearer to the mastoid process and as the head is brought back towards midline the transverse process moves away from the mastoid process.

Occipito-atlantal joint (flexion/extension)

Starting position

There is a small amount of movement in the nodding movement of the head. To feel this the patient lies supine with his head extending beyond the end of the couch. The physiotherapist cradles the patient's head in her lap holding his occiput in both hands and placing the tips of her thumbs in contact with the tip of each lateral mass of C1 and the antero-inferior border of the mastoid process (*Figure 2.21*).

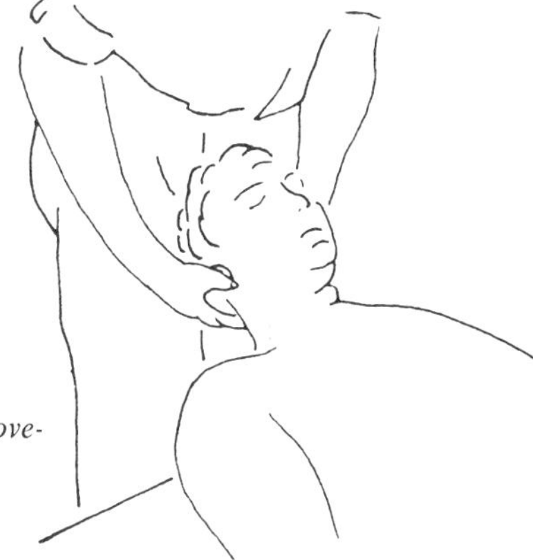

Figure 2.21. – Occipito-atlantal movement (flexion/extension)

Method

The physiotherapist rocks the base of the patient's skull back and forth through approximately 20 degrees reproducing the nodding movement. The crown of the head remains comparatively still. With the tips of her thumbs she assesses the small movement between the two bony points on each side.

C1/C2 (rotation)

Starting position

To examine the range of rotation to the left between the first and second cervical vertebrae the patient sits in a chair and the physiotherapist stands slightly behind the left shoulder. She places her left hand over the crown of his head with the little finger and thumb spreading over the right and left parietal areas respectively and the remaining fingers spreading backwards over the occiput. The hand should be spread to its maximum so that, with her left forearm pointing vertically, the physiotherapist has full control of the patient's head. With her right hand she grasps the spinous process of C2 in a pincer grip (*Figure 2.22a*) between the tip of of the index finger and thumb. The paravertebral muscles lie within the circle formed by the finger and thumb (*Figure 2.22b*).

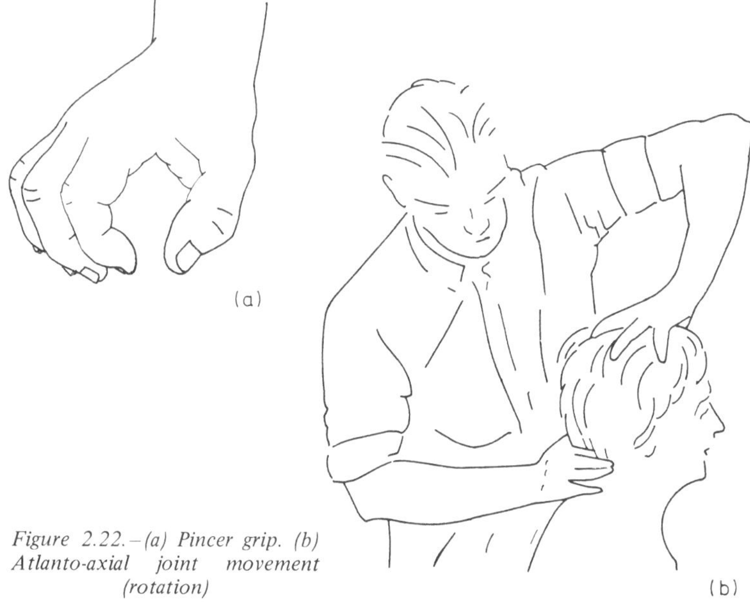

Figure 2.22.–(a) Pincer grip. (b) Atlanto-axial joint movement (rotation)

Method

Having taken up the position prior to testing the rotary movement between C1 and C2 the physiotherapist should, with her left hand, do small lateral flexion movements of the head on the neck through approximately 20 degrees, this being 10 degrees to each side. As she tips the patient's head to the left she should feel the spinous process of C2 move to the right. Similarly, as she laterally flexes his head to the right she will feel the spinous process of C2 move to the left. By assessing this movement she should stop at the point where the spinous process of C2 is in the midline. She then rotates the patient's head back and forth from the centre to the left up to the point where the spinous process is felt to move. The lamina of C2 on the left is felt to move backwards against her thumb and the right lateral surface of the spinous process moves against the pad of her index finger. Once this point has been reached the patient's head is held still and the range of movement assessed. Although the rotation to the right can be assessed by merely turning the patient's head the other way, it is far more accurate to change sides to repeat the technique to the right.

C2–C7 (flexion)

Starting position

The patient lies supine with his head beyond the end of the couch while the physiotherapist crouches at the head end of the couch, below the level of the patient. She holds the patient's occiput near the heel of her right hand while the fingers and thumb point forwards over the crown of the head. Her left hand is then placed against the left side of the patient's neck with the tip of the thumb between the sides of two spinous processes and the tip of the index and middle fingers reaching

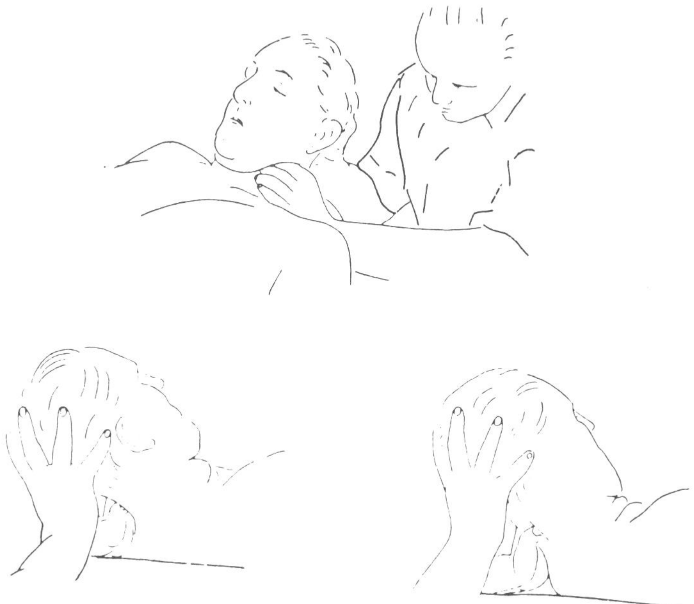

Figure 2.23. – Intervertebral movement. C2–C7 (flexion)

around the left sternomastoid muscle to the anterior surface of the cervical transverse processes. If movement is to be examined between C3 and C4 the thumb is placed laterally between the tips of the spinous processes of these vertebrae and the index and middle fingers are placed over the anterior surface of the left transverse process of C4 and C5 (*Figure 2.23*). If the ligamentum nuchae proves an obstacle to easy palpation the tip of the thumb is moved a little away from the centre line to palpate adjacent spinous processes from the side. This palpation can also be performed at the interlaminar area or at the apophyseal joint posteriorly.

Method

The patient's head is passively flexed by the physiotherapist's right hand with a 'chin on to chest' action, while with the tip of her left thumb she feels between the spinous processes for the amount of opening and closing which takes place as the head is moved backwards and forwards through a range of movement of 15–20 degrees. To produce the maximum movement between C3 and C4, the fourth cervical vertebra and those below it are stabilized by pressure against the anterior surface of their left transverse processes. The position of the 20 degree arc of oscillation within the full range of forward flexion varies with the joint being examined. To examine movement between C6 and C7 the oscillation is performed near the limit of forward flexion range, whereas movement between C2 and C3 must be sought in the first part of the range. Care must be exercised to ensure that movement is produced at the level being tested, and that the movement is the maximum available.

C2–C7 (lateral flexion)

Starting position

The patient lies supine with his head resting on the table, on a pillow, or in the physiotherapist's lap. The position chosen should facilitate relaxation and it should support the head and neck midway between flexion and extension for the joint being examined. In this position both lateral flexion and rotation are freest.

The physiotherapist places the tip of her index finger into the interlaminar space deeply enough to palpate adjacent laminae. With both hands, particularly the non-palpating hand, she gives support under his occiput. When the lower cervical movements are tested this support extends under his neck.

Method

Being careful to ensure that the joint tested is moving and not just the head on the neck, the physiotherapist first laterally flexes the joint towards her palpating finger and assesses the extent of closing of the interlaminar space. The opposite movement is then performed to assess the opening of the space. By this means the excursion of lateral flexion at that level on that side can clearly be evaluated. The palpating finger tip must remain motionless in the space so care must be exercised when that hand is used to produce the lateral flexion of the neck.

C2–C7 (rotation)

Starting position

The 'starting position' is identical with that described for lateral flexion except for the palpating finger. This is carried a fraction laterally

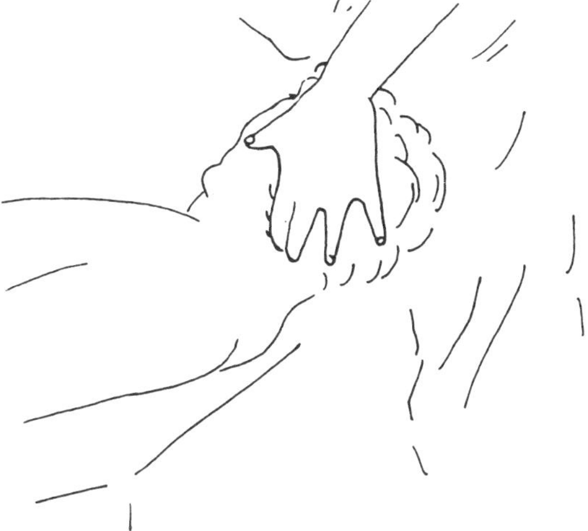

Figure 2.24. – Intervertebral movement. C2–C7 (rotation)

and a slightly broader contact is made. The tip and adjacent lateral margin of the index finger palpate the margin of the apophyseal joint (*Figure 2.24*).

Method

The head is pivoted, away from the side of palpation, around an imaginary central axis passing through the joint being tested. The physiotherapist's hands produce the movement in a steady oscillatory fashion producing movement down to the joint but not beyond it. Her palpating finger follows the movement of the joint, assessing the extent of sliding or opening between the two adjacent articular processes. It is not possible to assess the rotation towards the palpating finger because the muscles obstruct the palpation.

Occiput–C7 (extension)

Starting position

The patient lies supine with his head resting on the couch or in the physiotherapist's lap. The physiotherapist stands near his head, supporting under the patient's head and neck down to the level of the joint being tested. She placed the tip of both index fingers into the interlaminar space on each side, as described above for lateral flexion (*Figure 2.25*).

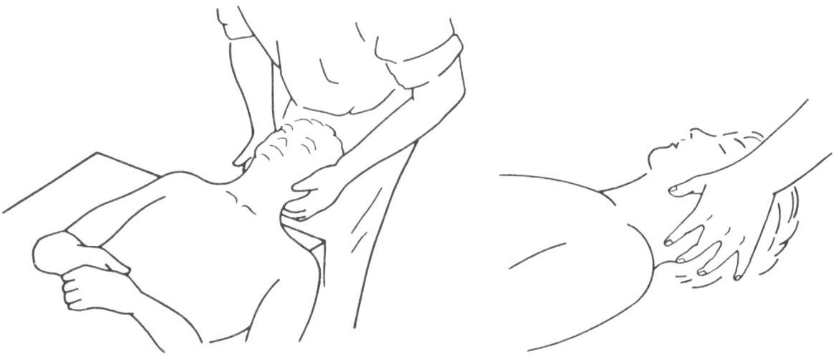

Figure 2.25. – Intervertebral movement. Occiput–C7 (extension)

Method

The physiotherapist extends the patient's head and neck down to the level being examined by lifting under his neck. At the same time she palpates for closing down of the interlaminar space with her finger tips.

C7–T4 (flexion)

Starting position

With the patient sitting the physiotherapist stands in front, slightly to the patient's right. She rests her left hand over his right shoulder with the middle finger positioned between two spinous processes while the index finger palpates the upper margin of the spinous process of the

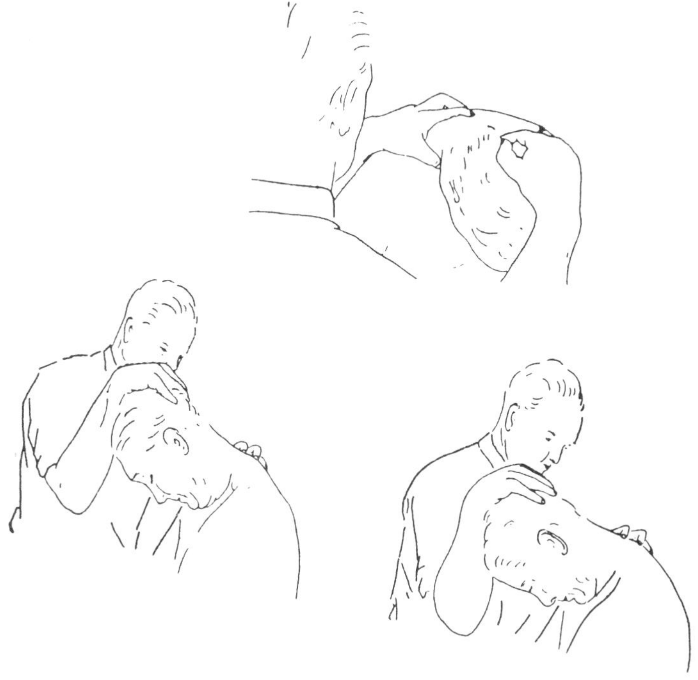

Figure 2.26. – Intervertebral movement. C7–T4 (flexion)

upper vertebra and the ring finger palpates the lower margin of the lower spinous process. To produce a firm yet comfortable grasp with the left hand, the pad of the thumb is placed in the supraclavicular fossa. The right hand and forearm are placed over the top of the patient's head so that they lie in the sagittal plane. The fingers and thumb grasp the occiput near the nuchal lines and the wrist is flexed to permit firm pressure on the front of the head by the forearm (*Figure 2.26*).

Method

Movement of the patient's head is controlled by the physiotherapist's right hand and forearm. All scalp looseness must be taken up by the grasp between the fingers and forearm to permit complete control of the patient's head, to make him feel that support of his head can be left to the physiotherapist.

As the amount of movement which can be felt at this level is much less than elsewhere in the vertebral column two complementary actions are necessary to produce the maximum intervertebral movement. Firstly, the oscillation of the head and neck needs to be through a range at least of 30 degrees performed near the limit of forward flexion. Secondly, because the lever producing movement is long, pressure by the three palpating fingers over the spine will help to localize movement as the head is moved back through a range of 30 degrees.

The intervertebral movement is felt by the ring, middle and index fingers as the spinous processes move away from and towards each other during the back and forth movements of the head and neck.

C7–T4 (flexion/extension)

An alternative method for testing flexion, which is more convenient if rotation and lateral flexion are also to be tested, is performed with the patient lying on his side.

Starting position

The patient lies comfortably on his right side, near the forward edge of the couch, with his head resting on pillows. The physiotherapist stands in front of the patient cradling his head in her left arm with her fingers covering the posterior surface of his neck, her little finger reaching down to the vertebral level being examined. She stabilizes his head between her left forearm and the front of her left shoulder. Next she leans across the patient, placing her right forearm along his back to stabilize his thorax and palpates the under surface of the interspinous space with the pad of her index or middle finger facing upwards (*Figure 2.27*).

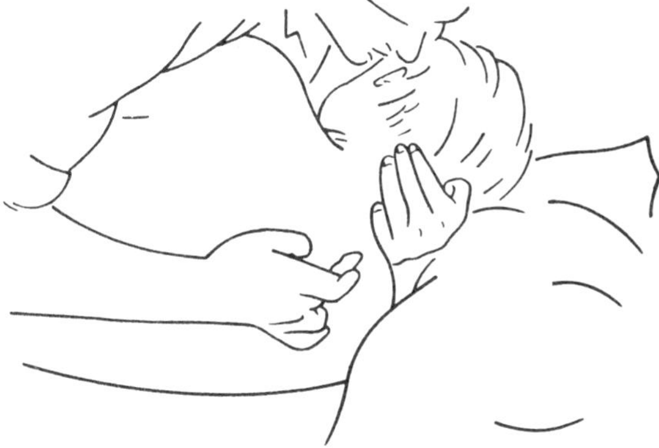

Figure 2.27. – Intervertebral movement. C7–T4 (flexion/ extension)

Method

With her left arm the physiotherapist flexes and extends the patient's lower neck as much as possible. The spine above C6 and the head are not flexed or extended because movement in this area makes movement in the test area less controlled and less isolated. The patient's head and neck are moved only until the particular joint tested has come to the limit of its range.

C7–T4 (lateral flexion)

Method

The starting position is identical to that described for flexion/ extension. The purpose of the method is to achieve lateral flexion at the particular joint being tested. Therefore the head does not laterally flex but rather is displaced upwards. Lateral flexion is produced by the physiotherapist lifting the patient's head with a hugging grip of his head, the majority of the lift being achieved by the ulnar border of her left hand against the underside of his cervicothoracic junction (*Figure 2.28*). To test lateral flexion in the opposite direction the patient must lie on his other side.

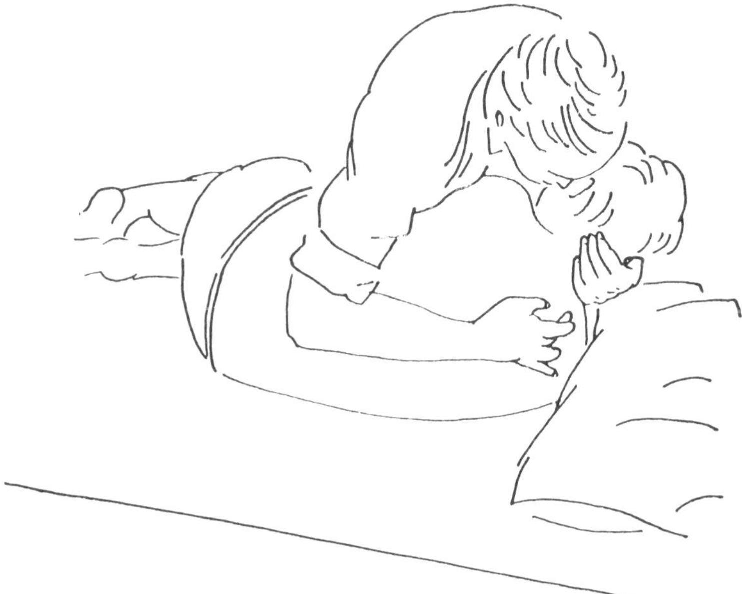

Figure 2.28. – Intervertebral movement. C7–T4 (lateral flexion)

C7–T4 (rotation)

Method

The starting position is again the same as for flexion/extension. To produce the rotation properly it is necessary to concentrate on moving the joint being examined without causing any tilting or flexing of the head and neck. Movement of the upper spinous process in relation to its distal neighbour is palpated through the pad of the physiotherapist's index or middle finger which is facing upwards against the underside of the interspinous space.

With the patient's head cradled between the physiotherapist's left forearm and shoulder, and his lower neck firmly gripped in the ulnar border of her hand between the little finger and the hypothenar eminence, she rotates his lower cervical spine towards her. This is achieved by elvating his scapula to its highest point while maintaining a stable thorax (*Figure 2.29*). As the movement is difficult to achieve accurately, more care is needed than with the other movements tested in this area.

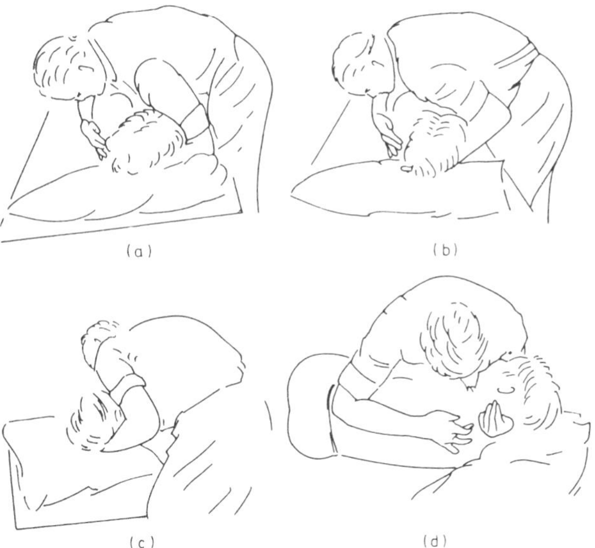

Figure 2.29. – Intervertebral movement. C7–T4 (rotation)

T4–T11 (flexion/extension)

Starting position

The patient sits with his hands clasped behind his neck while the physiotherapist, standing by his left side, places her left arm under his left upper arm and grasps his right upper arm in her supinated hand. She places her right hand across his spine just below the level being tested with the pad of the tip of the middle finger in the far side of the interspinous space to feel adjacent spinous processes.

Method

While the patient relaxes to allow his thorax to be flexed and extended the physiotherapist takes the weight of his upper trunk on her left arm.

To test flexion she lowers his trunk from the neutral position until movement can be felt to have taken place at her right middle finger, when the patient is then returned to the neutral position by lifting under his arms. The oscillatory movement through an arc of approximately 20 degrees of trunk movement is facilitated if the patient is held firmly and if the physiotherapist laterally flexes her trunk to the left as she lowers the trunk in flexion. This makes the return movement one of laterally flexing her trunk to the right rather than lifting with her left arm.

The extension part of the test is carried out in much the same way except that the physiotherapist assists the trunk extension with the heel and ulnar border of her right hand. In doing this she must be careful to keep the pad of her middle finger in a constant position between the adjacent spinous processes. Movement of the patient's trunk is from the neutral position into extension. It is important to remind oneself constantly that it is movement at only one joint which is being examined and that therefore large trunk movements are not necessary; in fact they detract from the examination.

T4–T11 (lateral flexion)

Starting position

The patient sits and holds his hands behind his neck while the physiotherapist stands side-on behind his left side reaching with her left arm to hold high around and behind his right shoulder. She grips his trunk firmly between her left arm and her left side in her left axilla. This high grasp with the left hand is necessary for examination of the higher levels. As the examination extends below T8 so the grasp needs to be taken down to the lower scapular area. She places the heel of her right hand on the left side of his back at the level being examined, spreads her fingers for stability and places the tip of the pad of her flexed middle finger in the far side of the interspinous space of the joint to be tested (*Figure 2.30*).

Method

The physiotherapist laterally flexes the patient's trunk towards her by displacing his trunk away from her with the heel of her right hand and her costal margin, and laterally flexing his upper trunk by lifting her left arm and pressing downwards with her left axilla. She palpates for the interspinous movement through the pad of her middle finger ensuring that, during the lateral flexion, her finger moves with the spine maintaining even contact against the spinous processes.

Lateral flexion in the opposite direction can be palpated without a change of position simply by laterally flexing the patient's trunk the other way. However it is more accurate to change sides and reproduce the technique on the opposite side.

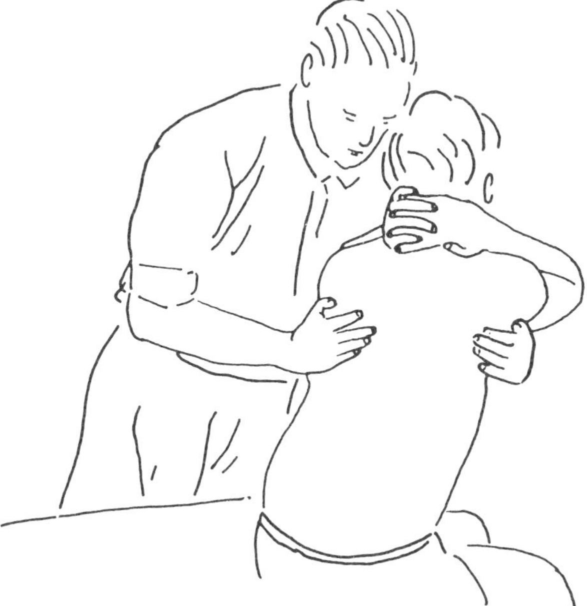

Figure 2.30. – Intervertebral movement. T4–T11 (lateral flexion)

T4–T11 (rotation)

Starting position

Though rotation can be tested in the sitting position it is more easily and more successfully tested when the patient is lying down. The patient lies on his right side with his hips and knees comfortably flexed while the physiotherapist, standing in front of the patient, leans over his trunk to cradle his pelvis between her right side and her right upper arm. This position stabilizes the patient's pelvis. The physiotherapist's forearm is then in line with the patient's spine and her hand reaches the level where movement is to be examined. She then places her right hand on his spine with the pad of her middle finger facing upwards against the under surface of the interspinous space to feel the bony margins of the adjacent spinous processes. With her left hand she grasps as far medially as possible over the patient's suprascapular area and places her forearm over his sternum (*Figure 2.31*).

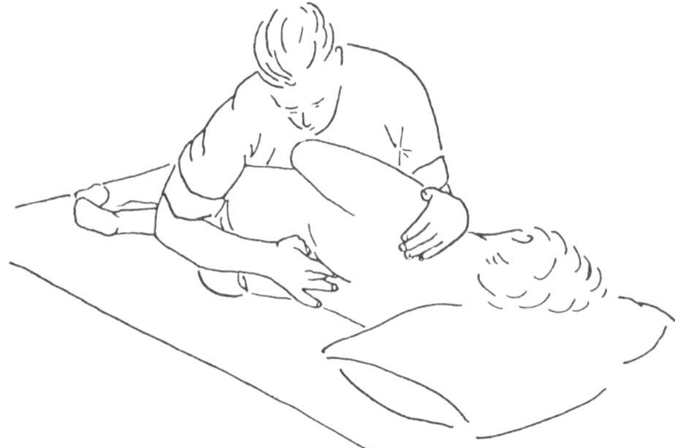

Figure 2.31. – Intervertebral movement. T4–T11 (rotation)

Method

The patient's trunk is repeatedly rotated back and forth by the physiotherapist's left forearm and hand through an arc of approximately 25 degrees. Care must be taken to ensure that the movement does not include scapulothoracic movement. To examine movement in the upper thoracic intervertebral joints the arc of movement should be performed just behind the frontal plane. As lower intervertebral joints are examined the arc of rotation used to assess movement moves backwards until an arc of rotation between 40 and 60 degrees from the frontal plane is used to examine the movement between T10 and T11. The palpating finger must follow the patient's trunk movement and when movement occurs at the joint being examined the upper spinous process will be felt to press into the pad of the middle finger which is facing upwards.

T11–S1 (lateral flexion)

Starting position

The patient lies on his right side with his hips and knees flexed to allow his lumbar spine to lie relaxed midway between flexion and extension. If the patient has unusually large hips compared with the size of the thorax, a pillow should be placed under the lumbar spine to prevent it sagging into lateral flexion. The physiotherapist, standing in front of the patient, facing his feet reaches across his left side resting her lower ribs against his side, with her left forearm, pointing caudad, along his spine and her right forearm grasping around his pelvis under the ischial tuberosity. She places the pad of her left middle finger facing upwards in the underside of the intraspinous space to feel the bony margin of the adjacent vertebrae (*Figure 2.32*).

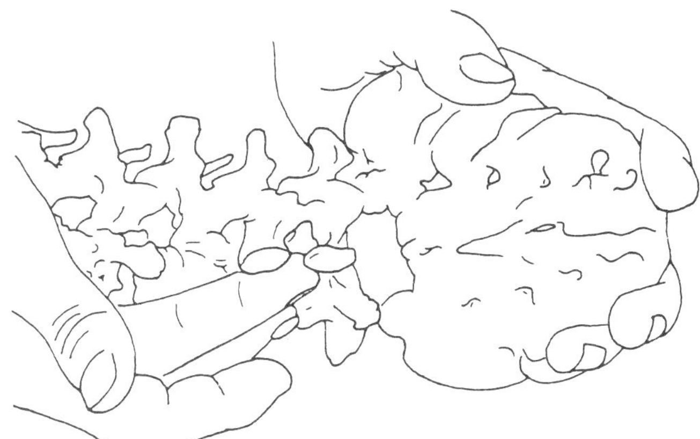

Figure 2.32. – Intervertebral movement. T11–S1 (lateral flexion). Position of palpating finger for lumbar spine

Method

With her grasp of the patient's pelvis and upper thigh with her right forearm and her right side, she laterally flexes his lumbar spine from below upwards by rocking his pelvis. She tips his pelvis cephalad on the left by pulling with her right forearm, and returns it by pushing against his thigh with her right side. An oscillatory movement produced in

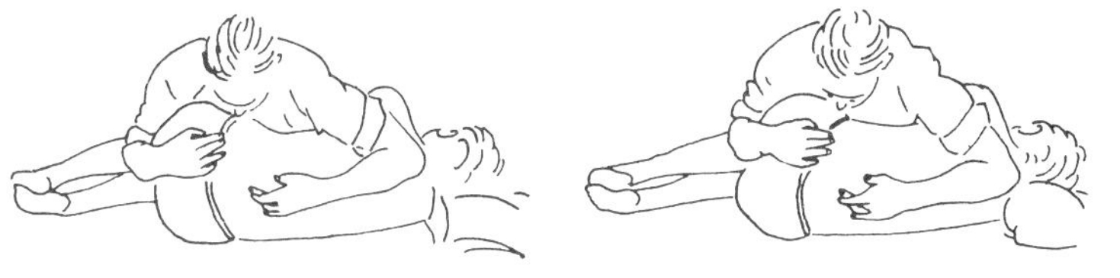

Figure 2.33. – Intervertebral movement. T11–S1 (lateral flexion)

this way rocks the pelvis with the underside hip and femur acting as the pivot. The movement is easy to produce and easy to palpate (*Figure 2.33*).

To test lateral flexion to the opposite side the patient should be asked to turn over.

T11–S1 (rotation)

Starting position

This starting position is similar to that described for lateral flexion but it is necessary to ensure that the patient's top knee will slide freely forwards over the underneath knee. The physiotherapist leans across the patient placing her left forearm along his back to palpate the interspinous space from underneath, while twisting her trunk slightly to face his hips. She holds over his left hip with her right hand, her fingers spreading out behind his trochanter and the heel of her hand anterior to the trochanter. Her right forearm holds along his left femur (*Figure 2.34*).

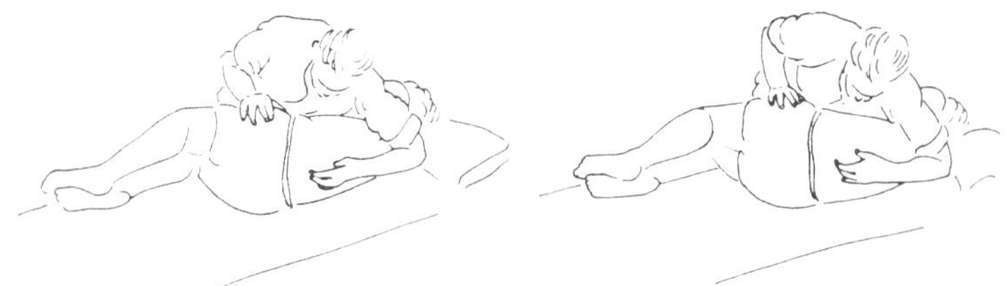

Figure 2.34. – Intervertebral movement. T11–S1 (rotation)

Method

While the physiotherapist stabilizes the patient's thorax with her left arm and side, she rotates his pelvis towards her by pulling with her right hand. As his top knee slides forwards over his right knee the pelvis, and lumbar spine, rotate forwards on the left side. Ensuring that her palpating finger keeps pace with this movement she will feel the displacement of the distal spinous process in relation to the proximal one. She effects the return movement of the pelvis with the heel of her right hand and her right forearm.

Rotation in the opposite direction can be tested without changing the patient to the other side. However, uniformity of 'feel' is best achieved by repeating the technique on the other side.

T11–S1 (flexion/extension)

Starting position

The patient lies on his right side with hips and knees flexed. The physiotherapist standing in front of the patient reaches behind and under the patient's flexed knees to grasp anteriorly around the right knee.

She then lifts them and rests the lower legs against her own upper thighs, placing the knees just beyond her left thigh. With her left arm stretched over the patient's lower scapular area to prevent any backward rotation of the thorax, the physiotherapist places the tip of the pad of the index or middle finger in the interspinous space to be tested where it can feel the adjacent margins of two spinous processes. To help palpate more deeply without losing sensibility, this finger can be reinforced over the nail by the middle finger (*Figure 2.35a*).

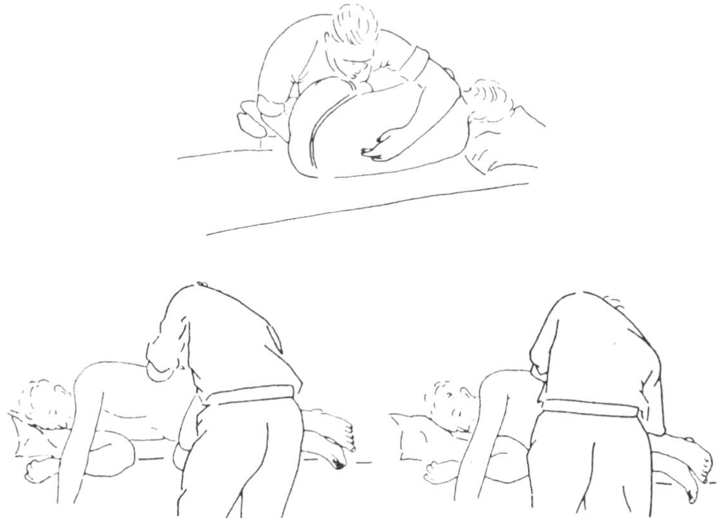

Figure 2.35(a). – Intervertebral movement. T11–S1 (flexion/extension)

Method

Passive movement of the spine is produced by rocking the patient's knees back and forth towards his chest through an arc of 30 degrees. Over-pressure should be applied at the limit of extension to assess any backward sliding of a vertebra which may indicate instability. The test movement is produced by a side to side movement of the physiotherapist's pelvis carrying the patient's legs with her. The palpating hand can help to increase the intervertebral range by pressing against the spine when the patient's legs are released from their flexed position. An opening and closing of the interspinous gap can be felt with the rocking of the patient's pelvis and legs.

T11–S1 (flexion/extension). Single-leg technique

As some physiotherapists find the technique using both of the patient's legs to produce the movement awkward, a single-leg technique is described. However, accurate positioning of the underneath leg becomes important.

Starting position

The patient lies on his right side and the physiotherapist stands in front of his upper chest facing towards his hips. She places her left forearm along his back to palpate between adjacent spinous processes from underneath with her middle finger while stabilizing his thorax between her left arm and left side. With her right hand she grasps his left upper tibia from in front (*Figure 2.35b*).

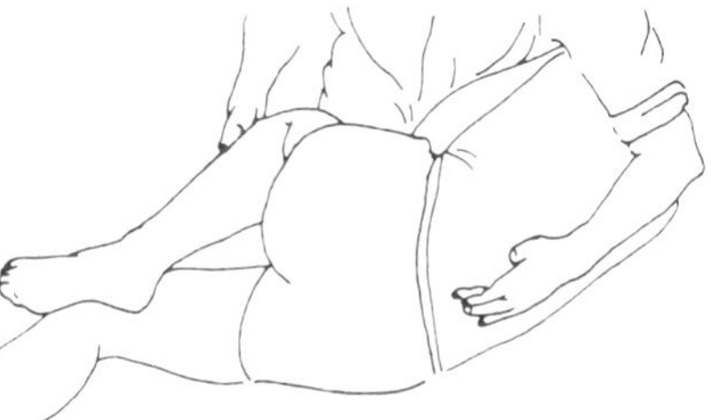

Figure 2.35(b). – Intervertebral movement. T11–S1 (flexion/extension). Single-leg technique

Method

The physiotherapist produces flexion and extension of the patient's lumbar spine by flexing and releasing the flexion of his left hip while she assists extension by pressure with the heel of her left hand against the lumbar spine.

Disturbances of spinal movements–These can be evaluated more clearly by study of the physiological and pathological changes which occur in the disc and apophyseal joints (Harris and Macnab, 1954). Similarly it is important to be familiar with the radiological appearance of the normal spine, for example, the contour and position of vertebrae, the size and appearance of disc spaces and intervertebral foraminae. This knowledge helps in the correlation of congenital and developmental abnormalities with physical findings.

It must be emphasized that abnormalities of position or movement of vertebrae which may be found during the foregoing examinations are not expected to be conclusive in themselves. They should however be informative when considered in relation to the whole examination.

Sacro-iliac joint

Mention was made earlier regarding palpation of the sacro-iliac joint (*see* page 34). Now passive movement of the sacro-iliac joints should be tested by laterally directed pressures against the medial surface of the anterior superior iliac spines to produce an opening effect of the anterior margin of the sacro-iliac joints. The movement should then be reversed by applying medially directed pressures against the lateral margin of the iliac crest. Small oscillatory movements of the sacro-iliac joints are produced by pressures being applied and relaxed repeatedly. These pressures should be gentle at first but should be gradually increased. Care must be taken to avoid lumbosacral movement.

The sacro-iliac test should be performed as part of the examination of every patient with back pain whether there is any likelihood of the symptoms arising from these joints or not, as pain with this movement can be the first sign of ankylosing spondylitis.

With the patient lying prone the sacro-iliac joint should be further tested by firm pressure through the centre of the sacrum. For the test to be positive, pain must be felt not in the centre of the back but in the sacro-iliac joint.

Two further tests which examine the rotary movements of the pelvis about the sacrum through a transverse axis should be used when the sacro-iliac joint is thought to be the source of pain. The first test tilts the upper pelvis backwards and the second tilts it forward.

Starting position

To test the left sacro-iliac joint the patient lies on his right side with his hips and knees comfortably flexed less than 90 degrees. The physiotherapist stands in front of his hips facing his shoulders and leans across the hips to place the heel of her right hand over the posterior surface of his left ischial tuberosity with the fingers and forearm pointing over his hip towards her face. She places the heel of her left hand over his anterior iliac spine with her fingers and forearm pointing over his pelvis towards her other hand. She then stretches over

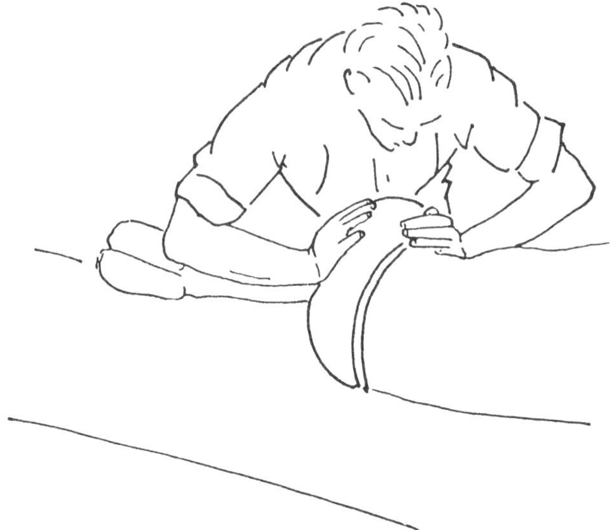

Figure 2.36. – Sacro-iliac joint movement in direction of lumbar flexion

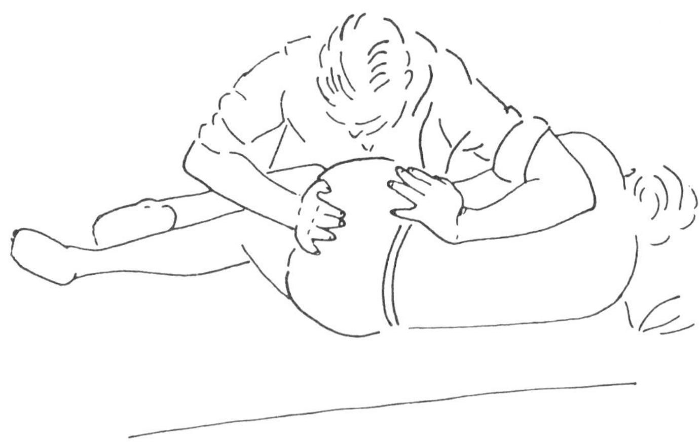

Figure 2.37. – Sacro-iliac joint movement in direction of lumbar extension

the patient's hip to be able to direct her forearms towards each other (*Figure 2.36*).

Method

By squeezing both arms towards each other and by simultaneously displacing her pelvis to the left the physiotherapist exerts a rotary strain on the sacro-iliac joint by pushing the anterior iliac spine upwards and backwards and the ischial tuberosity forwards.

The oppositely directed rotary movement is similarly effected.

Starting position

The patient adopts the same starting position but this time the physiotherapist stands in front of the patient's waist facing towards his hips and leans forwards across the patient to place the heel of her left hand against the posterolateral margin of the iliac crest. Her fingers point upwards continuing around the ilium. She cups the palm of her right hand over the left ischial tuberosity so that the heel of her hand, pressed into the patient's upper thigh, reaches as deeply as possible. Her fingers point backwards over the patient's buttock (*Figure 2.37*).

Method

By the same alternating pressures mentioned above a rotary strain is placed on the sacro-iliac joint.

Neurological tests

The physiotherapist must report to the doctor any deterioration in neurological changes which may occur during treatment. This means that the physiotherapist must examine for and repeatedly assess possible changes at the commencement of each treatment.

It is a well proven fact that referred pain can be caused by compression of the nerve root (Smyth and Wright, 1958) and by other sections of the intervertebral segment (Feinstein *et al.*, 1954). It is difficult

Harris, R. I. and Macnab, I. (1954). 'Structural changes in the lumbar intervertebral discs. Their relationship to low back pain and sciatica.' *J. Bone Jt Surg.* **36B**, 304

Smyth, M. J. and Wright, V. (1958). 'Sciatica and the intervertebral disc. An experimental study.' *J. Bone Jt Surg.* **40A**, 1401

Feinstein, B., Langton, J. N. K., Jamieson, R. M. and Schiller, F. (1954). 'Experiments on pain referred from deep somatic tissue.' *J. Bone Jt Surg.* **36A**, 981 to describe precisely the difference between a nerve root pain and a pain from other structures. Nerve root pain can frequently be identified by its character. It is not just an ache, but a pain, often severe. The severity of the pain frequently shows in the patient's facial expression, or in his description of the pain, or in the way he holds the limb. It is typically a very unpleasant pain and is often greatest in the distal part of the dermatome. The pain is not necessarily reproduced by normal movement tests but it frequently increases after a particular movement has been performed. The referred pain can often be reproduced however if certain movements are held at the limit of the range for some seconds (*see* page 27). Referred pain from other sources does not behave in this way.

Not all nerve root pain is severe but when it is severe the patients require especially careful neurological assessment and treatment must be gentle to avoid exacerbation and produce the best treatment result.

To refer to the many diagrams of dermatomes is confusing unless it is understood how different structures refer pain. It is now accepted knowledge that if the nerve root is the only source of the patient's pain, it will be felt only in the distal part of the dermatome. This explains the type of charts supplied by Cyriax (1975). Clinical examples of this are patients whose pain starts distally, or patients whose back or neck pain disappears and is replaced by distal limb pain. However, it is common to have patients referred with pain in the spine continuous with pain in the limb, which may or may not be worse distally. The reason for this may be that while the nerve root causes the limb pain, local pain may be present as a result of disc pathology (Cloward, 1959). The disc *may* in turn be irritating other pain-sensitive structures in the vertebral canal, for example the nerve root sleeve or dura. Supportive muscles and apophyseal joints, disturbed by the disc damage, may also give rise to some of the local pain. Pain of this kind of referral indicates the need for dermatome charts showing pain locally and throughout the limb (*see Figure 2.1*).

Muscle weakness resulting from nerve root compression is best assessed by static (isometric) tests and although each nerve root supplies more than one muscle, some muscles tend to be supplied by predominantly one root. The root or roots quoted are those found to have greatest clinical significance (*Figure 2.38*). While the patient lies supine the power of the appropriate arm muscles can be assessed quickly in the order shown in Table 2.1.

Cyriax, J. (1975). *Textbook of Orthopaedic Medicine.* 6th edn Vol. 1. London; Ballière Tindall

Cloward, R. B. (1959). 'Cervical diskography. A contribution to the etiology and mechanism of neck, shoulder and arm pain.' *Ann. Surg.* **150**, 1052

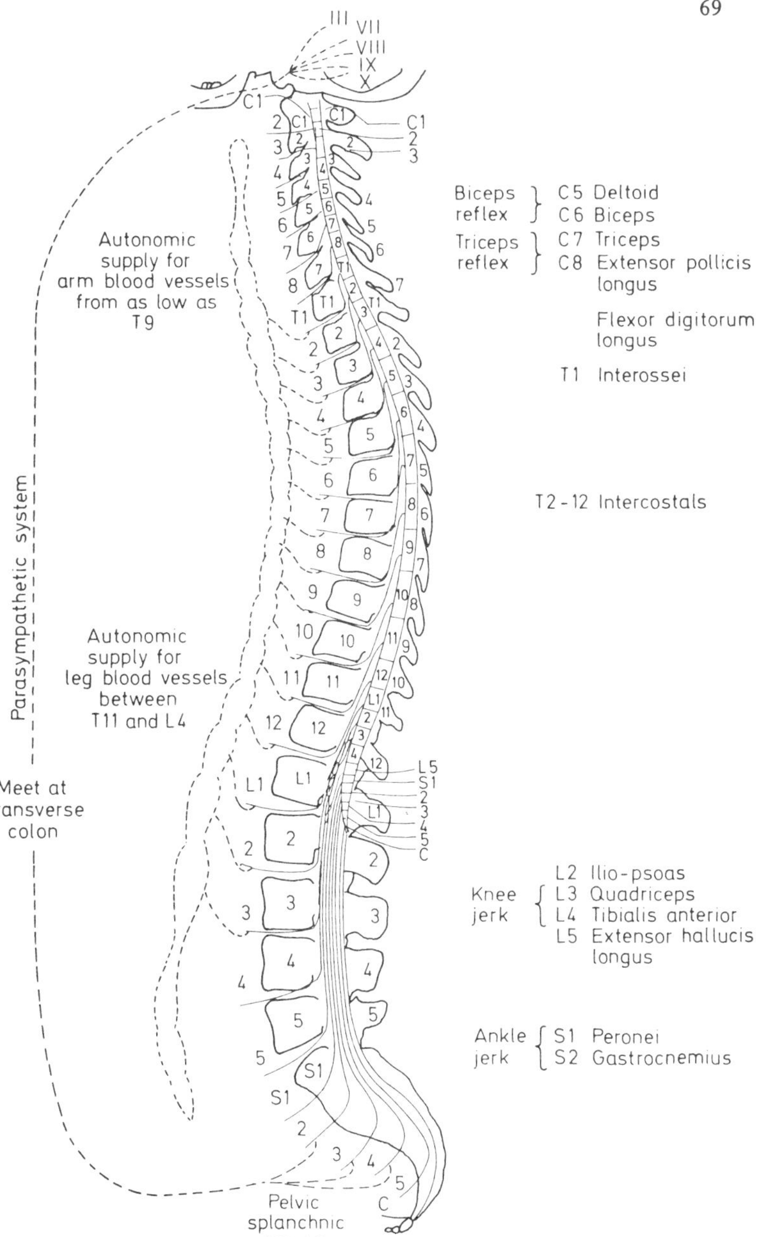

Figure 2.38. – Nerve roots and the spine

TABLE 2.1

Muscle	*Nerve root and reflexes*	*Method*
Flexion of head on upper neck, rectus capitis anterior	C1	The patient attempts to flex his head on his upper neck against the resistance applied by the physiotherapist's hand under the chin and on the forehead.
Extension of head on upper neck, rectus capitalis posterior major and minor with obliquus capitis superior	C2	While the patient attempts to extend his head on his neck the physiotherapist resists the movement by holding the occiput in one hand and the chin in the other.
Lateral flexion, scalene muscles	C3	The patient attempts to laterally flex his head and neck while the physiotherapist resists the movement by placing one hand on the shoulder and the other on the same side of the patient's head and face.
Hitching scapula, trapezius and levator scapula	C4	The physiotherapist applies resistance over the acromioclavicular joint area while the patient endeavours to elevate his shoulder girdle.
		SUPINE
Abduction of arm, deltoid	C5 Biceps jerk	The patient holds his arm abducted 45 degrees from his side and the physiotherapist applies resistance to the lateral aspect of the arm just above the elbow.
Elbow flexion, biceps	C6 Biceps and brachio-radialis jerks	The patient holds his supinated forearm flexed at the elbow to 90 degrees. Resistance is applied against the anterior surface of the forearm just above the wrist.
Elbow extension, triceps	C7 Triceps jerk	The patient holds his elbow flexed to 90 degrees and resistance is applied against the dorsum of the forearm just above the wrist.

Extension of thumb, extensor pollicis longus	C8	The patient flexes his elbow to 90 degrees and supinates his forearm to mid-position and holds his extended thumb away from the palm pointing towards his face. Resistance is directed against the thumb-nail towards the little finger.
Interphalangeal flexion, flexor digitorum profundus	C8	The patient flexes his elbow to 90 degrees and supinates his forearm to mid-position. The physiotherapist stablizes his forearm and curls his fingers into his palm so that the patient in clenching his fist squeezes the physiotherapist's fingers. She tests the power of his long finger flexors by resisting terminal interphalangeal flexion.
Intrinsic action of the fingers	T1	The patient flexes his elbows to 90 degrees, extends his fingers at the interphalangeal joints and flexes them at the metacarpophalangeal joints. The physiotherapist places her finger between adjacent fingers in turn while the patient squeezes his extended fingers together to prevent the physiotherapist sliding her finger out along the length of the patient's fingers.

Motor supply in the leg is tested standing, supine and prone lying.

		STANDING
Plantar flexion, gastrocnemius	S1	The patient stands on one leg rising onto his toes and lowering while the physiotherapist holds his hands to maintain balance.
		SUPINE
Hip flexion, iliopsoas	L2	The patient holds his flexed hip and knee at 90 degrees while resistance is applied just above the knee.

Knee extension, quadriceps	L3 Knee jerk	The physiotherapist threads one arm under the patient's lower thigh to place her hand on the opposite thigh. While the patient holds his leg just short of the fully extended position, resistance is applied against the front of the leg just above the ankle.
Dorsiflexion with inversion, tibialis anterior	L4 Knee jerk	The patient holds his foot in dorsiflexion and inversion while the physiotherapist applies resistance against the the dorsomedial surface of the proximal end of the first metatarsal.
Big toe extension, extensor hallucis longus	L5	The patient holds his foot and toes dorsiflexed while resistance is placed against the nail of the big toe.
Toe extension, extensor digitorum longus	L5 (and S1)	The patient holds his foot and toes dorsiflexed whilst resistance is applied against the dorsal surface of all toes.
Eversion, peroneus longus and brevis	S1 Ankle jerk	The patient is asked to keep his heels together and hold the soles of his feet twisted away from each other. The physiotherapist applies resistance against the lateral borders of the feet, pushing them towards each other.
		PRONE
Knee flexion, hamstrings	L5 and S1	The patient holds his knee flexed to 90 degrees while the physiotherapist applies resistance behind the patient's heel.
Hip extension, gluteus maximus	L4 and L5 (S1 and S2)	The patient holds his hip extended with the knee bent while the physiotherapist applies a downward resistance just above the knee with one hand and palpates the gluteal mass medially with the other hand to assess firmness.

OTHER NEUROLOGICAL TESTS (as applicable)
1. Babinski; 2. Clonus

The relationship of sensory disturbance to nerve root involvement is simplified by remembering that the thumb and index finger are supplied by C6, the index, middle and ring fingers by C7 and the ring and little fingers by C8. Dermatomes of C5 and T1 reach to the wrist on the lateral and medial aspects respectively. In the foot the dorso-medial aspect of the foot to the big toe is supplied by L4, the dorsum

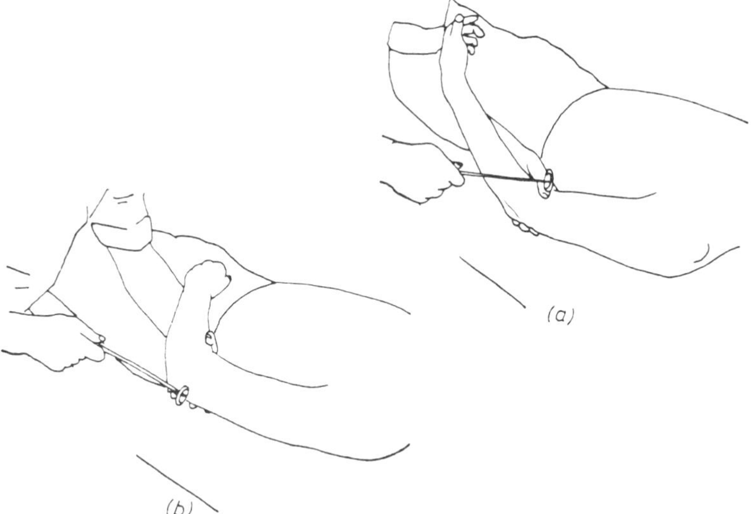

Figure 2.39. – Testing: (a) biceps reflex; (b) triceps reflex

of the foot over the top of all toes to the ball of foot by L5, and the lateral aspect of the foot and the little toe by S1 (*see Figure 2.1*).

The biceps and triceps reflexes are the main reflexes in the arm tested to elicit disturbances caused by nerve root compression, although this test can be extended to the supinator, finger flexors and deltoid. To test the biceps reflex the patient's slightly flexed arm must be fully supported and completely relaxed. The thumb, placed firmly over the biceps tendon at the elbow, is then tapped with the percussion hammer. The triceps reflex is tested by tapping the triceps tendon behind the elbow while the patient's hand rests on his abdomen and his flexed elbow is supported in the physiotherapist's hand (*Figure 2.39*).

To test the knee jerk with the patient lying supine the physio-therapist must slightly flex the patient's knee approximately 30 degrees and ensure that the quadriceps is relaxed before tapping the patellar tendon. When the response is weak some reinforcement may be gained by asking the patient to grip his hands together in a monkey-grip and pull strongly. If the ankle jerk is tested while the patient lies prone the distal end of his tibia should be supported to flex his knee approximately 30 degrees. The tendo-Achilles is then trapped. This reflex activity is increased when the patient kneels erect on fully supported lower legs with his feet over the edge of the couch.

From the physiotherapist's point of view the examination cannot be considered complete unless certain facts have been clarified. For example, if radiographs have been taken the physiotherapist should endeavour to see them so as to be more aware of the state of the spine being treated. It is important to be familiar with the radiological appearance of the normal spine, for example, the contour and position of vertebrae, the size and appearance of disc spaces and intervertebral foramina. This knowledge helps the correlation of congenital and developmental abnormalities with physical findings. The physiotherapist should find out if the patient has had an extended course of steroid therapy and should know the extent of any osteoporotic changes caused by such treatment. Although it is the province of the medial practitioner to exclude from manipulative treatment patients with signs of cord or cauda equina compression, it is our responsibility to be aware of these dangers. Finally, as a result of our interpretation we should realize that although nerve root signs involving two roots can be due to benign pathology in the lumbar area, dual root signs are unlikely to have a benign origin in the cervical area.

All of the text in this chapter on examination is summarized in the following tables.

TABLE 2.2

Planning the Examination

A. The sources of the symptoms

1. Name as *possible* source of *any part* of the patient's pain every joint and muscle which must be examined:

Joints which lie under the painful area	**Joints** which refer pain into the area	**Muscles** which lie under the painful area

2. Are you going to do a **neurological** examination? Yes/No

B. Influence of symptoms and pathology on examination and first treatment

1. Is pain 'severe'? Yes/No

2. Does the subjective examination suggest an easily irritable disorder? **Local pain** Yes/No **Referred pain** Yes/No

   Give the Example

   Part (*i*) Activity causing pain . . . .
   Part (*ii*) Severity of pain so caused . . . .
   Part (*iii*) Duration before pain subsides . . . .

3. Does the 'nature' of the pain indicate caution?
   (*i*) pathology (osteoporosis, RA etc.)
   (*ii*) easy to cause bouts
   (*iii*) imminent nerve root compression Yes/No

C. **The kind of examination**

   1. Do you think you will need to be gentle or moderately vigorous with your examination of movements?

   2. Do you expect a comparable sign { to be easy or to be hard } to find?

D. **Provocative factors leading to the cause of pain**

   What associated factors must be examined
   (*a*) as reasons why the joint or muscle has become painful?
   or
   (*b*) why the joint or muscle pain may recur?
   (e.g., posture, muscle imbalance, muscle power, obesity, stiffness, hypermobility, instability, deformity in a proximal or distal joint etc.)

E. *In planning the TREATMENT* (after the examination) *what measures would you use to prevent or lessen recurrences?*

TABLE 2.3
Cervical Spine

A. Subjective examination

1. *Area of symptoms*

   (*a*) Record on 'body chart'
   (*i*) area and depth of pain indicating areas of greatest intensity and stating type of symptoms;
   (*ii*) paraesthesia;
   (*iii*) anaesthesia.
   (*b*) Check for pain all other areas which are relevant to the cervical spine.

2. *Behaviour of symptoms*

(*a*) When are they present or when do they fluctuate and why?
(*b*) What effect does rest have on the local pain and the referred pain. (What pillow is used–size and content?) Does the patient need to get up during the night because of pain (severe intractable pain indicative of acute inflammatory process or Ca.)
What is the pain like on rising in the morning; is the neck stiff?
(*c*) What aggravates the symptoms? What positions ease the symptoms?
(*d*) What is the pain like with activities involving sustained neck flexion or other sustained positions?

3. *Special questions*

(*a*) Does the patient have any associated dizziness (vertebral artery)?
(*b*) Does the patient have bilateral tingling in hands and/or feet, or any disturbance to gait (cord signs)?
(*c*) General health and relevant weight loss.
(*d*) What tablets are being taken for this and other conditions (osteoporosis from extensive steroid therapy)?
(*e*) Have recent radiographs been taken?

4. *History*

(*a*) of this attack;
(*b*) of previous attacks, or of associated symptoms.
(*c*) Are the symptoms worsening or improving?
(*d*) Prior treatment.

Highlight important findings with asterisks

5. *Plan*

(*a*) Which joints and muscles must be examined as a possible cause of the symptoms? (Remember G/H and cuff, also ribs.)
(*b*) What other factors should be examined?
e.g., muscle weakness, imbalance or shortening; posture, etc.
(*c*) What is your assessment of the patient's symptoms in regard to:
(*i*) severity;
(*ii*) 'irritability' of the condition;
(*iii*) nature of the referred symptoms, or ease of recurrence?

B. Objective examination

Observation

Posture, willingness to move head and neck

Movements

Other joints (quick tests)
(Move to pain or move to limit)
F(flexion), E(extension), LF Ⓛ and Ⓡ (lateral flexion to left and right) Rot^{n} Ⓛ and Ⓡ (rotation to left and right); pain and its behaviour, range, protective deformity, localizing, overpressure, intervertebral movement (repeated movement and increased speed)

When Applicable

Differentiating between upper and lower cervical
Passive intervertebral movement (PPIVM) C1/2 rotation
Sustained E, LF towards pain, Rot^{n} towards pain (when necessary to reproduce referred pain)
Q, upper and/or lower, and sustained (if F, E, LF and Rot^{n} are negative)
Compression and distraction (if F, E, LF and Rot^{n} and Q are negative)
Compression in slight LF towards pain and minimal E (when necessary to reproduce referred pain)
Sustained Rot^{n} each side and E or Q (vertebral artery)
Other vertebral artery tests
Active peripheral joint tests

Supine

Neurological examination
Isometric tests for muscle pain
Passive physiological intervertebral movements (PPIVM) F, E, LF, Rot^{n}
First rib
Passive peripheral joint tests

Prone

'Palpation'
  Temperature and sweating
  Soft tissue palpation
  Position of vertebrae
  Passive intervertebral accessory movement
Examination of other relevant factors (*see* A, 5b)

C. Other tests

Check 'case notes' for reports and relevant tests
(radiographs, blood tests)

Highlight important findings with asterisks

D. After treatment

(*i*) Warning of possible exacerbation
(*ii*) Request to report details
(*iii*) Instruction in 'neck care' if required

TABLE 2.4

Thoracic Spine

A. Subjective examination

1. *Area of symptoms*

(*a*) Record on 'body chart'.
  (*i*) area and depth of pain indicating areas of greatest intensity and stating type of symptoms;
  (*ii*) paraesthesia;
  (*iii*) anaesthesia.
(*b*) Check for pain all other areas which are relevant to the thoracic spine.

2. *Behaviour of symptoms*

(*a*) When are they present or when do they fluctuate and why?
(*b*) What effect does rest have on the local pain and the referred pain? (What type of bed is used?)
Does the patient need to get up during the night because of pain? (Severe intractable pain indicative of acute inflammatory process, ankylosing spondylitis or Ca.)
What is the pain like on rising in the morning; is the back stiff?
(*c*) What aggravates the symptoms; What positions ease the symptoms?
(*d*) What is the pain like with activities involving sustained bending or other sustained positions?
(*e*) Is pain felt on full inspiration or full expiration?

3. *Special questions*

(*a*) Does the patient have bilateral tingling in the feet, or any disturbance to gait (cord signs)?
(*b*) General health and relevant weight loss.
(*c*) What tablets are being taken for this and other conditions? (Osteoporosis from extensive steroid therapy)?
(*d*) Have recent radiographs been taken?

4. *History*

(*a*) of this attack;
(*b*) of previous attacks, or of associated symptoms.
(*c*) Are the symptoms worsening or improving?
(*d*) Prior treatment.

Highlight important findings with asterisks

5. *Plan*

(*a*) Which joints and muscles must be examined as a possible cause? (Remember C/V, and I/C).
(*b*) What other factors should be examined, e.g. muscle weakness, imbalance or shortening, posture, etc?
(*c*) What is the assessment of the patient's symptoms in regard to:
(*i*) severity;
(*ii*) 'irritability' of the condition;
(*iii*) nature of the referred symptoms?

B. Objective examination

Observation

Posture, willingness to move

Movement

(Move to pain or move to limit)
F,E,LF Ⓛ and Ⓡ, Rot^{n} Ⓛ and Ⓡ; pain and behaviour, range, protective deformity, localizing, overpressure, intervertebral movement (repeated movement and increased speed).

When applicable

Neck movements should be tested for upper thoracic pain.

Cervical rotation may need to be superimposed onto thoracic rotation for testing upper thoracic joints.

Rotation may require testing in F and E.

Sustained E, LF towards pain, Rot^{n} towards pain (when necessary to reproduce referred pain)

Tap test (when F, E, LF and Rot^{n} are negative)

Compression and distraction (when F, E, LF and Rot^{n} and tap are negative)

Active peripheral joint tests

First rib

Passive physiological intervertebral movement (PPIVM) F, E and LF

Supine

Passive neck F; range, pain (back and/or referred)

SIJ (sacro-iliac joints)

Neurological examination (sensation)

Passive peripheral joint tests

Side lying

Passive physiological intervertebral movement (PPIVM) rotation

Prone

'Palpation'

Temperature and sweating

Soft tissue palpation

Position of vertebrae and ribs especially first rib

Passive intervertebral accessory movement, costovertebral and intercostal movement

Isometric tests for muscle pain

Examination of other relevant factors (*see* A, 5b)

C. Other tests

Check 'case notes' for reports of relevant tests
(radiographs, blood tests)

Highlight important findings with asterisks

D. After treatment

(*i*) Warning of possible exacerbation
(*ii*) Request to report details
(*iii*) Instruction in 'back care' if required

TABLE 2.5
Lumbar Spine

A. Subjective examination

1. *Area of symptoms*

(*a*) Record on 'body chart'
   (*i*) area and depth of pain indicating areas of greatest intensity and stating type of symptoms;
   (*ii*) paraesthesia;
   (*iii*) anaesthesia.

(*b*) Check for pain all other areas which are relevant to lumbar spine.

2. *Behaviour of symptoms*

- (*a*) When are they present or when do they fluctuate and why?
- (*b*) What effect does rest have on the local pain and referred pain? (What type of bed is used? What is the effect of supine, prone and side lying?) Does the patient need to get up during the night because of pain? (Severe intractable pain indicative of acute inflammatory process, ankylosing spondylitis or Ca.)
  What is the pain like on rising in the morning; is the back stiff?
- (*c*) What aggravates the symptoms? What positions ease the symptoms?
- (*d*) What is the pain like with activities which involve the lower back (particularly flexion)?
- (*e*) What effect does sitting have on the back pain and the leg pain?
  Does the patient have any difficulty standing from sitting?
- (*f*) What effect on the symptoms has coughing or sneezing (back and/or leg pain)?

3. *Special questions*

- (*a*) Does the patient have any bladder retention, or anaesthesia in this area? (cauda equina compression)
- (*b*) General health and relevant weight loss.
- (*c*) What tablets are being taken for this and other conditions (osteoporosis from extensive steroid therapy)?
- (*d*) Have recent radiographs been taken?
- (*e*) Cord signs for L1 level.

4. *History*

- (*a*) of this attack;
- (*b*) previous attacks, or of associated symptoms.
- (*c*) Are the symptoms worsening or improving?
- (*d*) Prior treatment.

Highlight important findings with asterisks

5. *Plan*

- (*a*) Which joints and muscles must be examined as a possible cause?
- (*b*) What other factors should be examined, e.g. muscle weakness, imbalance or shortening, posture, etc?
- (*c*) What is your assessment of the patient's symptoms in regard to:
  - (*i*) severity;
  - (*ii*) 'irritability' of the conditions;
  - (*iii*) nature of the referred symptoms, or ease of recurrence?

B. Objective examination

Observation

Getting out of the chair, willingness to move, gait, posture

Movements

Other joints (quick tests)
(Move to pain or move to limit)
F, E, LF Ⓛ and Ⓡ, Rot^n Ⓛ and Ⓡ; pain and behaviour, range, protective deformity, localizing, over-pressure, intervertebral movement. (Repeated movement and increased speed).

When applicable

Sustained E and LF towards pain, (when necessary to reproduce referred pain)
Quadrants (if F, E, LF and Rot^n are negative)
Tap test (if F, E, LF, Rot^n and Q are negative)
Compression and distraction (if F, E, LF, Rot^n, Q and Tap are negative)
Neurological (calf)
Active peripheral joint tests

Supine

Passive neck F; range, pain (back and/or leg pain) (may require combining with slouch sitting and SLR)
Passive SLR (straight leg raising); range, pain (compare supine with standing)
SIJ
Neurological examination
Resisted isometric tests for muscular pain
When applicable compare F (and/or SLR) in standing with supine
Passive peripheral joint tests

Prone

Passive PKB (prone knee bend)
Neurological examination
Resisted isometric tests for muscular pain
'Palpation'
- Temperature and sweating
- Soft tissue palpation
- Position of vertebrae
- Passive intervertebral accessory movement

Examination of other relevant factors (*see* A,5b)
Passive peripheral joint tests

Side lying

Passive physiological intervertebral movement (PPIVM); F, E, LF, Rot^n

C. Other tests

Check 'case notes' for reports of relevant tests
(radiographs, blood tests)

Highlight important findings with asterisks

D. After treatment

(*i*) Warning of possible exacerbation
(*ii*) Request to report details
(*iii*) Instructions in 'back care' if required

3 Techniques of Mobilization

Techniques of mobilization must be mastered before manipulation is attempted. They are presented here as simply as possible. The techniques, therefore, have been kept to a minimum, those more easily handled being described first and each one is described in such a way that it forms a natural step towards the manipulative techniques described later. As skill develops with practice and experience, the physiotherapist sometimes finds that other starting positions are easier, and she may make changes to suit her own needs. For descriptive purposes the spine is divided into cervical, thoracic and lumbar regions. As in the previous chapter the patient is referred to as 'he' and the physiotherapist as 'she' for the reasons given on page 10, despite the fact that in the figures both patient and physiotherapist are males.

The most important factor in achieving effective mobilization is learning to sense or 'feel' movement. It can be likened to the way in which one feels for the meshing of cogs in the gearbox of a car when changing gears; the movements taking place inside cannot be seen but can be sensed. Until this feel is learned by practice, treatment by mobilization will not be fully effective. Many people seem to believe that treatment by passive movement necessarily involves stretching but this is not always so. However, treatment always involves movement whether it is stretching or not; hence the importance of feeling movement. All of the techniques involve oscillatory movements but if the rate of oscillation is too quick or too slow it will be impossible to gain any feel of movement at the joint. Instead the movement will feel like shaking or stretching. Although it would be wrong to try to establish any set rate, some guiding figure seems reasonable and therefore a rate of two or three oscillations per second is offered as a guide. The importance of learning to feel movement cannot be emphasized too much for without this feel examination will be less informative and treatment less effective.

To produce movement of a joint in any one direction, it is easier to gain the fullest range, with least effort for the physiotherapist and without strain to the patient, if this joint is positioned approximately in the mid-position of all its other ranges. A clear example of this is seen in the metacarpophalangeal joint of the index finger. If the maximum distraction movement with least effort is desired the starting position should be midway between the normal limits of flexion, extension, abduction, adduction and the rotations. To put the joint at the limit of any one of these ranges will severely limit the range of distraction movement. When applying this principle to the cervical spine it is clear that if the head and neck are kept in normal alignment the lowest cervical intervertebral joints will be much nearer their extended than their flexed position. Therefore, when using the techniques of longitudinal movement, rotation, lateral flexion or traction (and in a smaller measure this applies to the techniques involving pressures to the vertebrae) it is necessary to position the neck in some degree of flexion in order to gain the mid-position between the limits of flexion and extension for the lowest cervical intervertebral joints. Exactly the same principle applies to the techniques of traction, longitudinal movement and rotation in the lumbar spine. When movement is desired in the lower joints the lumbar spine should be positioned towards flexion and when the upper lumbar joints are being mobilized the position of the lumbar spine as a whole is towards extension.

In Chapter 2, watching for disturbances in the normal rhythm of movement was emphasized (page 20). This is equally important when performing cervical and lumbar rotation techniques. During treatment mobilization is directed to the faulty joint even though the adjacent joints are also rotated. Therefore, during the rotary mobilization distortion of the movement should be watched for and if the faulty joint is the cause of such distortion the movement should be performed only up to this point and not carried beyond it.

Techniques which involve pressure against some part of the vertebra require special care. The thumbs or the hands are only the medium through which the physiotherapist's bodyweight is transmitted to the vertebrae to produce movement. If the intrinsic muscles of the hands are used to produce the pressure, the technique will immediately become uncomfortable to both patient and physiotherapist, the hands will become tense and all possibility of 'feeling' the movement will be lost. A study of the diagrams will show how the shoulders are positioned above or behind the hands, and how the joints from the shoulders downwards act as a series of springs. Every effort should be made at the beginning to observe these points.

When performing techniques which involve direct pressure on palpable parts of an individual vertebra two basic sets of circumstances can exist.

(*a*) The technique may be used in the treatment of a stiff joint with the intention of increasing its range. Movement is produced by thumb pressures against the vertebrae (*see* pages 34–42) and the direction chosen should be in the direction which is stiff.

(*b*) These same techniques can be used in the treatment of pain rather than stiffness. Under these circumstances the method is to produce as large an amplitude of movement as is possible with the gentlest of pressure and without feeling any degree of stiffness. If postero-anterior pressures are used on the spinous process care must be exercised to find the right position for the supporting fingers as well as the right direction for the arms and thumbs to be on top of the movement. This can be likened to applying pressure on top of one of a series of balls set in rubber (*Figure 3.1*). If the direction of the pressure or the point of contact of the pressure is off centre the movement produced will not be a pure postero-anterior movement. During performance of the technique this will be felt as uneven pressure under the thumbs or sliding on the spinous process.

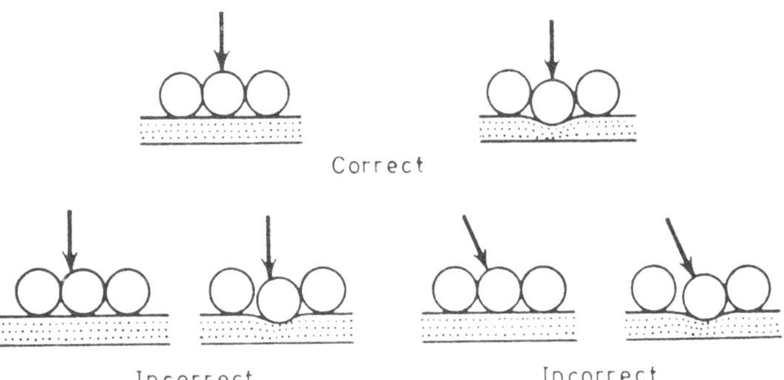

Figure 3.1. – Direction of pressure on spinous processes

The starting positions are also important since they must allow the patient to relax completely and the physiotherapist to work effectively with the minimum of effort. Relaxation of the physiotherapist's hands is essential, for it is impossible to feel through hands which are tense.

When using the cervical techniques of lateral flexion and rotation, relaxation and finer control will be obtained if the physiotherapist cradles the patient's head between her arm and chest so that she hugs it.

Each of these techniques when practised on the normal spine or when used in treatment can be performed in different positions in the range using movements of small or large amplitude. Application of technique in treatment will be discussed in Chapter 4 but for the sake of learning the techniques on the normal spine the types of movement are divided into four grades.

Grade I is a tiny amplitude movement near the starting position of the range.

Grade II is a large amplitude movement which carries well into the range. It can occupy any part of the range but does not reach the limit of the range.

Grade III is also a large amplitude movement but one which reaches to the limit of the range.

Grade IV is a tiny amplitude movement at the limit of the range.

These grades can be depicted diagrammatically against a line representing a range of movement from the starting or resting position to the limit of the range. This line can be representative of any chosen movement and although the end of the range is always the same the starting position can be any position of choice. For example, cervical rotation of the supine patient is most easily considered as starting from the position where the face faces forwards. Obviously the end position will be full rotation with the face looking approximately over the shoulder (*Figure 3.2*):

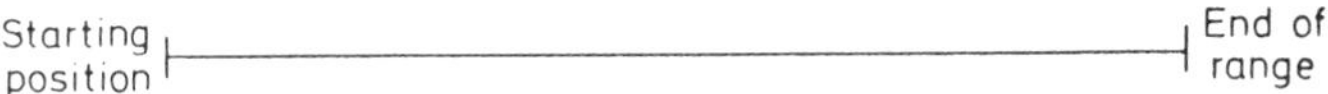

The arrows, marked for each of the four grades, depict the amplitude of each of the movements and the position they occupy in the range (*Figure 3.3*):

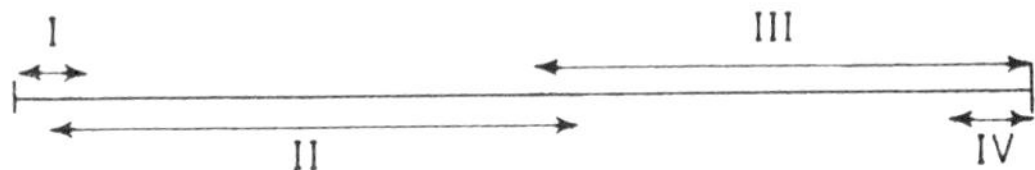

When pathology limits the range of movement the grades are reduced in range also (*Figure 3.4*):

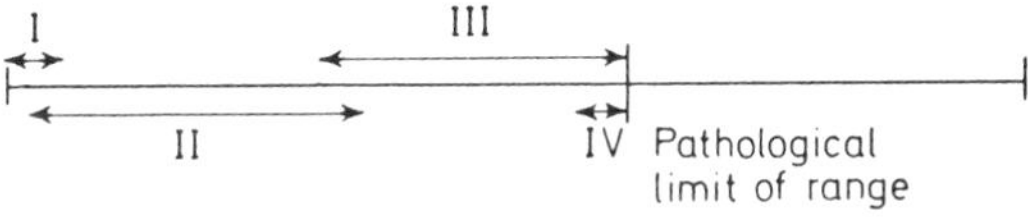

Learning to control the gentleness of Grade I is as important as learning to control the smoothness of rhythm with Grades II and III, and all of these need far more emphasis than Grade IV. The oscillatory movement is applied for 20 or more seconds at a time.

Longitudinal movement (↔)

Starting position

The patient lies supine, his neck level with the end of the couch. His head, supported in the physiotherapist's hands, rests with the joint being treated in a neutral position, approximately midway between full flexion and full extension or as near to it as pain permits.

The physiotherapist stands at the head of the couch with the back of the patient's head cradled in her right hand so that the fingers are spread over the left side of the patient's occiput to behind the left ear while the thumb is placed behind the right ear. The palm of the right hand is so positioned that the palmar surface of the metacarpo-phalangeal joint of the index finger lies over the superior nuchal line. This then forms a good grasp of the occipital area of the head. If the lower cervical spine is the only section requiring mobilization, the right hand grasps around the neck immediately above the level being treated. The physiotherapist comfortably grasps the patient's chin with her left hand from the left side being careful to avoid any pressure on the throat. The left forearm lies along the left side of the patient's face.

The physiotherapist, with her feet in a position of walking and her arms flexed at the elbows, crouches over the patient's head to hold the crown of his head against the front of her left shoulder (*Figure 3.5*).

Method

The oscillatory movement, elongating the patient's neck, is produced at the intervertebral joints by a gentle longitudinal pulling through the physiotherapist's forearms combined with a slight backward movement of her body, followed by an equally controlled relaxation to the starting position. This is repeated continuously to produce the oscillation.

As the technique is gentle, friction between the patient and couch is sufficient to prevent any sliding of the patient.

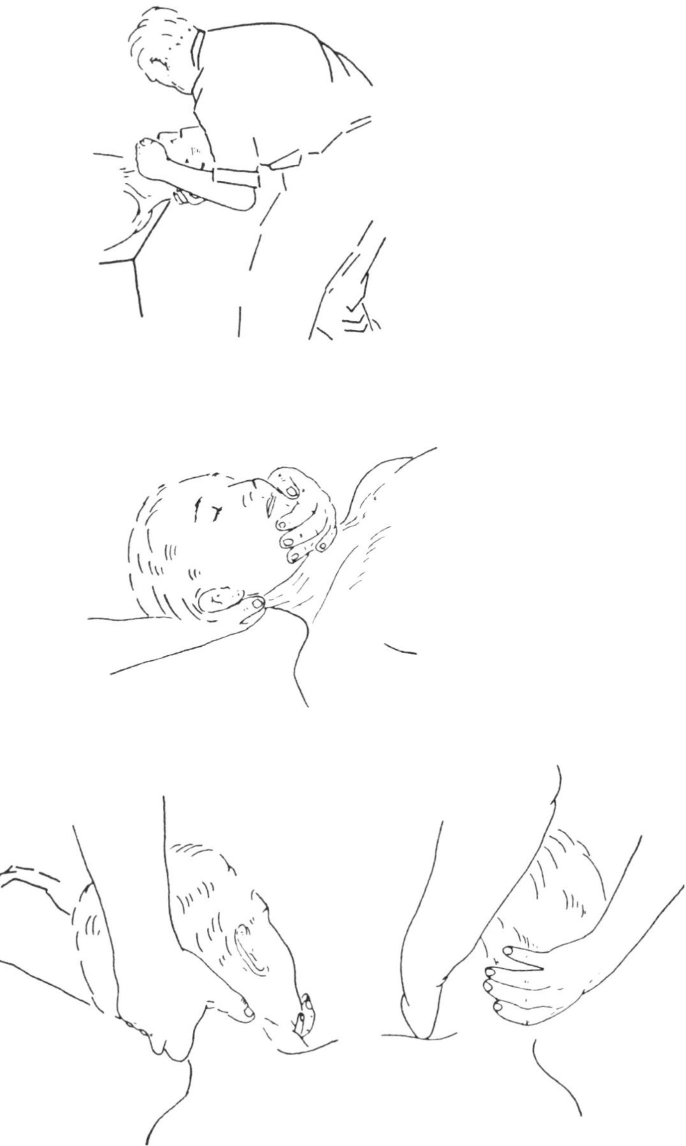

Figure 3.5. – Cervical region. Longitudinal movement (↔)

Local variations

When this technique is used in treatment of the lowest cervical intervertebral levels the neck should be positioned in approximately 30 degrees of flexion. Mid-cervical treatment requires a neck position approximately in line with the body. For upper cervical problems it is the head–neck relationship rather than the angle of the neck which is important. Again the position must be midway between flexion and extension.

Precautions

Pain can be produced in the mid-thoracic spine if the pull is strong or if it is carried out with the spine in too much extension. This over-extended position must be avoided if the patient has an abnormal kyphosis, and consideration must be given to these factors when positioning the patient. A strong pull can irritate an existing thoracic condition and may in fact cause thoracic pain in a previously pain-free area.

Uses

This procedure is of particular value in gaining the confidence of the patient. By the assessment of the patient's symptoms and signs afterwards, it can serve as a useful guide as to whether or not it will be easy to relieve the symptoms. Those patients whose symptoms or signs improve markedly with this procedure are likely to respond easily and quickly. It will effect initial improvement in a neck exhibiting a protective deformity such as a wry neck.

Postero-anterior central vertebral pressure (↕)

Starting position

The patient lies face downwards. It is usually satisfactory for him to rest his forehead in the palms of his hands, but it may be necessary for the chin to be tucked well in. This is particularly necessary for mobilization of the first and third cervical vertebrae because of their relative inaccessibility. When a patient has a limited range of extension

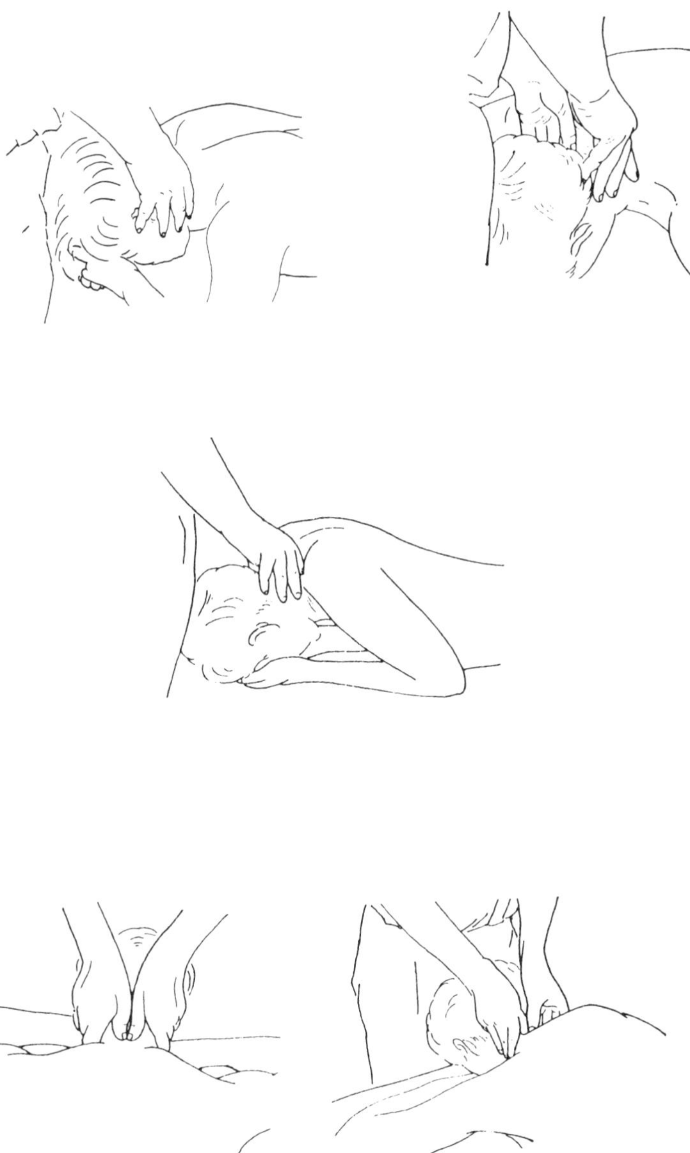

Figure 3.6. – Cervical region. Posterior-anterior central vertebral pressure (↓)

or the movement is painful an alternative starting position is for him to cradle his forehead in his palms with the arms partially under the chest.

The physiotherapist stands at the head of the patient with her thumbs held in opposition and back to back with the thumb tips on the spinous process of the vertebra to be mobilized. The fingers straddle the sides of the patient's neck and head. Balance and steadiness of the physiotherapist's thumbs are gained through the finger position, but it is unnecessary for the fingers to grip tightly.

If too much of the pad is used the localizing ability will be lost because the spinous processes are so small. However with strong pressure the bone to bone contact may be uncomfortable and it is then advisable to use more of the pad of the thumb near the tip.

The best position is to have the thumbs in contact with each other on the tip of the same spinous process. A method using one thumb to reinforce the other can be used but this tends to make very gentle technique difficult to achieve and it certainly detracts from the ability to feel small movements. In the case of the second cervical vertebra the thumbs can be placed on the upper and lower margins of its spinous process (*Figure 3.6*).

Method

Extremely gentle pressures will produce a definite feeling of movement but the tendency always is to use too much pressure.

The alternating pressure should be applied by the arms combined with the trunk. It is impossible to carry out the technique successfully or comfortably by the action of the intrinsic hand muscles. If the patient has considerable pain, thus making this technique difficult to perform, the palmar surfaces of the pads of the fingers can be used to lift the neck into a degree of flexion. This will make the technique possible in a pain-free range.

Local variations

The degree of pressure required to feel movement in the mid-cervical area is much less than that required at either the second or the seventh cervical vertebra. The first cervical vertebra is rarely able to be palpated in the midline as a bony surface; however, it is possible to produce movement by pressure through the overlying muscles and ligaments. The third cervical vertebra is often difficult to palpate due to the large and sometimes overhanging spinous process of the second cervical vertebra. Palpation of the two vertebrae is enhanced by asking the patient to tuck his head into slightly more flexion.

As was mentioned in the chapter on examination (*see* page 36) the direction of the central pressure can be angled towards the head or towards the feet. Such changes in direction may be required by pain or stiffness found with these movements.

Precautions

Excessive mobilizing in the region of first and second cervical vertebrae, both in regard to the length of time and the strength of the pressure, can produce a feeling of general weakness and nausea and can, on rare occasions, cause vomiting at the time of the mobilization or shortly afterwards. The technique must never be used if it causes giddiness.

Uses

Postero-anterior central vertebral pressure is of most benefit to those patients whose symptoms of cervical origin are situated either in the midline or distributed evenly to each side of the head, neck, arms or upper trunk.

This technique is valuable for patients who have considerable bony degenerative changes in the cervical spine, irrespective of the area to which the pain of cervical origin is referred. While carrying out this procedure on these patients however, the degree of movement felt is noticeably less than that felt in the normal cervical spine.

The technique is of particular value when pressure over the vertebrae produces even small amounts of muscle spasm. Under these circumstances the pressure used, and the depth of mobilization produced, should be just less than that which causes spasm. After using this technique it will be noticed that a greater depth of pressure can be applied before spasm reappears.

In cases where arm pain is particularly severe and active movements are only moderately limited, this technique usually aggravates the pain.

Postero-anterior unilateral vertebral pressure (•↴)

Starting position

The patient lies prone with his forehead resting comfortably on his hands. The physiotherapist stands towards the side of the patient's head. She places the tips of her thumbs, held back to back and in opposition, on the posterior surface of the articular process to be mobilized.

Her arms should be directed 30 degrees medially to prevent them from slipping off the articular process. The fingers of the uppermost hand rest across the back of the patient's neck and those of the other hand rest around the patient's neck towards his throat. Most of the contact is felt with the underneath thumb (*Figure 3.7*).

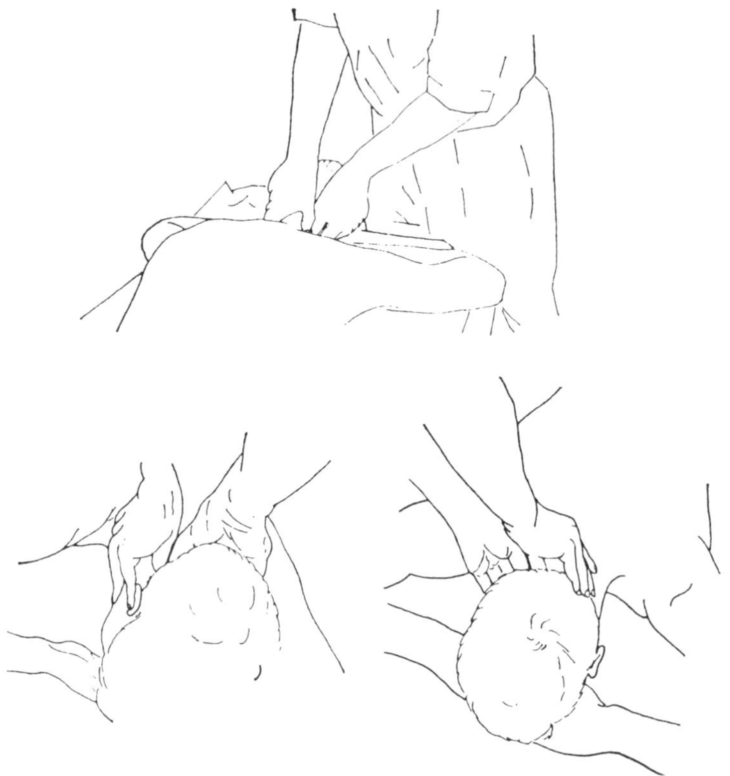

Figure 3.7. – Cervical region. Postero-anterior unilateral vertebral pressure

Method

Oscillatory pressure directed postero-anteriorly against an articular process if done very gently will produce a feeling of movement but to prevent any lateral sliding at the point of contact a gentle constant pressure directed medially must be maintained. If the movement is produced correctly there will be small nodding movements of the head but no rotary or lateral flexion movement.

As with other techniques involving pressures through the thumbs this movement must not be produced by intrinsic muscle action.

Local variations

When mobilizing the first cervical vertebra, the physiotherapist needs to lean over the patient's head so as to direct the line of her thumbs towards the patient's eye. In the lower cervical area the line is directed more caudally.

The second, third and fourth articular processes are far easier to feel accurately than are the remainder. The first cervical vertebra can be felt laterally and the lower articular processes can be felt if the thumbs are brought in under the lateral border of the trapezius.

The symbol indicates that the unilateral pressure on the vertebra is directly postero-anterior in direction. There are two common variations to this direction which are used in treatment. Under circumstances where pain is quite severe the direction is angled slightly away from postero-anterior as indicated by the symbol . The second variation, used when the joint is stiff and pain is minimal, is to angle the pressure more medially endeavouring to increase the range. The angle is indicated by the symbol . Also, as was mentioned in the chapter on examination (*see* page 36) these directions can be varied still further by inclining them cephalad and caudad as indicated by the requirements of pain or stiffness.

Precautions

The only precaution is to perform the techniques very gently especially in the upper cervical region. It is seldom realized how effective these techniques can be while still being performed very gently.

Uses

Application of this technique is the same as for the previous technique except that it is used for unilateral symptoms on the side of the pain.

Postero-anterior unilateral vertebral pressure (C1/2)

When postero-anterior unilateral vertebral pressure is applied to C2 with the patient's head straight it is the C2/3 joint which is being examined or mobilized. If however the patient's head is turned to the left and postero-anterior unilateral vertebral pressure is applied to the left side of C2 it is C1/2 rotation which is being examined or mobilized. This is because when the prone patient turns his head to the left, C1 is fully rotated to the left on C2 and postero-anterior pressure on the left articular pillar of C2 further increases this rotation.

Starting position

The patient lies prone with his head turned approximately 30 degrees to the left. He places his forehead in his palms. The physiotherapist stands at his head. She places the tips of both thumbs, their nails back to back, against the articular pillar of C2 on the left. The articular pillar is found in relation to the spinous process of C2, which will be unchanged from the position it held when the head was straight, and the left lateral mass of C1. Her fingers spread to each side to stabilize the hands. She holds her thumbs in opposition and directs the long axis of each thumb in a postero-anterior direction and inclined slightly towards the head (*Figure 3.8*).

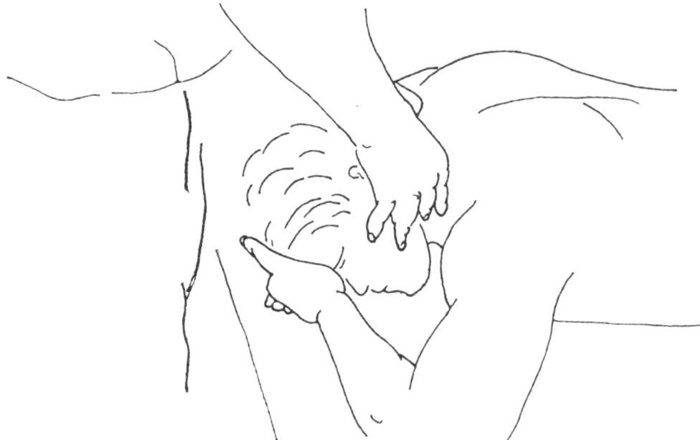

Figure 3.8. – Testing for abnormalities of C1/C2 rotation on the left side (↻)

Method

The movement is produced by a trunk and arm action transmitted to the thumbs which act as springs. Although the mobilization is created by a postero-anterior pressure against C2, it is in fact increasing the rotation between C1 and C2.

Uses

This technique is of value for suboccipital symptoms or headaches arising from the C1/2 joint. It is usually performed on the side of the pain or restriction.

Anteroposterior unilateral vertebral pressure (⌐↑)

Starting position

The patient lies supine. A pillow is not used unless the patient has a 'poking-chin' postural abnormality. The physiotherapist stands by his head and makes a broad contact with the transverse process of the vertebra to be mobilized with both thumbs. The thumbs should be used with care as direct bone to bone contact can be uncomfortable. She spreads her fingers around the adjacent neck area for stability while positioning her shoulders above the joint being treated (*Figure 3.9.*).

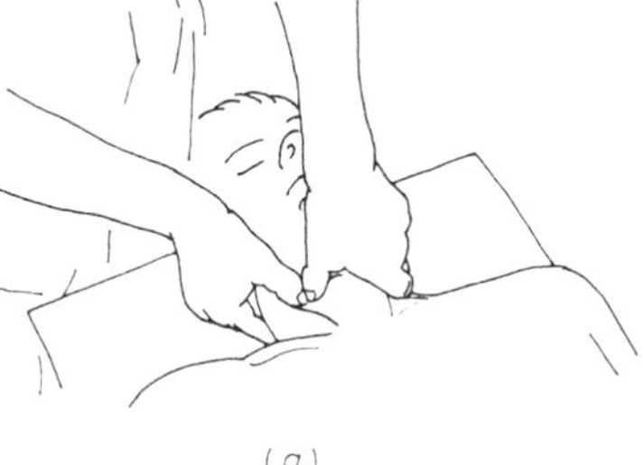

Figure 3.9(a). – Unilateral anteroposterior vertebral pressure

Method

The oscillatory anteroposterior pressures are performed very gently and the movement must be produced by the physiotherapist's arms and trunk. Any effort to produce the movement with intrinsic thenar muscle action will produce discomfort immediately.

This technique is not a comfortable one to use unless great care is taken. Also, the muscles lying over the area make direct contact rather difficult and care should be taken to see that the thumbs are positioned immediately over the transverse process. This means that at some levels the muscle belly needs to be moved to one side.

Local variations

This technique can be performed either unilaterally or bilaterally as is shown in the diagrams (*Figures 3.9a* and *b*). The intervertebral level to which one can reach varies enormously from person to person. In the stocky, heavily built patient with a short, thick neck extending down into the thoracic area is almost impossible. Conversely in the long-necked, slim person enough space is allowed to reach down to approximately T3 and sometimes even T4 (*Figure 3.9c*). With all patients the technique can be used as high as C1.

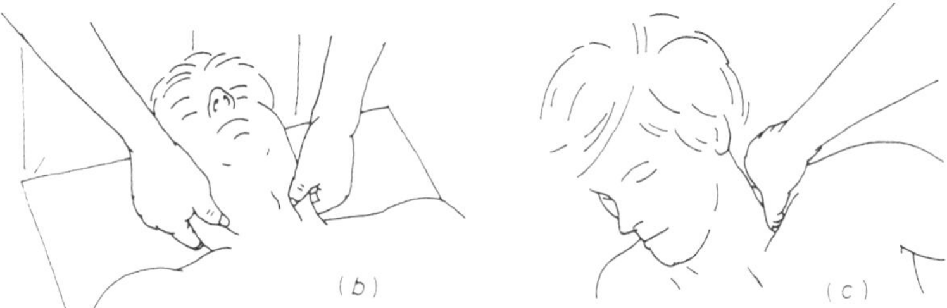

Figure 3.9. – (b) Bilateral anteroposterior vertebral pressure. (c) Anteroposterior unilateral vertebral pressure in upper thoracic area

Anteroposterior movement can be produced with the patient lying prone. The patient rests his forehead in his palms and the physiotherapist grasps around the sides of the neck to hook the palmar surface of the pads of her fingers onto the transverse process area. It is easy to localize the joint to be mobilized by the accurate placement of the fingers (*Figure 3.9d*).

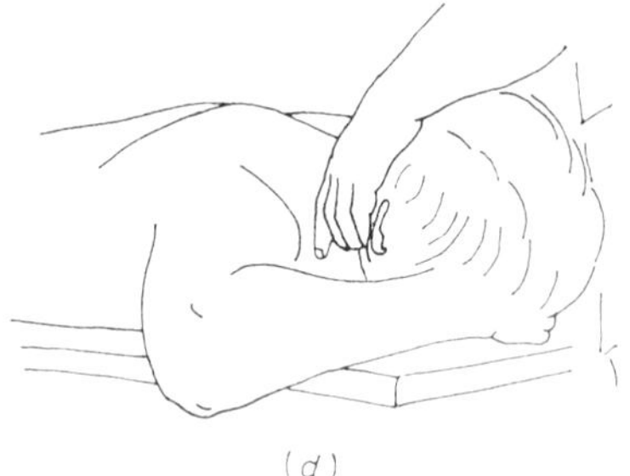

Figure 3.9. – (d) Anteroposterior unilateral vertebral pressure

Precautions

The only precaution necessary is to avoid discomfort from undue pressure.

Uses

Application of this technique is reserved for patients whose symptoms, felt anterolaterally, can be reproduced by anteroposterior pressure on the side of the pain. Pain referred to the ear or throat can often be reproduced by this technique. Under these circumstances it could be treated by the described technique.

Transverse vertebral pressure (←•—)

Starting position

The patient lies face downwards with his forehead resting on the backs of his fingers or hands, with a moderate degree of 'chin-in' position to lessen the cervical lordosis slightly.

The physiotherapist stands at the patient's right side with her hands placed over the patient's neck, so that the distal part of the pad of the

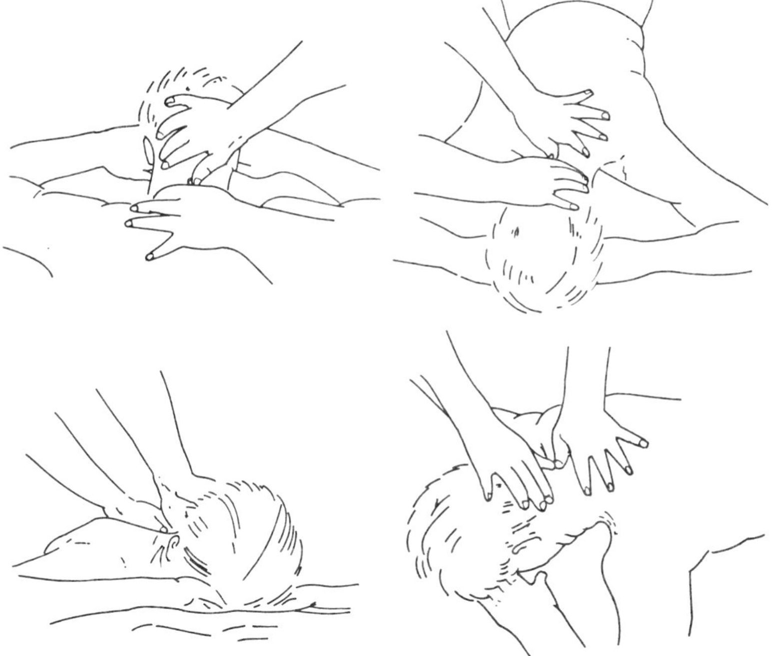

Figure 3.10. — Cervical region. Transverse vertebral pressure (←•—)

left thumb is against the right side of the spinous process, with the right thumb giving a reinforcing pressure against the left thumb-nail. The fingers of each hand spread out over the adjacent body surfaces to provide stability for the thumbs. The part of the thumb in contact with the lateral surface of the spinous process should consist of as much of the pad of the thumb near its tip as it is possible to use. The hard tip of the thumb causes too much discomfort to the patient and should be avoided. It is essential that the physiotherapist's wrists be in a position to allow for a horizontally directed pressure to be imparted to the spinous process through the thumbs (*Figure 3.10*).

Method

Only very gentle pressure should be used here because movement is produced very easily. For the same reason the amplitude of the oscillations should also be very small. It is necessary, therefore, to judge the direction and pressure finely if a feeling of movement is to be gained.

Local variations

When applying pressure in this position there is a moderate degree of natural tenderness which must be considered. This makes it necessary to use as much of the thumb pad as possible to produce the movement without jeopardizing the ability to localize the pressure to the one spinous process.

The second and the seventh cervical vertebrae are the most easily palpated. However, although the lateral surface of the seventh cervical spinous process is superficial, to reach the lateral surface of the second cervical spinous process it is sometimes necessary to get under the paravertebral muscles. The spinous processes of the third to the sixth cervical vertebrae are much smaller but can be reached by reducing the cervical lordosis with a slightly increased chin-in position of the patient's head. It is sometimes necessary to use each thumb against the same side of adjacent spinous processes to gain sufficient feeling of movement.

Uses

As with the postero-anterior central vertebral pressure, transverse vertebral pressure is of most value in cases where the cervical spine shows marked degenerative radiological changes. Its greatest application is with unilateral symptoms of cervical origin. This is particularly so if the symptoms do not extend very far from the vertebrae or are ill-defined in their area of distribution when no neurological changes are evident.

When this technique is used with patients whose symptoms of cervical origin are unilaterally distributed, it is more likely to produce an improvement if the direction of the pressure is performed from the non-painful side towards the painful side.

Variations

There are two variations of 'transverse vertebral pressure' which can be used effectively. Both involve pressure at the most lateral aspect of the vertebrae. The first description is for the method applied to the second to the sixth cervical vertebrae, and the second is for the first cervical vertebra.

Alternative transverse vertebral pressure C2–C6 (←•—)

Starting position

With the patient lying prone and his forehead resting on the backs of his fingers or hands, the physiotherapist stands to the patient's right and places the pad of the left thumb against the lateral border of the apophyseal joint, while the pad of the right thumb reinforces the left thumb-nail. The fingers of each hand spread out over the left side of the patient's neck onto the head and thorax respectively (*Figure 3.11*).

Method

With this technique the supporting fingers are used to apply a lateral flexion movement of the neck around the fulcrum of the thumbs.

The oscillating movement is produced through the thumbs with the fingers either acting as stabilizers or supplying a counter pressure by laterally flexing the neck. This counter pressure is produced by adduction of both glenohumeral joints and ulnar flexion of both wrists. It is poor technique to attempt to produce this counter pressure by finger flexion. Also, the thumb flexors must not be used as prime movers.

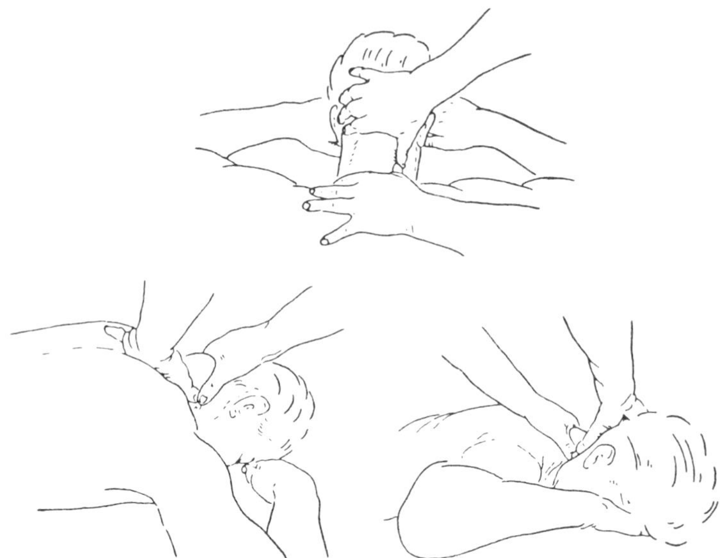

Figure 3.11. – Cervical region. Alternative transverse vertebral pressure (C2–C6 ←•–)

Local variations

This technique can only be used from the second to the sixth cervical vertebrae, and any sense of movement which can be felt is more general than that felt with the former method.

Uses

These are the same as for the former method.

Transverse vertebral pressure C1 (–•→)

Starting position

The patient lies prone with his head turned comfortably to the left. The physiotherapist stands facing the patient's head and places the tip of her left thumb over the tip of the left transverse process of the first cervical vertebra. The tip of the transverse process is found situated deeply between the angle of the mandible and the mastoid process just distal and anterior to the mastoid process. The right thumb points towards the crown of the head and is placed tip to tip with the left thumb over C1. The fingers of each hand are spread out over the adjacent surface of the crown of the head and back of the neck to stabilize the action of the thumbs (*Figure 3.12*).

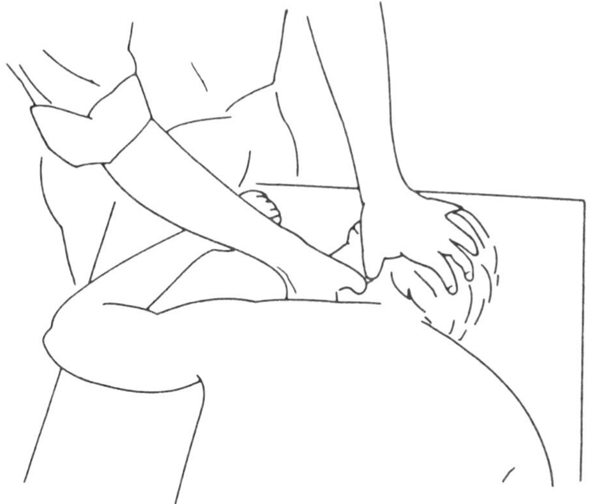

Figure 3.12. – Cervical region. Transverse vertebral pressure (C1→)

Method

As with the previous mobilizations, the pressure must be transmitted through the body and arms to the thumbs and not by thumb movement only.

The bony prominence is sometimes very difficult to find and it is normally a particularly sensitive area which sometimes prevents any deep pressure. The sense of movement with mobilization in this area is very small, and frequently it is impossible to feel any movement at all because of stiffness in the joint.

Uses

It is used for symptoms about the head or upper neck which arise from this level of the cervical spine, whether they are distributed evenly to both sides or unilaterally. If the symptoms are unilateral the technique should be carried out on the non-painful side as the first choice. If the symptoms are bilateral the mobilization should be performed on both sides.

Rotation (⟲)

Starting position

The position described is for a 'rotation' to the left. This particular starting position is chosen because it is the most suitable position for learning feel and because it is the starting position for the manipulative technique described later (*see* page 197).

The patient lies on his back so that his head and neck extend beyond the end of the couch.

The physiotherapist stands at the head of the couch and places her right hand under the patient's head and upper neck with the fingers spread out over the left side of the occiput and adjacent neck. The thumb extends along the right side of the neck with the thenar eminence over the right side of the occiput. She grasps the chin with the fingers of her left hand while the palm of the hand and the forearm lie along the left side of the patient's face and head just anterior to the ear. The patient's head should be held comfortably yet firmly between the left forearm and the heel of the right hand, and also between her left hand and the front of her left shoulder.

When oscillatory movements are being performed near the beginning of the rotation range the physiotherapist stands head-on to the patient and the occiput is centred in the palm of her right hand. When the movements are performed at the limit of the range she moves her body to the right until she is facing across the patient, and moves her hand further around the occiput towards the ear. The head should at all times be comfortably supported from underneath. The physiotherapist should crouch over the patient so that she hugs the patient's head. The position of the patient's head and neck may be raised or lowered to position the joint being treated approximately midway between its flexion and extension limits. A position of flexion is shown in the diagrams.

The starting position finally adopted should be the one where the grasp with either arm should be able to perform the movement on its own (*Figure 3.13*).

Method

The position is taken up by turning the head to the left with a synchronous action of both hands. It is most important that the fingers of the right hand should produce as much movement of the occiput as the left hand produces with the chin. This turning movement of the patient's head can be likened to the movement of a barbecue chicken as it revolves on a spit. In most other techniques the

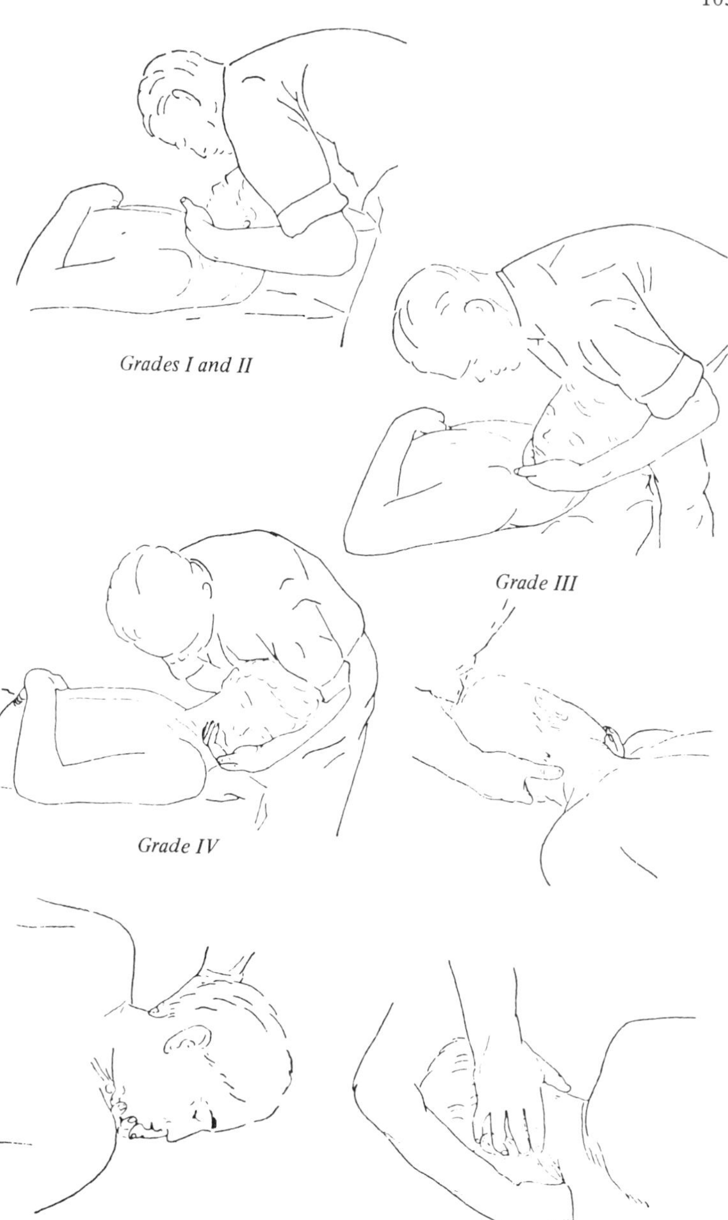

Figure 3.13. – Cervical region. Rotation

oscillatory movement is produced by body movement but with rotation the physiotherapist's trunk remains steady and the rotation is produced purely by the physiotherapist's arm movement. *The movement of the left arm is glenohumeral adduction with the elbow passing in front of the trunk.*

Particular care needs to be exercised to be sure that a normal rotation is being produced and not a rotation distorted by deformity or muscle spasm. The range at which the oscillation is done should be kept at the extreme of the normal movement obtainable.

Local variations

The upper cervical vertebrae are more readily mobilized with the head and neck in the same plane as the body. To mobilize the lower cervical vertebrae the neck needs to be held in a degree of neck flexion. The lower the cervical level being mobilized, the greater the angle of neck flexion required for successful movement of that intervertebral joint. The level being mobilized can be isolated somewhat by using the index finger of the occipital hand to hold around the vertebra above the joint.

Precautions

If a patient feels neck discomfort on the side of the neck to which the head is turned during or following this technique, it will readily disappear in a few minutes with active neck movements.

Although it may seem reasonable at times, when the technique is very gentle and symptoms are localized to the neck, to do rotation towards the side of pain, it should never be done in this direction as a strong procedure or when pain is referred from the neck. In general it is wiser to adhere to the rule that rotation should not be done towards the side of unilateral pain.

Rotation should never be used in treatment if it produces any sign of dizziness and to this end it is wise to do an exploratory rotation before carrying out rotary treatment.

Uses

Rotation is one of the most valuable mobilizing procedures for the cervical spine. It is frequently the first technique chosen when treating symptoms of cervical origin, and is of greatest value in any unilateral distribution of pain of cervical origin. In such cases the procedure is carried out with the patient's face being turned away from the painful side.

Lateral flexion (⤴)

Starting position

The position described is for a 'lateral flexion' mobilization on the right. This technique is one of the most difficult to do well and the starting position is best reached in three stages.

The patient lies on his back, with his head and neck beyond the end of the couch.

Initially the physiotherapist should stand at the head end and take up the head and arm position adopted for rotation. This position should then be altered so that her left forearm lies behind the patient's left ear almost under the occiput, and the right hand is brought forwards so that the palm covers the whole of the ear. Slight left rotation of the patient's head will balance it more comfortably until the next stage is adopted.

Without permitting any lateral flexion of the patient's head or allowing any movement of the heel of the right hand away from the patient's ear, the physiotherapist moves round alongside the patient's right shoulder to face diagonally across his head. If the right hand is kept in position, the physiotherapist's right arm will lie across the front of the patient's right shoulder and her right elbow will be almost in her right iliac fossa.

The final stage involves crouching to hug the patient's head while adopting the required degree of lateral flexion by displacing his neck to the left with the right hand and laterally flexing the head with the left hand and arm. The movement can be localized to a particular intervertebral level by the pressure of the palmar surface of the index finger, just distal to the metacarpophalangeal joint, on the relevant level of the articular pillar. Head rotation is prevented by the action of the left hand and arm and the right hand. It is imperative that the palmar surface of the right hand remain in contact with the patient if the technique is to be comfortable.

If the physiotherapist is properly crouched over the patient her right forearm will be fixed between her side and the front of the patient's shoulder (*Figure 3.14*).

Method

The oscillatory movement is produced entirely by body movement, which is a combination of movements in two directions. The physiotherapist rocks her hips gently from side to side to laterally flex his

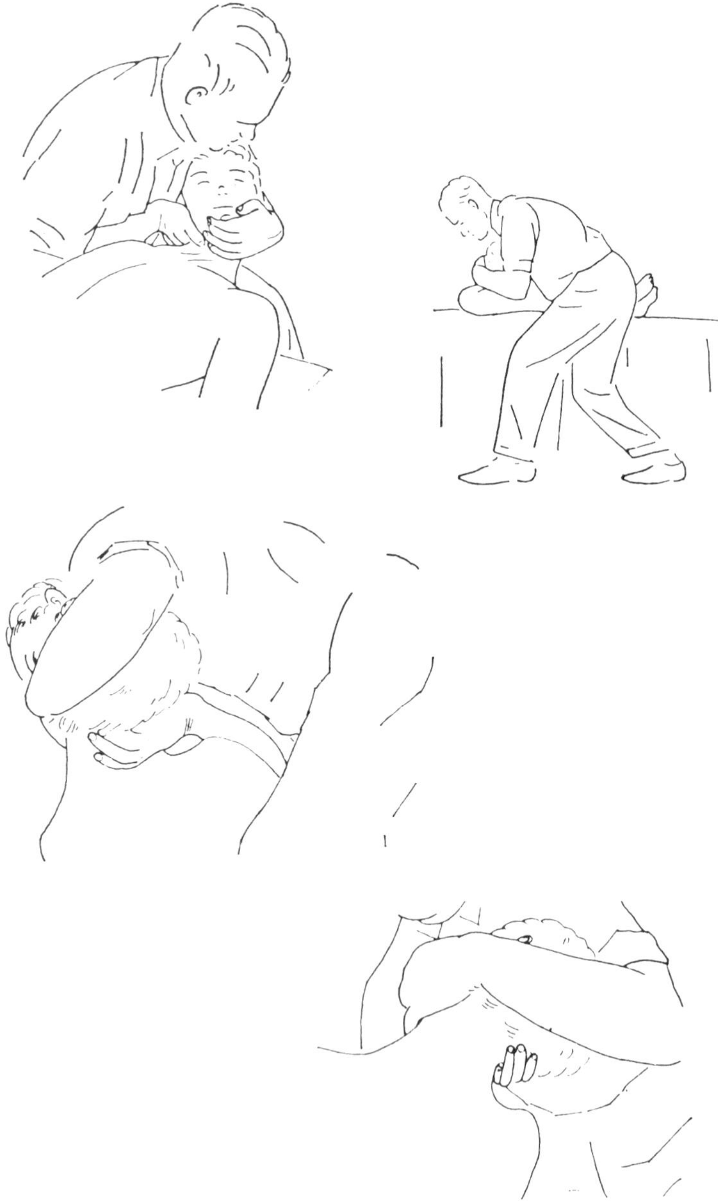

Figure 3.14. – Cervical region. Lateral flexion

neck, and at the same time employs a forward movement of her right pelvis to displace his neck away from her. These movements are transmitted to the patient's head by a very localized pressure against the articular pillar while his head is firmly hugged.

It is very easy to give an unbalanced pull on the patient's chin which will result in the patient's face being pulled out of its coronal plane. Care must be taken to control this with the heel of the right hand. If the position of the lateral flexion in the range is correctly maintained the head will not be any nearer the shoulder at the end of the procedure than it is at the beginning.

Local variations

Variations in the position of the patient's head in relation to the right shoulder are necessary when localizing the movement at the different vertebral levels. When carrying out lateral flexion at C5 or C6 the neck is taken further into lateral flexion. It may be necessary to depress the patient's shoulder to obtain sufficient space in which to work. When localizing the movement to the first cervical vertebra, the movement becomes a lateral flexion of the head without any marked curving of the neck into lateral flexion.

If lateral flexion is being localized to any of the lower levels, the neck should be flexed, and for the upper cervical levels the neck should be nearer the neutral or straight position.

The feeling of movement is greater in the mid - cervical spine than it is in either the upper or lower cervical spine, although in all positions the feeling of movement is small.

Care must be taken to stabilize the localizing index finger adequately. This is necessary because sliding on the articular pillar causes discomfort. Because of natural tenderness, pressure must be moderate and the palmar surface of the index finger must be used.

Uses

Lateral flexion is used in patients whose symptoms of cervical origin are unilaterally distributed, either cranially or in the neck, scapula or arm. In such cases, when this mobilization is being used for the first time, it is done with the patient's head laterally flexed away from the painful side. It can be used towards the painful side but this is usually only of value when the painful limitation of lateral flexion is away from the painful side.

Mobilizing in lateral flexion is often of value in improving a limitation of the patient's active range of rotation.

Cervical flexion (F)

Starting position

The patient lies supine with his head near the end of the couch. The physiotherapist, standing by his left shoulder, places her left hand over his sternum and her right hand under the occipital area. She then gently flexes his chin towards his chest and directs her right hand so that the heel of her hand is under his occiput and the fingers spread forwards over the occipital area.

The position of the right hand depends upon the level of the cervical spine being treated. The lower the level being treated the more the heel of her right hand is extended down his neck (*Figure 3.15a*).

If the high cervical area is being treated she places the occiput in the palm of her right hand and her left hand is placed over his chin (*Figure 3.14b*).

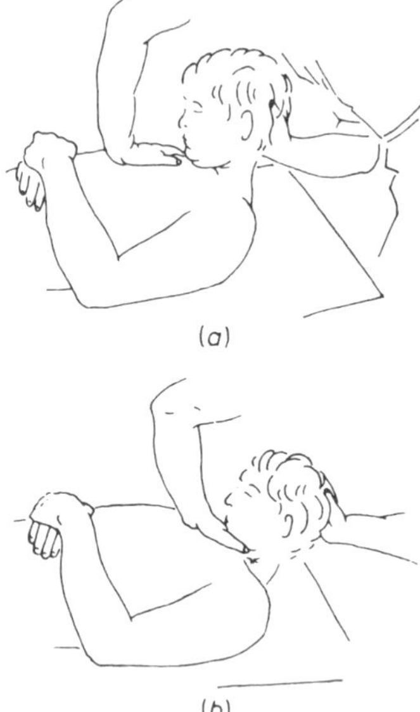

Figure 3.15. – Cervical flexion: (a) lower; (b) upper

Method

The right hand is used to flex the head and neck in a small amplitude oscillatory fashion while she directs her forearm in whatever direction is required to emphasize the flexion at particular intervertebral levels.

For example, if the middle cervical area is being treated her forearm is directed approximately horizontally whereas if the lower cervical level is being treated her elbow points slightly towards the floor. When the upper cervical area is being mobilized she places her left hand on his chin and raises her right forearm so that her elbow points slightly towards the ceiling. Under these circumstances she works both hands in an equal and opposite direction to emphasize the stretch in the upper cervical area.

Precautions

This technique is not one selected early in treatment particularly in the presence of disc pathology, neither is it a technique which should be used strongly.

Uses

The main indication for this technique is stiffness in forward flexion in the absence of pain or when pain is only minimal. It can also be used as a technique when this movement reproduces the patient's pain in any area associated with the vertebral column. This means that if left buttock pain is reproduced by neck flexion in the supine position then it can be used to mobilize the faulty structures in the lumbar vertebral canal.

Cervical traction

Although cervical traction can be administered by hand it is more efficient if this is done by means of a halter, thus enabling longer periods of traction to be maintained with less effort.

There are many types of cervical traction halter in use today but those which support under the patient's chin and occiput must be adjustable in two of their relationships. When applied to the patient it must be possible to alter the height of the occipital band in relation to the band which supports the chin. It must also be possible to adjust the strap at the side of the patient's head to control distance between the chin band and the occipital band. Once the adjustments are made they must not be able to slip. Any halter used for different patients which is not adjustable in these two directions must inevitably result in some patients being given traction with too much flexion or extension of the head. Few halters have these two adjustments, and some that do are inadequate because they are not stable when the adjustments are made. For example, one variety has the occipital strap and chin strap constructed out of one piece of material which is continuous through a metal ring from which the halter is suspended. Though the patient's position may be adjusted with his head in the frontal plane the position may be lost during treatment because the harness material is able to slide through the rings.

The two adjustments which must be possible are firstly, the vertical length of the occipital and chin straps, and secondly, the horizontal distance between them. It is necessary to be able to fit the patient who has a long or short jaw as well as the patient who has a small or large head. If the head is small it will be necessary to bring the chin strap closer to the occipital strap in its horizontal direction, and if the chin is small it will be necessary to bring the chin strap closer to the occipital strap in its vertical direction. *Figure 3.16* shows the occipital strap and chin strap each with its own pair of buckles for adjustment in the vertical direction. It is more convenient to have both sections adjustable, although the occipital strap can be of fixed length with a more widely variable length of chin strap, or vice versa. The other adjustment is made by the pair of horizontally directed straps from the occipital strap to the chin strap. They pass on each side of the patient's jaw and buckle under the chin to avoid the patient's hair becoming entangled during adjustment.

Discussion surrounding the advisability of giving traction in flexion or in a neutral position is common. However, the amount of flexion or extension of the head on the upper cervical spine during traction treatment should also be considered. This consideration is particularly relevant when the upper cervical spine is treated. It must therefore be possible to adjust the halter, not only to fit the various shapes of head and jaw but also for different 'head–neck' relationships. This is achieved by vertical adjustment of the occipital strap in relation to the chin strap.

A swivel hook in the spreader bar, as shown in *Figure 3.16,* is not an essential requirement but is very convenient. The traction is applied best through double pulley blocks and a rope. With a mechanical advantage of four, small adjustments are possible without losing any feel of the tractive pressure.

Treatment may be administered in three ways. Constant traction requires continuous bedrest for the patient with the traction applied 24 hours of the day, or in cycles of 1 hour traction followed by ½ hour rest repeated throughout the day. This type of traction is mainly used for patients with severe nerve root pain. The second method is intermittent traction, administered once or twice a day for short periods.

This is the more common variety used in physiotherapy practice and is used for patients with less severe nerve root and other intervertebral joint conditions. Thirdly, there is the method, also administered only

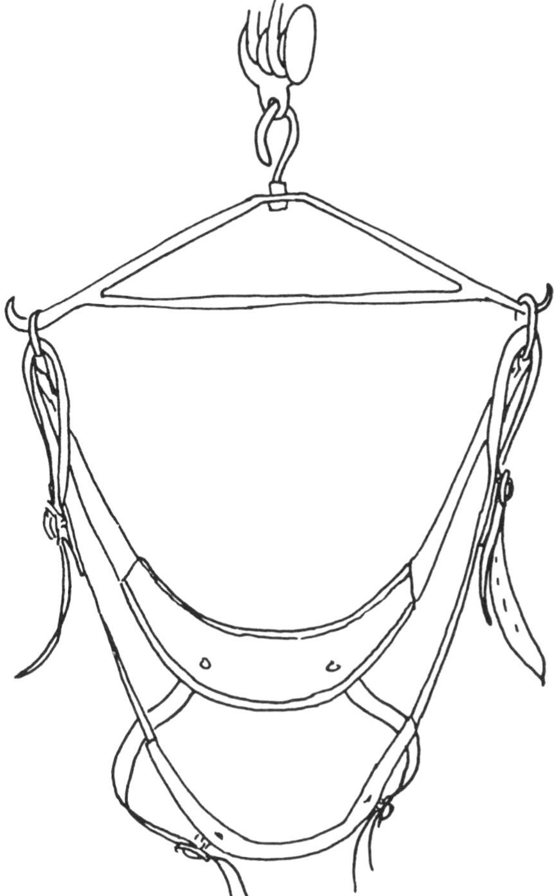

Figure 3.16. – Cervical traction halter

once or twice a day, which comprises a gradual application of traction to a certain weight which is held momentarily and then gradually released; this is followed by momentary rest before reapplication of the traction. This cycle is repeated for varying periods and the times for the 'hold' and 'rest' periods, as well as treatment times, can be varied. This 'intermittent variable traction' has a wide application among patients whose joint condition requires movement.

A patient with severe nerve root pain, if he is to be treated conservatively, requires cervical traction. A choice needs to be made between cervical traction administered in a hospital or at home on the one hand and in physiotherapy rooms alone or in conjunction with self-administered traction at home on the other. The former method seriously restricts the patient's daily movements and this must be borne in mind but the severity of the pain may demand it as the treatment choice. If traction is to be given in hospital the method is as follows.

Hospital traction

The patient is comfortably supported by pillows in a half-lying position with a pillow supporting the head and neck in the correct position. If the traction is being administered for a lower cervical nerve root pain the neck is flexed slightly on the trunk and the head is supported in a neutral position on the upper neck. If traction is being given for a high cervical nerve root pain the neck is supported in a neutral position of comfort for the patient, his head is supported in a position midway between flexion and extension of the upper cervical spine. The halter is then adjusted on the patient's head so that the chosen position will be maintained when the tractive force is applied. The direction of the pulley rope should be in line with the longitudinal axis of the joint to be treated. For the patient with lower cervical nerve root pain the rope will form an angle of some 30 degrees with his trunk whereas for high cervical nerve root pain the angle is much shallower. Initial weights used are low, approximately 2–3 kg; these can be increased by from 0.5 to 1 kg per day up to a maximum of 5 kg. The patient's build and general joint mobility on the one hand and the severity of the pain on the other govern weight. Patient tolerance governs the periods spent on traction but one hour on traction followed by half an hour's rest repeated throughout the waking periods is usually all that is required in the most severe nerve root pain if it is going to respond to this type of management. Ten days is usually sufficient time for the traction to be maintained and if there is no improvement in the first seven days it is unlikely that the patient will be helped by the constant traction. Traction at home may be used intermittently following the hospital traction.

There are many positions described in the literature for applying traction to the cervical spine varying between full flexion and extension. Basically the position chosen should be one which positions the joint being treated approximately midway between limits of flexion and extension for that joint. This position may vary from patient to patient because of structural joint changes due to disease, congenital anomalies or trauma. It may also vary in the same patient as treatment effects improvement of a painful restriction (for example, extension). As has been discussed earlier (*see* page 83) the neck should be positioned in flexion for a lower cervical intervertebral joint and towards the neutral position for an upper cervical joint.

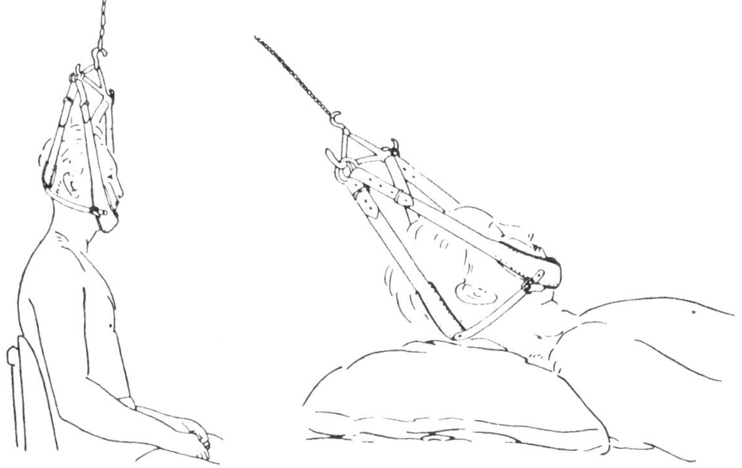

Figure 3.17. – Cervical traction

Whether a patient is treated sitting or lying is governed by factors related to comfort and ease of administering the traction and not by whether the flexed or neutral position is desired. For example, when traction is being applied in the neutral position the patient is usually more comfortable in the sitting position. If the traction is applied in the supine position the thoracic spine is more extended and can become uncomfortable during treatment. However, when the supine position is used for traction in flexion the thoracic spine is not extended so it then becomes the position of choice. Although the sitting position can be used for traction in flexion it has the disadvantage that the trunk is less stable than when supine and does not give the same counter-resistance to stronger tractive forces. For these reasons the following text describes traction in neutral for the upper cervical spine performed in sitting and traction in flexion for the lower cervical spine performed in lying (*Figure 3.17*).

Traction in neutral (CT ↑)

Starting position

The patient sits in a comfortable chair which has adequate support for his back, and if possible for his arms, to encourage complete relaxation. This is an important consideration. For this reason it is advisable to ask the patient to slide his buttocks forwards on the seat to produce slight slumping and therefore better relaxation.

The head halter is applied and the necessary adjustments are made so that when the traction is applied the head, in relation to the neck, will be lifted in the neutral position. The occipital strap must lift under the occiput and must not include suboccipital structures.

Method

Before applying any traction the physiotherapist should know the area and severity of the patient's symptoms at that moment. The physiotherapist then places the tip of her index or middle finger against the side of the interspinous space of the joint to be treated. Then the traction is applied and relaxed in an oscillatory movement very gently at first but gradually increasing until movement can be felt by the finger in the interspinous space. This oscillatory traction should continue until the right pressure is found which is the minimum amount required to produce movement at the intervertebral level being treated. When this pressure has been sustained for approximately 10 seconds the patient's symptoms are reassessed. The following changes in symptoms will indicate how the pressure should be further altered and how long it should be sustained.

1. When severe symptoms are completely relieved by this gentle pressure the pressure must be reduced by half and the traction time kept within 5 minutes as the patient is likely to have a severe exacerbation later unless this reduction is made.

2. If symptoms have been partly relieved the traction should be kept at this level and sustained, for 5 minutes if the pain was severe before traction and for 10 minutes if it was moderate.

3. If the symptoms have not altered, the traction can be increased a little and a further assessment made. The new pressure should be sustained for 10 minutes.

4. Symptoms made worse by this gentle traction should be given half the pressure and reassessed. If the symptoms are still worse, changes of position of the head–neck relationship by alteration of the harness or sitting position should be carried out and the gentler traction reapplied. If the symptoms are still worse then one of two courses remains open. If the aggravation is not too great the gentlest traction can be maintained for 5 minutes or less but if the aggravation is more than minimal, traction should be discontinued. On reassessing next day, only if the response to the gentle pressure shows improvement can traction be continued.

For the initial treatment one point must be emphasized. The angle or direction of the pull is not altered in response to changes in the patient's symptoms during treatment. It is the strength and duration which is modified by changes in the symptoms. The angle of the pull must be as near to the neutral position (midway between the intervertebral joint's ranges of flexion, extension, lateral flexion and rotation) as possible so as to achieve the maximum longitudinal movement for that joint with the minimum strength of traction.

Method of progression

The importance of continually assessing symptoms and signs for changes resulting from treatment will be discussed in Chapter 4, but it is by these methods that treatment is guided. As with techniques of mobilization, changes in techniques are guided by checking the patient's movements after the use of a technique and also by the amount of change which is retained from one treatment to the next. When the traction is released the patient's movements should be reassessed but it is also important to assess the symptoms and the signs on the day following treatment.

Follow-up treatment can be considered in two categories: those patients with severe pain and those with moderate pain. Treatment of a patient who has severe pain should be progressed very slowly, as circumstances allow, until the symptoms become moderate. At first the progression should be by small increases in duration of the traction rather than strength. When there is little or no reaction from treatment the strength can be increased in small stages also. Progression can be by both strength and duration when symptoms are moderate. With the exception of treatment for severe nerve root pain the total time required for traction is not greater than 15 minutes. Results which cannot be obtained with traction of this duration will not be achieved with longer periods, and tractive forces rarely need to be heavy. Traction, as a form of treatment, should be discarded when symptoms and signs remain unchanged after four treatments.

No mention has been made regarding strength and it is assumed that the amount of traction given will be governed by careful assessment of symptoms and signs before, during and following traction. As has been indicated, the application of pressure at first is governed by movement produced at the intervertebral level being treated. It is obvious that 4 kg traction applied to a 102 kg patient will produce less movement than if applied to a 42 kg patient. Therefore, although scales which indicate strength of traction are necessary in research projects and in hospital departments where staff changes occur, it is essential to realize that tractive forces should be governed by assessment and not by the scale.

There is one time when knowledge of the weights which can be considered normal for cervical traction is valuable. People of middle age have some aches which do not worry them and which they class as normal. Examination of their movements frequently exhibits slight pain at the limit of range but again this is considered normal. However, if this pain increases, these people seek treatment. With these thoughts in mind, a person's cervical spine, even with a degree of symptoms and signs which might be classed as being within normal acceptable limits, should be able to accept traction of up to approximately 10 kg (22 lb) without discomfort or after-effect. Similarly, minor discomfort felt with a traction force in excess of 10 kg may, under the circumstances mentioned, be classed as normal. These facts should be borne in mind when treating patients who have discomfort during traction.

Traction in flexion (CT ➶)

Starting position

The patient lies comfortably on his back, with one or two pillows to support his neck in slight flexion in relation to his trunk, so that the joint being treated will be midway between flexion and extension, and to support his head neutrally on his upper cervical spine. If he has at any time had any lower back symptoms, it is advisable to have him flex his hips and knees to allow the lower back to rest. The halter is applied and the occipital strap is positioned first. Because the patient rests his head on this strap on the pillows, it will remain in position while the side straps and chin strap are being adjusted. To ensure that the harness is correctly adjusted, the physiotherapist applies some traction via the spreader bar while he watches to see that the head–neck relationship is neutral.

Method

Knowing the area and the severity of the patient's pain, the operator alternately applies and relaxes pressure through the pulley system while watching and palpating for movement at the intervertebral level being treated. The pressure is sustained at that amount which is the smallest required to produce movement at the joint. After approximately 10 seconds the patient's symptoms are reassessed. From this point onwards the procedure is identical with that described for traction in neutral.

Precautions

A frequent problem with strong cervical traction is discomfort or pain in the patient's temporomandibular joints. This pain may be relieved by an alteration of the position of the straps, or by placing a pad between the patient's molars. However, traction of this magnitude is to be avoided unless absolutely essential.

It is surprising how often pre-existing, but possibly dormant, thoracic or lumbar symptoms are irritated by cervical traction. Traction in neutral can irritate either thoracic or lumbar conditions but traction in flexion only irritates the lumbar spine. Therefore, when traction is being used, the patient should be questioned as to the existence of such symptoms, and care should be taken to avoid any aggravation of them.

When traction in neutral is given with the patient sitting, it is as well to be aware of the fact that a patient can experience nausea, but this usually only occurs with prolonged or very strong traction or with excessively apprehensive patients. On releasing traction, patients can experience a feeling of giddiness if the traction has been very strong.

Traction in flexion can cause a burning feeling or pain in the vicinity of the first cervical vertebra. In such a case it is advisable to alter the harness so that the head is extended more on the upper neck while the lower neck is maintained in flexion.

Uses

A patient whose neck movements of lateral flexion and rotation towards the painful side are markedly limited by arm pain should be treated by traction only, and it is traction in flexion which should be used. Traction should always be the first choice in treatment when recent neurological changes are present.

Traction is of value in almost any distribution of pain arising from the cervical vertebrae. However, the rapidity with which complete relief of symptoms and signs is obtained is usually slower than with mobilization. When intervertebral joints are stiff, traction may be ineffective if not preceded by manipulation.

Intermittent variable cervical traction (IVCT), referred to on page 110, can be applied in neutral or in flexion for the same reasons as have been given already. Weight and duration are governed in exactly the same manner also. The only factor not already covered is the mode of establishing or progressing the hold and rest periods. When symptoms are severe the amount of movement should be less, which means that the hold and rest periods should be long. As symptoms become less severe the rest period can become minimal. When symptoms can be classed as an ache rather than a pain the hold period should be approximately 3–5 seconds with minimal rest periods.

THORACIC REGION

Postero-anterior central vertebral pressure (↓)

Starting position

The patient lies prone with either his forehead resting on the backs of his hands, or with his head comfortably turned to one side and his arms lying by his sides on the couch. The position depends on the amount of chest tightness created by the 'arms up' position, which is usually reserved for upper thoracic mobilization.

If the patient is on a low couch the physiotherapist's position for mobilizing the upper thoracic spine (approximately from T1 to T5) needs to be at the head of the patient, with her shoulders over the area to be mobilized to enable the direction of the pressure to be at right angles to the surface of the body. The pads of the thumbs are placed on the spinous process pointing transversely across the vertebral column, and the fingers of each hand are spread out over the posterior chest wall to give stability to the thumbs. As the spinous processes are large, the thumbs may be positioned tip to tip or with the tips side by side in contact with upper and lower margins of the same spinous process. To gain the best control and feel of movement with the least discomfort to the patient the pressure should be transmitted through the thumbs so that the interphalangeal joints are hyperextended enabling the softest part of the pad to be flat over the spinous processes and with a slight degree of flexion in the metacarpophalangeal joints. Not only is this more comfortable for the patient, but it hinders the physiotherapist's intrinsic muscles from producing the pressure.

To mobilize the mid-thoracic spine (T5–T9) the physiotherapist should stand at the patient's side with her thumbs placed longitudinally along the vertebral column, so that they point towards each other. The fingers can then spread out over the posterior chest wall, to each side of the vertebral column above and below the thumbs.

It may be more comfortable (and this is far easier to do if the patient is lying on a low couch) for the physiotherapist to stand to one side of the patient, approximately at waist level, facing his head, and place the pads of the thumbs on the spinous process pointing across the vertebral column. The fingers of each hand can then spread over opposite sides of the posterior chest wall for stability.

For the lower thoracic spine (T10–T12) the physiotherapist's position depends upon the shape of the patient's chest. Either of the last two positions described may be used but the essential factor is that the direction of the pressure must be at right angles to the body surface at the level. This means that the shoulders may need to be anywhere between vertically above the lower thoracic spine and vertically above the sacrum (*Figure 3.18*). If the patient has difficulty lying prone because extension is painful a small pillow under the chest will assist.

Method

The mobilizing is carried out by an oscillating pressure on the spinous processes produced by the body and transmitted through the arms to the thumbs. It is important that this pressure be applied by the bodyweight over the hands and not by a squeezing action with the thumbs themselves. The fingers, which are spread out over the patient's back, should not exert any pressure but only act as stabilizers for the thumbs. It is easy to dissipate the pressure and lose the effectiveness of the thumbs by faulty use of the fingers.

If the physiotherapist's elbows are kept slightly flexed, and the thumbs maintained in the position of hyperextension of interphalangeal joints and slight flexion of metacarpophalangeal joints, the pressure

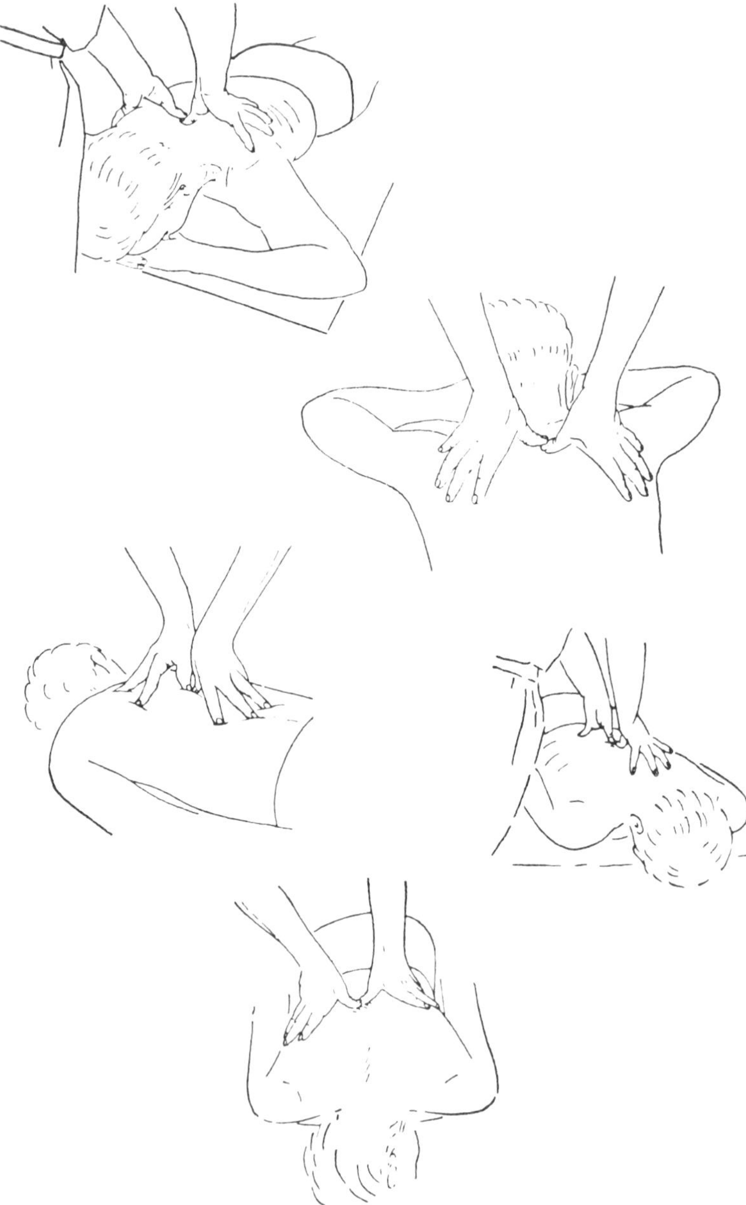

Figure 3.18. – Thoracic region. Postero-anterior central vertebral pressure (↓)

can be transmitted to the pads of the thumbs through this series of strong springs. This springing action at the joints can readily be seen as the bodyweight is applied during the mobilizing.

Local variations

The degree of pressure required in the upper thoracic spine to produce movement is far greater than that required in the cervical spine and slightly stronger than that required for the remainder of the thoracic spine.

The degree of movement possible in the middle and lower thoracic spine is considerable, and it is here that it is easiest to learn a feeling of movement. The degree of movement possible in the upper thoracic spine is considerably limited, and this is particularly so between T1 and T2.

Uses

Postero-anterior central vertebral pressure is as useful for the thoracic spine as rotation is for the cervical spine. In all symptoms arising from the thoracic vertebrae it is worth trying this procedure first.

'Central pressure' is more likely to be successful with symptoms which are situated in the midline or evenly distributed to each side of the body, but it should be tried also for unilateral symptoms, particularly if they are ill defined or widespread in their distribution.

Transverse vertebral pressure (←•→)

Starting position

When the middle and lower thoracic vertebrae are to be mobilized with transverse pressures the patient lies prone with his arms hanging over the sides of the couch or by his side to aid relaxation of the vertebral column. The head should be allowed to rest comfortably by being turned to one side, preferably towards the side to which the physiotherapist stands. However, as this head position tends to produce some degree of rotation in the upper thoracic vertebrae, it is better for the patient to adopt the 'forehead rest' position, when these vertebrae are to be mobilized, to eliminate any rotation.

The physiotherapist stands at the patient's right side at the level of the vertebrae to be mobilized, and places her hands on the patient's back so that the pads of the thumbs are adjacent to the right side of the spinous processes while the fingers are spread over the patient's left ribs. The left thumb acts as the point of contact, and is fitted down into the groove between the spinous process and the paravertebral muscles, so that part of the pad of the thumb is pressed against the lateral aspect of the spinous process on its right-hand side. It is essential to have as much of the pad in contact with the spinous process as is possible. To prevent the thumb sliding off the spinous process the palmar surface of the metacarpophalangeal joint of the index finger must be firmly brought down on top of the interphalangeal joint of the thumb. This is a valuable position to learn to adopt as its stability is of value in other techniques. The right thumb, acting as reinforcement, is placed so that its pad lies over the nail of the left thumb. This thumb relationship is chosen because considerable effort is required to keep a single thumb comfortably against the spinous process.

The fingers of both hands should be well spread out over the chest wall to stabilize the thumbs, and the wrists need to be slightly extended to permit the pressure to be transmitted through the thumbs in the horizontal plane. Because of the slightly different functions required of the left and right thumbs, the left forearm is not as horizontal as the right forearm (*Figure 3.19*).

Method

The pressure is applied to the spinous process through the thumbs by movement of the trunk: alternate pressure and relaxation is repeated continuously to produce an oscillating type of movement of the intervertebral joint. For the gentler grades of mobilizing very little pressure is needed. When stronger mobilizing is used movement of the patient's trunk is involved and timing of pressures should coincide either with the patient's rolling or, in order to make the technique stronger, the pressure should go against the rolling.

Local variations

The upper thoracic spinous processes (T1–T3 or T4) are readily accessible but have a limited amount of movement, T1 being almost immovable. The lower thoracic vertebrae (T8 or T9–T12) are more

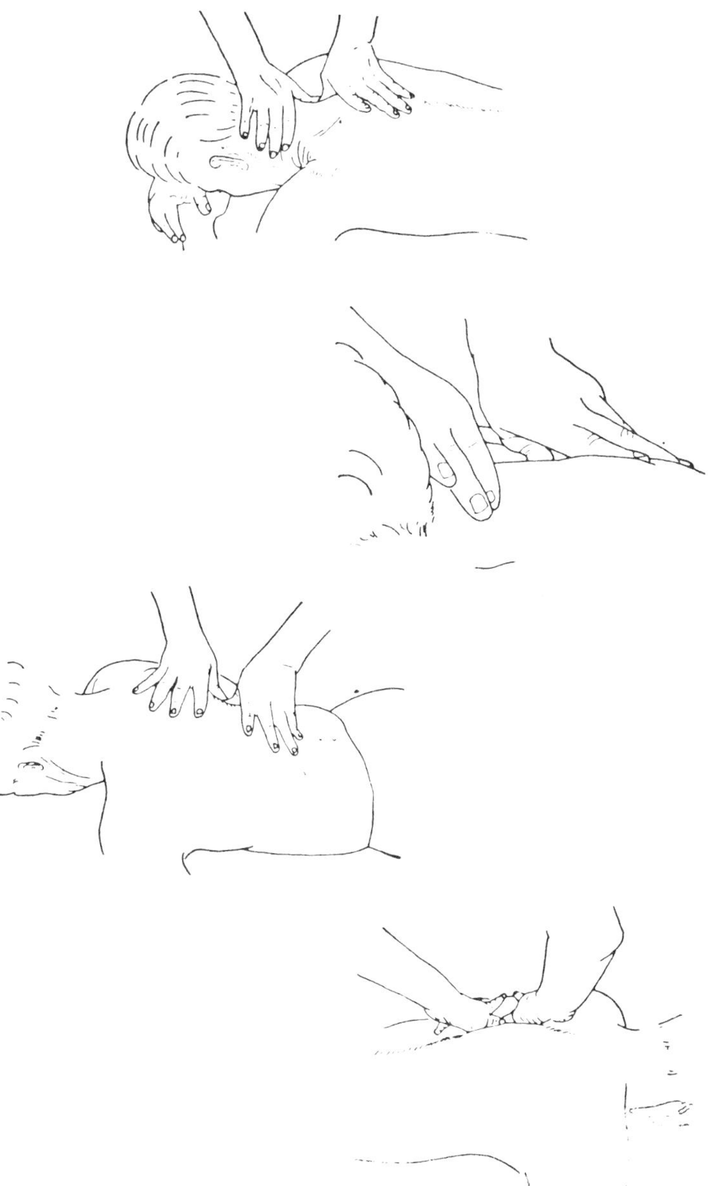

Figure 3.19. – Thoracic region. Transverse vertebral pressure (←•– *)*

easily moved and do not require great pressure. Local tenderness in these two areas is comparatively negligible. Mobilization of the mid-thoracic spine is made difficult by the relative inaccessibility of the spinous processes and natural tenderness. When a painful condition is superimposed on this natural tenderness adequate mobilization may be very difficult.

Uses

This technique is particularly useful for pain of unilateral distribution in the thoracic area. In such cases the pressure is best applied against the side of the spinous process which is away from the pain, applying the pressure towards the patient's painful side. When using this technique it is frequently necessary to mobilize the rib cage by a postero-anterior pressure directed through the angle of the rib.

Postero-anterior unilateral vertebral pressure (↓‾•)

Starting position

The patient lies prone with his head turned to the left and his arms hanging loosely over the sides of the couch or by his side.

To mobilize the left side of the middle or lower thoracic spine (approximately T5–T12) the physiotherapist stands on the left side of the patient and places her hands on the patient's back so that the pads of the thumbs pointing towards each other, lie over the transverse processes. The fingers of the left hand spread over the chest wall pointing towards the patient's head while the fingers of the right hand point towards his feet and the thumbs are held in opposition. By applying a little pressure through the pads of the thumbs they will sink into the muscle tissue adjacent to the spinous processes until the transverse process is reached. The metacarpophalangeal joint of the thumb needs to be slightly flexed and the interphalangeal joint must be hyperextended to enable the pad of the thumb to transmit the pressure comfortably. When a much finer degree of localization of the pressure is required the thumb-nails should be brought together so that the tips of the thumbs make a very small point of contact. In this position the metacarpophalangeal joints of the thumbs are brought much closer together to lie directly above the thumb tips. The physiotherapist's shoulders and arms, with slightly flexed elbows, should be in the direct line through which the pressure is to be applied and this is at right angles to the plane of the body surface.

Because of the curve of the thoracic spine it is necessary, when mobilizing the upper levels (T1–T4), to stand either at the patient's head or towards the shoulder of the side being mobilized to accommodate the necessarily altered angle of the physiotherapist's arms. It is advisable to use the largest amount of the pad of the thumb that can be brought into contact with the transverse process to enable the pressure to be administered as comfortably as possible (*Figure 3.20*).

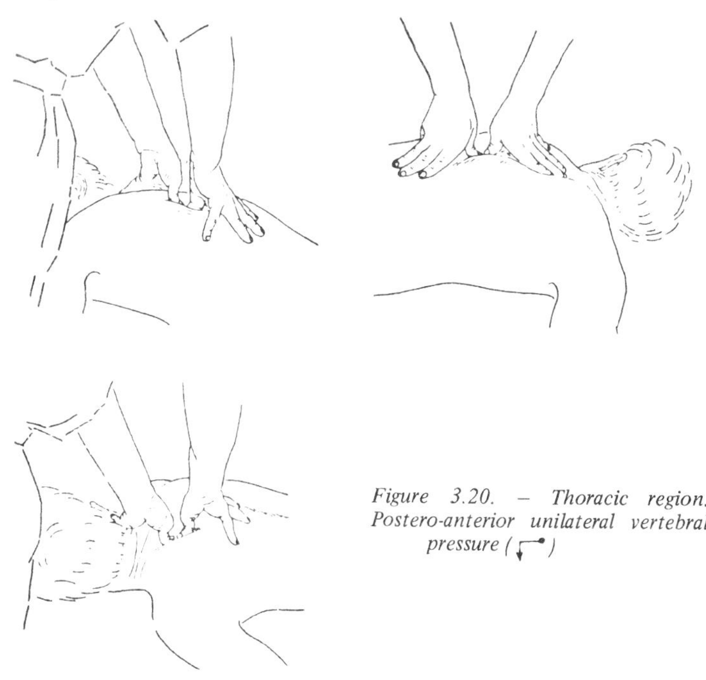

Figure 3.20. – Thoracic region. Postero-anterior unilateral vertebral pressure (⌐•)

Method

A very steady application of pressure is necessary to be able to move some of the muscle belly out of the way and make bone to bone contact. As this procedure can be quite uncomfortable for the patient, care must be given to the position of the arms and hands to enable a spring-like action to take place at the elbows and the thumbs. This reduces the feeling of hardness and soreness between the physiotherapist's thumbs and the patient's transverse process which is present if the pressure is applied by intrinsic muscle action.

Once the required depth has been reached the oscillating movement at the intervertebral joint is produced by increasing and then decreasing the pressure produced by trunk movement.

Local variations

Because of the structure and attachments of the rib cage it is not possible to produce very much movement with this mobilization.

Some people may find it easier to carry out the mobilization using the hands (as described for the lumbar spine) instead of the thumbs, but this should be discouraged as the thumbs have a greater degree of feel and they can localize the mobilization more accurately. They also cause much less discomfort to the patient, a factor of considerable importance. When the hands are used the technique is frequently more vigorous than is required.

Uses

Postero-anterior unilateral vertebral pressure is used, almost entirely, for unilaterally distributed pain arising from the thoracic spine, and the technique is done on the painful side. Unless the patient's pain is severe it is less likely to produce a favourable change in the patient's signs and symptoms if it is done on the side away from the pain. When this technique is used in the presence of spasm, the pressure must be steadily applied and not hurried, in order to allow time for the spasm to relax.

Postero-anterior unilateral costovertebral pressure ([symbol])

Starting position

The patient lies prone with his arms by his side or hanging over the sides of the couch.

The physiotherapist stands at the side of the patient where the mobilization is to be effected. The physiotherapist's thumbs are placed along the line of the rib at its angle. Thus the maximum area of contact can be made between the thumbs and the rib (*Figure 3.21a*). Alternatively the whole ulnar border of the hand and little finger may be used to produce the movement (*Figure 3.21b*).

Method

As oscillatory movement is transmitted to the rib by the thumbs or hands. The range of movement produced at one rib angle is compared with that produced at the rib angles above and below. The pain produced

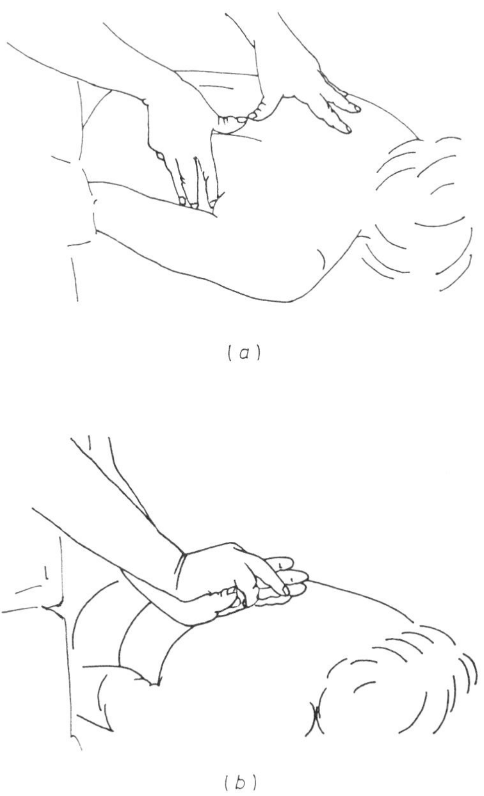

Figure 3.21. – (a) Postero-anterior unilateral costovertebral pressure using thumbs. (b) Postero-anterior unilateral costovertebral pressure using hands ( )

by the movement of the faulty rib is also compared with the pain (if any) produced at the rib above and the rib below. Similarly both the range of the movement and the pain should also be compared with the ribs on the opposite side of the body.

Local variations

First rib Examination of the first rib is somewhat different from that of the other ribs as the technique can be applied in three ways due to a greater area of the rib being palpable.

1. The pressure can be applied against the rib posteriorly through the trapezius muscle, and the direction of the pressure is not only postero-anteriorly but is also inclined towards the feet (*Figure 3.22*).

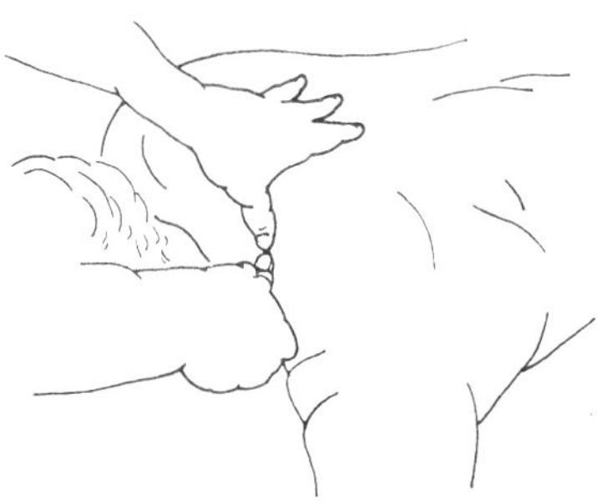

Figure 3.22. – Pressure applied against the first rib posteriorly through the trapezius

2. Alternatively the physiotherapist can place her thumbs underneath (anterior to) the muscle belly of the trapezius and the direction of the pressure can be inclined a little more towards the feet as well as being postero-anteriorly directed (*Figure 3.23*).

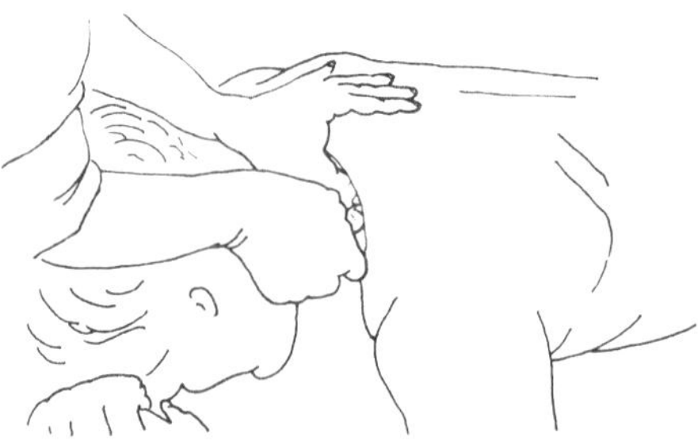

Figure 3.23. – Pressure applied against the first rib posteriorly under the trapezius

3. For this next technique which mobilizes the first rib the patient lies supine while the physiotherapist, standing at the patient's shoulder level of the side to be treated, applies the pressure to produce the oscillatory anteroposterior and caudad movement on all parts of the first rib which are palpable (*Figure 3.24*). The symbol for this technique is ⤴ R1

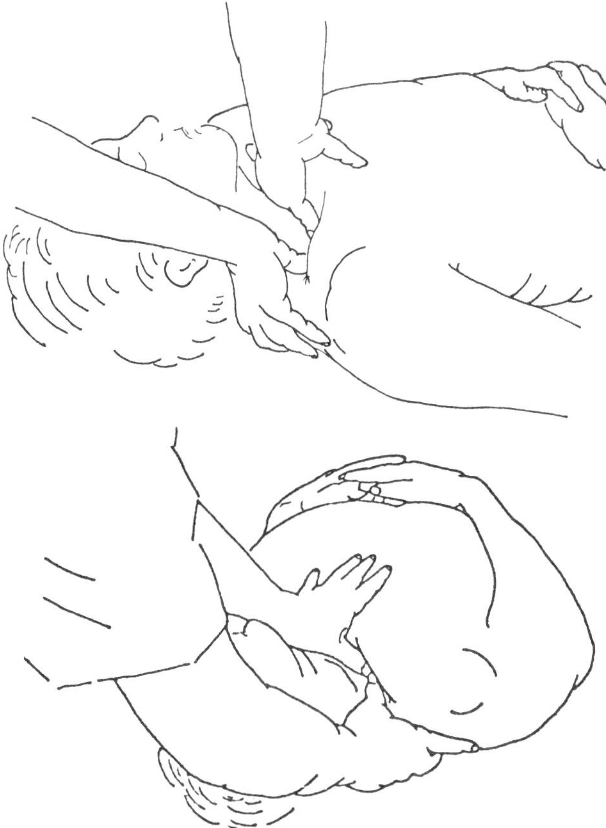

Figure 3.24. – Pressure applied to the first rib anteriorly

Other ribs All of the ribs can be examined throughout their entire length by thumb palpation. This includes costochondral junctions and the junction with the sternum. The freedom of movement between adjacent ribs can also be tested. As these are not part of the vertebral column they are not described in this book. They are described however in *Peripheral Manipulation* (Maitland, 1970).

Uses

Whenever treatment is applied to the thoracic intervertebral joints, the inclusion of mobilization of the ribs should be considered, for two reasons.

Firstly, it is frequently difficult to assess whether a patient's pain arises from the intervertebral joint, the costovertebral joint or the costotransverse joint. Therefore, if mobilization of the thoracic intervertebral joint is not producing adequate improvement when used on a patient, mobilization of the rib at its angle should be added to the intervertebral mobilization.

Secondly, if the rib is moved as a treatment technique it must also create some movement at the intervertebral joint. This combination may hasten the rate of progress.

If pain is in a referred area of the rib cage the symptoms may be arising from some abnormality between adjacent ribs. Palpation will reveal abnormalities of position and of movement between adjacent ribs. This aspect of treating costal pain is described in *Peripheral Manipulation* (Maitland, 1970).

Thoracic traction

Traction can be administered to the thoracic spine just as readily as it can in the cervical and lumbar areas, and the guiding principles are exactly the same. However, it is true to say that it is less frequently successful than it is in either of the other two areas and this may be due, at least in part, to the presence of the thoracic cage.

The principle is to position the vertebral column so that the particular joint to be treated is in a relaxed position midway between all ranges. Then the amount of pressure to be used is guided firstly by movement of the joint, with further changes in tension made in response to changes in the patient's symptoms as outlined for cervical traction. Further treatments are guided by changes in symptoms and signs as already discussed with cervical traction (*see* page 115).

Maitland, G. D. (1970). *Peripheral Manipulation*. London; Butterworths

Upper thoracic spine (TT ➚)

Starting position

The patient lies on his back with one or two pillows under his head to flex the neck until the intervertebral level to be treated is positioned midway between flexion and extension. A cervical halter is then applied in the same way as has been described for cervical traction in flexion

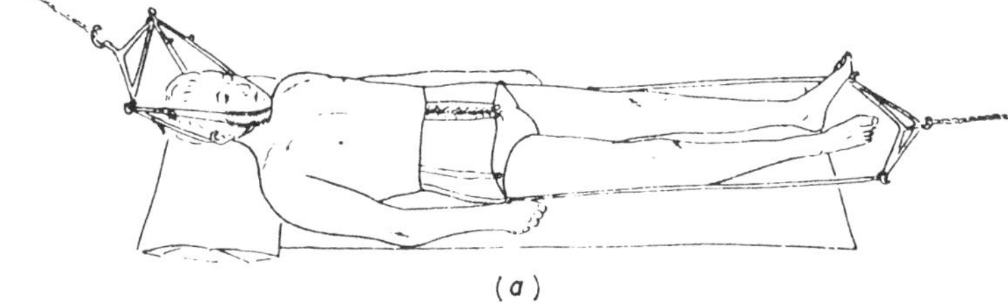

(a)

Figure 3.25 (a). – T1–T10 traction with counter-resistance (TT ➚)

(*see* page 116). If a lower level is to be treated and if the strength of the traction needs to be very firm it may become necessary to apply some form of counter-traction. A belt is fitted around the pelvis and is attached to the foot end of the couch to stablize the distal end of the vertebral column. The halter is then attached to its fixed point so that the angle of the pull on the neck will be approximately 45 degrees from the horizontal. The actual angle used varies with the amount of kyphosis present in the upper thoracic spine. It should be an angle which will allow the thoracic intervertebral joint to be stretched longitudinally while in a position mid-way between its limits of flexion and extension. To relieve strain on the patient's lower back during the period when the traction is being applied his hips and knees may be flexed (*Figure 3.25a*).

Method

The traction can be adjusted from either end or from both ends, but whichever method is used, care must be taken to ensure that friction between the patient's trunk and the couch is reduced to a minimum. This can be done while the traction is being applied by gently lifting the weight of the patient's thorax or pelvis off the couch, allowing it to relax back into a new position. Friction is almost completely eliminated by a couch whose surface is in two halves which are free to roll longitudinally (*see* page 133). Releasing the traction does not present any problem, but it is advisable to release slowly.

Lower thoracic spine (TT→)

Starting position

For the lower thoracic spine a thoracic belt similar to that used for lumbar traction is used in place of the cervical halter. Traction is usually more effective if it is carried out with the patient supine, but it can be done with him prone.

The thoracic belt is applied to hold the chest above the level of the spine to be treated and it is then attached to its fixed point. After this the pelvic belt is applied and attached to its fixed point. The direction of the pull is then longitudinal in the line of the patient's trunk but pillows may be needed to adjust the position of the spine so that the joint being stretched is relaxed midway between flexion and extension (*Figure 3.25b*).

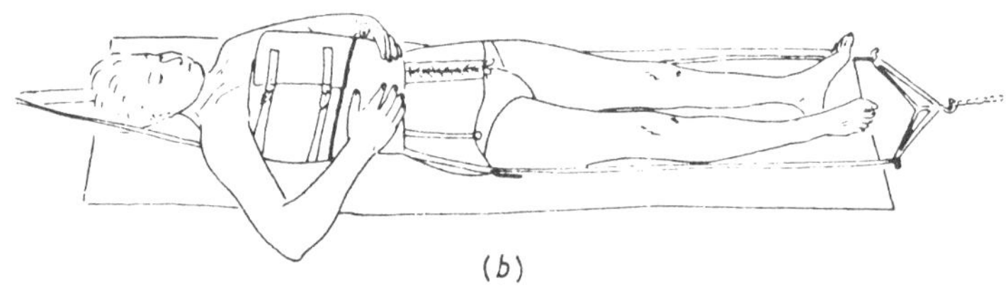

Figure 3.25 (b). – T10–T12 traction (TT→)

Method

Traction is applied from either end or from both ends, but again care is required to reduce friction to a minimum at both thoracic and pelvic levels. As mentioned previously a roll-top couch eliminates friction. A simple, cheap and extremely effective roll-top couch is described below (*Figure 3.26*).

Releasing the traction should be done steadily and the patient should rest for a short time before standing.

Intermittent variable traction can also be used in this area of the spine and the details of times for 'rest' and 'hold' periods are the same as have been discussed for the cervical spine.

Local variations

The thoracic kyphosis varies considerably from person to person and the positioning of the patient is controlled by this curve. Theoretically the direction of the pull may be thought of as being at right angles to the upper and lower surfaces of the intervertebral disc at the level which is being stretched. The kyphosis usually influences the position for upper thoracic traction more than for the lower thoracic spine.

Precautions

A check must be kept on the patient to ensure that the traction does not cause any low-back pain.

As with the cervical traction in flexion it is possible for the head halter in upper thoracic traction to cause occipital headache but this can be eliminated by means already described (*see* page 117).

Uses

Traction is of greatest value in patients who have widely distributed areas of thoracic pain, particularly if they are associated with radiological degenerative changes in the thoracic spine. It is also of value for the patient whose thoracic symptoms do not appear to be aggravated by active movements of the spine or when neurological changes are present. Similarly it is the treatment of choice for the patient with severe nerve root pain. Whenever mobilizing techniques have been used in treatment without achieving the desired result, traction should be tried.

A friction-free traction couch

There are many different ways in which lumbar traction treatment can be applied. Essentially, a belt is fixed around the patient's thorax and another around the pelvis, and these are attached to fixed points at the foot and head ends of the treatment couch. A scale to measure poundage of traction is inserted in the apparatus and the traction is applied by ropes and pulleys, or a screw thread with a wheel. Some couches have a free-running top to eliminate friction, while others have the normal fixed top.

A friction-free couch is not an essential requirement for traction therapy but the advantages to both patient and physiotherapist are considerable. These advantages can only be appreciated fully by the comparative use of traction with and without the friction-free top. The time saved in eliminating friction when applying traction on a friction-free couch is valuable, but probably the most important factor is the ease and accuracy with which small increases and decreases in the tractive force can be made, knowing that they are immediately effective in the spine. Another important factor is that a scale used during traction provides a more true measure of the tractive force between the thoracic and pelvic belts.

Many varieties of patented friction-free couch are available, but mostly they have a mobile lumbar section and a fixed thoracic section. This is not satisfactory because the thorax moves when traction is applied, even though the movement may sometimes be small. If the thoracic part of the couch is not free to move, some of the tractive force will be taken up by friction between the patient's thorax and the couch. Therefore, both lumbar and thoracic sections must be free to move. It must also be possible to fix the friction-free roll top in a stable position to allow the patient to get on and off the couch, and to enable it to be used for other treatments. These requirements are met in the couch described, and the modifications can be adapted to any couch which has a wooden top, or wooden edges to its top.

The friction-free top is formed by placing two sections of 1.85 cm (¾ inch) plywood end to end on top of a normal couch with dowelling to act as rollers between the plywood and the top of the couch. The thoracic plywood section is 76 cm (30 inches) long and the lumbar section 107 cm (42 inches) long, and their widths equal the width of the couch. If the top of the couch measures 1.98 m (6.5 feet) in length, and both plywood sections are placed end to end with the head end of the thoracic section level with the head end of the couch, there will be 15 cm (6 inches) of the couch uncovered by plywood beyond the foot end of the lumbar plywood section. Four pieces of dowelling 1.85 cm (¾ inch) in diameter and equal in length to the width of the couch are placed across the couch under the plywood. Two dowels are used to support each plywood section.

To prevent the sections of plywood from rolling off the head end of the couch, a piece of timber is nailed to the end of the couch so that the top of the timber is level with the top of the plywood when it is in position on top of the dowels (*Figure 3.26a*). To prevent the plywood from rolling off the foot end of the couch, a 'U' piece is made to fit into an 'L'-shaped hole cut out of the table top immediately below the foot end of the lumbar section of plywood (*Figure 3.26b*).

To lock the friction-free top into a stable position against the piece of timber nailed to the head of the couch, the 'U' piece is lowered into the largest part of the cut-out section of the couch, pushed forwards to clamp over the top of the plywood and under the top of the couch,

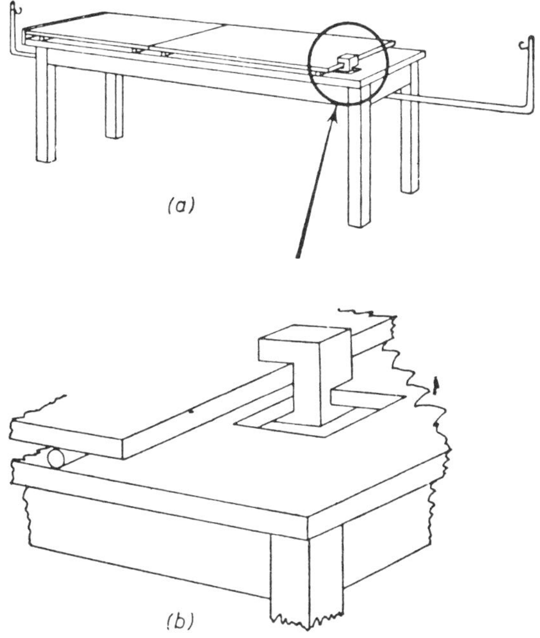

Figure 3.26. – (a) Roll-top traction table; (b) enlargement of the end

and then pushed sideways to lock the 'U' piece into the smaller part of the hole. When in this position the 'U' piece also prevents the foot end of the lumbar section of plywood from lifting when a patient sits in the middle of the couch. This lifting must be prevented if the couch is to be used for treatments other than traction. When the 'U' piece is removed, both plywood sections are free to roll independently towards the foot end of the couch.

The four dowels must be carefully positioned to enable each plywood section to roll far enough for traction treatments and for the friction-free top to be made stable enough for use with other forms of physiotherapy. One dowel should be positioned under each plywood section 12.7 cm (5 inches) from the head end, and the other should be level with the foot end. Each plywood section can then roll 27.5 cm (12 inches) before each head-end dowel reaches the end of its plywood section. The position of the dowel under the foot end of the thoracic section also allows the patient to sit in the middle of the couch where the two plywood sections meet, without the head end of the thoracic section lifting. The foot end of the lumbar section is prevented from lifting, as would be the case if the patient sat on the lumbar section nearer its head end than the dowel, by the locking effect of the 'U' piece.

The total cost of material for converting a normal treatment couch into a stable and efficient friction-free couch is minimal, and labour costs are very small.

Because many physiotherapists are deterred from acquiring friction-free lumbar traction equipment by high prices and by equipment which is too cumbersome to be used for routine physiotherapy, a cheap and simple method for providing the two fixed points required for traction on a normal treatment couch is described. The tractive force is effected by a system of ropes and pulleys. The ropes and pulleys are attached to one end, usually the foot end, and a scale is inserted at the opposite end. This method is preferable to wheel-operated traction on a screw thread because of its quicker action. Also, the rope and pulley system gives the operator some feel of the tractive force during application. Accommodating for the stretch of the harness during the first few moments of treatment is also far easier with the pulley system.

If a tube having an internal diameter of 3.17 (1.25 inches) is fixed under a normal treatment couch by metal straps at each end, two tubes having a slightly smaller external diameter than 3.17 cm can slide inside the fixed tube from each end. Each inner sliding tube should be half the length of the outer fixed tube. A strut should be welded at right angles to one end of each inner tube, and a length of this end strut should be such that when it is positioned vertically, with the inner tube within the fixed outer tube, its top is approximately 13 cm (5 inches) above the level of the top of the couch. When the couch is not being used for lumbar traction these sliding tubes can be slid out of the way inside the fixed tube. When they are in use they should be extended a distance of approximately 36 cm (14 inches) at the head end and 81 cm (32 inches) at the foot end, and are held with the end struts upright by a pin inserted through holes appropriately placed through the outer and inner tubes at each end of the couch. These distances allow the ropes and pulleys to be fitted to the foot end, and the scale at the head end.

LUMBAR REGION

Postero-anterior central vertebral pressure (↕)

Starting position

The patient lies face downwards with his arms by his side or hanging over the sides of the couch and his head turned comfortably to one side.

When extremely gentle mobilizing is being performed the starting position and method is identical with that described for postero-anterior central vertebral pressure for the middle and lower thoracic area (*see* page 119). However, as the need for stronger pressure arises the thumbs are inadequate because the technique becomes uncomfortable for the patient and the physiotherapist loses the degree of feel which she should have. It is better to change to using the hands as the means for transmitting the pressure.

The physiotherapist stands at the left side of the patient and places her left hand (this one is chosen for convenience) on the patient's back so that that part of the ulnar border of the hand between the pisiform and the hook of the hamate is in contact with the spinous process of the vertebra to be mobilized. For this bone to be the major point of contact while the physiotherapist's shoulders are positioned directly above the vertebra, it is necessary to extend the left wrist fully and hold the forearm midway between full supination and full pronation. If complete wrist extension is not maintained the whole of the ulnar border of the hand will become the contact area and accurate localization will be lost. This left hand is then reinforced by the right by fitting the carpus of the right hand, cupped by the approximation of the thenar and hypothenar eminences, over the radial aspect of the left carpus at the base of the left index finger (*Figure 3.27a*). Then, by allowing the right middle, ring and little fingers to lie between

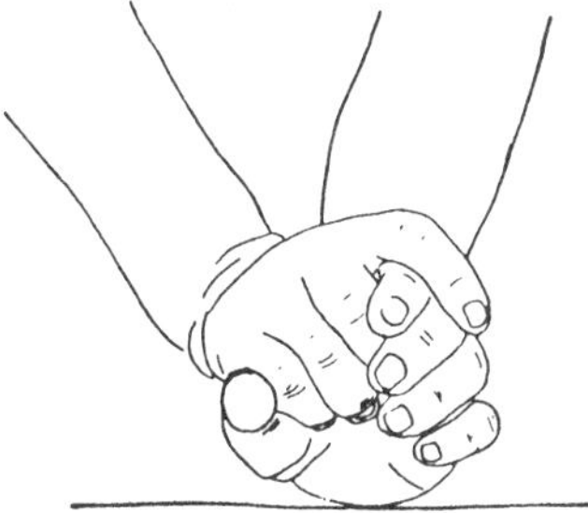

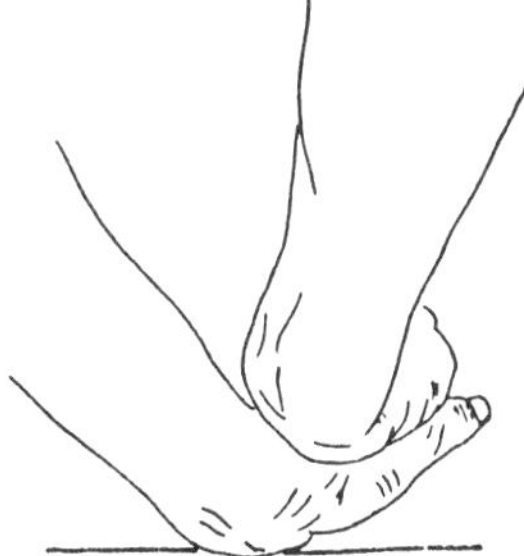

Figure 3.27 (a). – Lumbar region postero-anterior central vertebral pressure (↕)

the left index finger and thumb, and by allowing the right index finger and thumb to lie over the back of the left hand, stability is gained by grasping the palm of the left hand between the thenar eminence and the middle, ring and little fingers of the right hand. To hold this right-hand position with the physiotherapist's bodyweight over the hands, the right wrist must be extended.

The physiotherapist's shoulders are balanced over the top of the patient, and the elbows are allowed to flex slightly (*Figure 3.27b*).

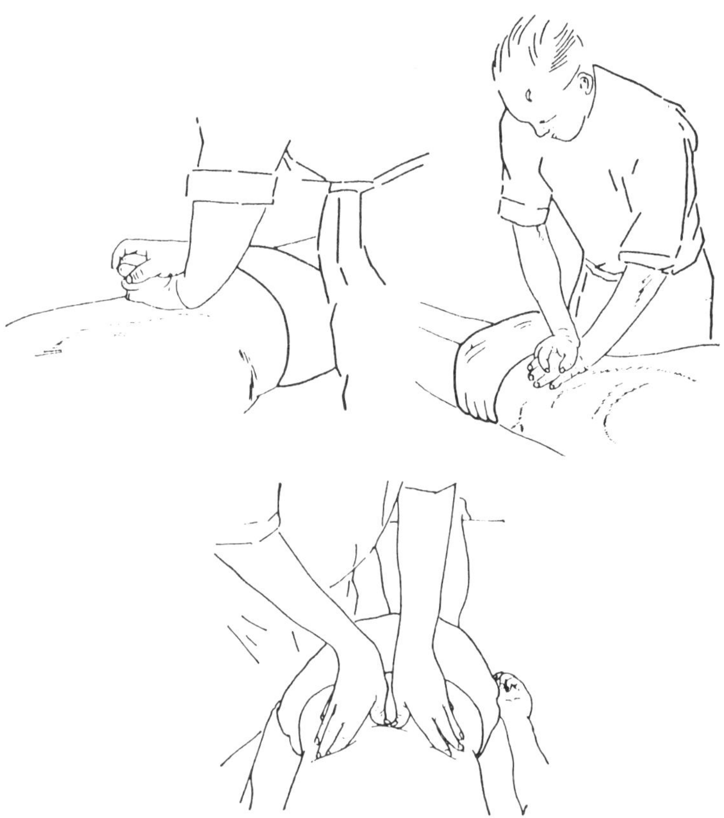

Figure 3.27 (b). – Lumbar region. Postero-anterior vertebral pressure (↨)

Method

The position is taken up by gradually moving the bodyweight forwards more directly over the patient's vertebral column and the oscillating movement of the vertebra is obtained by a rocking movement of the upper trunk up and down in the vertical plane. The pressure is transmitted through the arms and shoulders which act as strong springs.

Local variations

There is no natural tenderness to be felt when mobilizing the lumbar spine. Movement can be felt readily but is noticeably less at the level of the fifth lumbar vertebra than it is above this level.

When a patient has an excessive lordosis a small firm pillow placed under the abdomen may be necessary for joint positioning. Whether a pillow is used or not, the physiotherapist often needs to alter the direction of her arms to enable the push to be at right angles to the surface of the body.

Uses

Postero-anterior central vertebral pressure is best used in conditions of the lumbar spine which cause a pain which is evenly distributed to both sides of the body.

As in the cervical spine this technique is of value in patients whose symptoms arise from an area of the lumbar spine which has marked bony changes, whether these changes arise from degeneration, an old injury, or are structural changes associated with faulty posture.

This technique is indicated when pain or protective muscle spasm is felt with movement in this direction but under these circumstances it is performed in such a way that the pain or spasm is not provoked.

Postero-anterior unilateral vertebral pressure (⌐•)

Starting position

The patient lies prone with his arms by his side and his head can be turned to the side. If the technique is to be performed on the left side of the spine the physiotherapist stands by the patient's left side and places her thumbs on his back, pointing towards each other, immediately adjacent to the spinous process on the left. It is wise not to reinforce one thumb with the other as this destroys the feel which can be obtained through the pad of the thumb. The fingers are spread around the thumbs to provide stability. The base of the thumb is brought as near directly above the tip of the thumb as possible. This position is governed by the ability to hyperextend the thumbs (*Figure 3.28*).

Because the muscle bulk in this area is large it is difficult to feel clearly the transverse process. However if the points of the pads of the thumbs are used and the pressure is applied slowly, the majority of the muscle bulk can be penetrated, to reach a firm bony base.

Method

The physiotherapist positions her shoulders above her hands and transmits the pressure of her trunk through her arms to her thumbs. The thumbs act as springs as the pressure is applied and in no way do the thumb flexors act as prime movers.

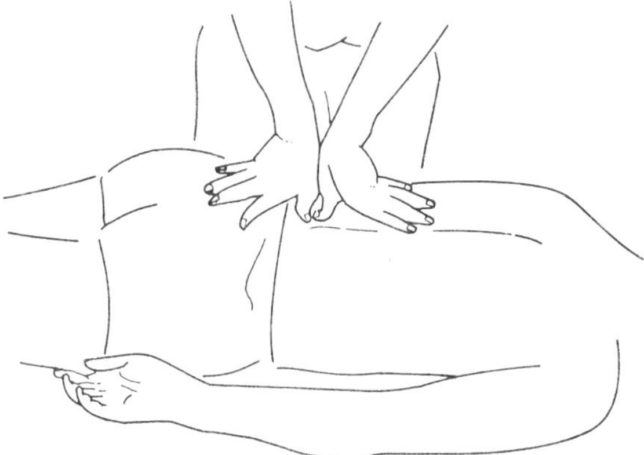

Figure 3.28. – Lumbar region. Postero-anterior unilateral vertebral pressure (⌐•)

The hands can be used to perform this technique and when using this method the position of the hands is the same as that described for postero-anterior central vertebral pressure (*see* page 137). However the disadvantage of using the hands is that the pressure cannot be localized as well, nor can there be as much feel for the very localized abnormalities of movement which can be palpated with the thumbs.

Local variations

In the upper and middle lumbar areas it is easy to palpate the lateral margin of the transverse processes as they are quite long. In the lower lumbar spine however the technique must be performed near the spinous process and time must be taken over penetrating the muscle bulk to reach the bony base.

Uses

This technique is extremely valuable when muscle spasm of the deep intrasegmental muscles can be felt. The technique is carried out on the side of the muscle spasm or the pain and its angle can be varied as indicated by the response to the technique.

Transverse vertebral pressure (←•—)

Starting positions

The patient lies prone with his arms by his side or hanging over the sides of the couch and his head comfortably turned to the side.

The physiotherapist stands by the patient's right side and places her hands on the patient's back so that the thumbs are against the right side of the spinous process of the vertebra to be mobilized. As much as possible of the pad of the left thumb is placed against the right lateral surface of the spinous process. The right thumb is used as reinforcement by placing the pad of the right thumb over the nail of the left thumb. It is necessary to hyperextend the interphalangeal joint of the thumb and hold the metacarpophalangeal joint in a position of slight flexion. The left thumb is then wedged into position by the palmar surface of the base of the index finger to prevent the thumb sliding up and over the spinous process. The fingers of both hands are then spread out over the patient's back to help stabilize the position of the thumbs. Pressure is applied to the thumbs through the forearms held near the horizontal plane (*Figure 3.29a*).

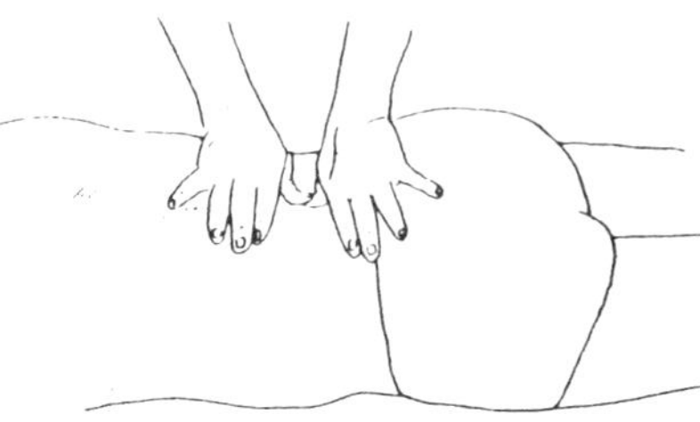

Figure 3.29 (a). – Lumbar region. Transverse vertebral pressure (←•—)

Method

When applying body pressure through the thumbs against the one spinous process, a certain amount of care is necessary to differentiate between the intervertebral joint movement and the rolling movement of the patient's trunk. The pressure is applied and relaxed repeatedly ro produce an oscillating type of movement, small movement being produced by small pressures and larger movement by stronger pressures.

Local variations

Movement is much greater at L1 than it is at L4 and in fact is felt readily at L1. The spinous process is far more accessible at L1 and L2 than it is at the lower levels.

Uses

This technique is of greatest value when used with symptoms which have a unilateral distribution. Under these circumstances it is more likely to produce an improvement in the patient's symptoms and signs if it is done from the painless side, pushing the spinous process towards the painful side. In this way the joint on the painful side is opened.

When used in the lower lumbar spine this mobilization is less valuable than either rotation or postero-anterior central vertebral pressure. It is useful, however, when used for conditions of the upper lumbar spine, and the higher the lumbar level causing the symptoms the more likely this technique is to succeed.

If a strong technique is required for the purpose of stretching the joint which is not painful the following technique may be adopted.

Starting position

A position similar to the above is adopted but with the right thumb pad placed against the spinous process of the vertebra being mobilized. The patient's right knee, flexed to a right angle, is then cradled in the physiotherapist's left hand so that the grasp is around the medial aspect of the knee (*Figure 3.29b*).

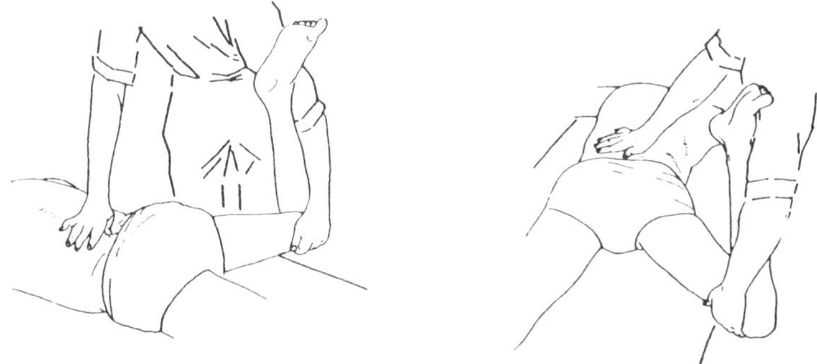

Figure 3.29(b). – Lumbar region. Transverse vertebral pressure (←•—)

Method

When the leg is used as a lever, care is needed in taking up the slack because of the movement which takes place at the hip joint. With the right thumb against the spinous process, the left arm abducts the patient's right leg until movement is felt to take place at the vertebra under the right thumb. The oscillating movement is then produced by a combined action of the right thumb against the spinous process and the left arm acting on the patient's leg. The range through which the femur is moved to assist with mobilizing after the slack has been taken up is quite small.

Local variations

Movement is much greater at L1 than it is at L4 and is readily felt at L1. The spinous process is far more accessible at L1 and L2 than it is at the lower levels.

Uses

This technique is of greatest value when used with symptoms which have a unilateral distribution. Under these circumstances it is more likely to produce an improvement in the patient's symptoms and signs if it is done from the painless side, pushing the spinous process towards the painful side.

When used in the lower lumbar spine this mobilization is less valuable than either rotation or postero-anterior central vertebral pressure. It is useful, however, when used for conditions of the upper lumbar spine, and the higher the lumbar level causing the symptoms the more likely this technique is to succeed.

Rotation (⟳)

Starting position

For this mobilization the patient should be lying on his right side with pillows supporting his head. While the patient remains relaxed the physiotherapist moves the patient around to adopt the position required. The patient's left arm is adjusted so that his hand rests on the left side of the abdomen with the shoulder extended and the elbow flexed. When the gentlest rotation is being used the patient's thorax is kept in the side-lying position while both hips and knees are flexed, the top one slightly more than the right. The physiotherapist then stands behind the patient and with her hands grasps the patient's pelvis. Positioning of the intervertebral joint being treated, so that it is midway between flexion and extension, is achieved by the degree of hip flexion and the grasp of the pelvis. This grasp enables the physiotherapist to tilt the pelvis towards flexion or extension and the pelvis carries the lumbar spine with it.

If the rotation is to be performed further into the range the physiotherapist rotates the patient's thorax to the left by lifting the patient's right arm towards the ceiling so that the chest faces upwards. This range of rotation is governed by the flexibility of the patient. His underneath leg (right leg) is slightly flexed in relation to his trunk. However, this leg can be extended slightly or flexed more depending upon whether the rotation is to be applied with the lumbar spine towards extension or flexion. The left leg is positioned so that the hip and knee are flexed with the medial tibial condyle resting just over the edge of the couch. When additional pressure is required during mobilization this top leg can hang over the side of the couch.

The physiotherapist then stands behind the patient and places the palms of her hands over the patient's pelvis and left shoulder with the fingers pointing forwards. The hand on the shoulder is cupped over the head of the humerus with the fingers spreading forward over the pectoral muscles. In some cases where the shoulder itself is painful it is necessary for the patient's shoulder to be in a lesser degree of extension and for the physiotherapist's hand to be moved further

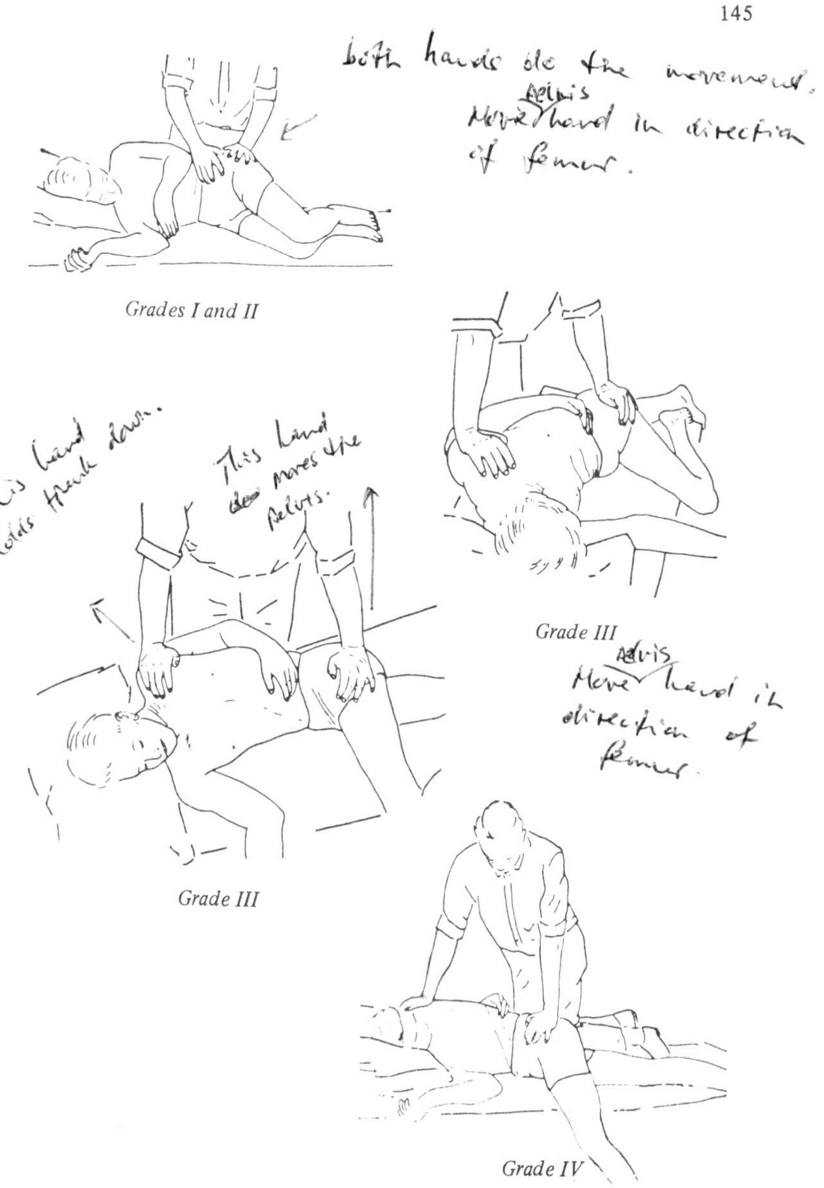

Grades I and II

Grade III

Grade III

Grade IV

Figure 3.30. – Lumbar region. Rotation

towards the pectoral area to apply the pressure. The hand over the pelvis is placed near the crest if the rotation is to be carried out with the lumbar spine towards extension, or over the greater trochanter if the rotation is to be carried out towards flexion.

When the technique is being carried out as a general rotation with the patient's lumbar spine midway between flexion and extension, the physiotherapist's shoulders are placed over the patient's body midway between the hand positions. The elbows should be minimally flexed. If the rotation is to be performed with the lumbar spine tending towards extension, the physiotherapist should move slightly towards the patient's shoulder to enable the line of the left arm operating on the patient's pelvis to encourage extension by its altered position. Similarly, if the rotation is to be done in some degree of flexion, it is necessary for the physiotherapist to move towards the patient's pelvis to enable the left arm operating on the pelvis to encourage flexion with the rotation.

When a stronger mobilization is required the patient's position remains unchanged but the physiotherapist kneels on the couch behind the patient. The physiotherapist can then carry her weight directly over the patient and use her knee under the patient's buttock to assist the rotation (*Figure 3.30*).

Method

Because the leverage is long the physiotherapist must at all times be in a position to see the patient's back to watch the movement taking place.

With the gentle techniques the small oscillatory movements are produced through the physiotherapist's left hand which has a double function. Firstly, by its grasp of the pelvis the intervertebral joint is positioned midway between flexion and extension. Secondly, while the pelvis is held in this position, the left hand imparts the rotary movement to the pelvis. No counter-pressure to prevent thoracic movement is required but great care is necessary to be sure that the movement is purely rotary. The physiotherapist should endeavour to produce a rotary movement round an axis through the lumbar vertebrae like the chicken-on-a-spit action mentioned in relation to cervical rotation.

Even with the change of starting position required for stronger techniques, the rotary movement is still a movement of the pelvis (not the thorax) about a central axis. There is a need for the thorax to be stabilized by the hand on the shoulder, but this counter-pressure is not one which pushes the shoulder and thorax backwards, but is rather a holding action which allows the thorax to follow the direction of the pelvic movement but only to a limited degree.

During the oscillation it is often desirable from time to time to roll the patient's trunk back and forth, without attempting any increase in the amount of rotation, to be sure that maximum relaxation is being obtained and that all slack has still been taken up.

Local variations

The sense of movement which can be obtained here is quite marked, and a noticeable degree of feel can be acquired despite the fact that the leverage is so great. This is aided by watching the patient's lumbar area of movement throughout the procedure.

Rotation with the lumbar spine towards extension is better used when mobilizing the middle or upper lumbar spine, and rotation towards flexion is best reserved for the lowest joints.

Precautions

Occasionally a patient will develop cervical discomfort following treatment by lumbar rotation. It is preferable, therefore, not to alter the head position from that which he feels is comfortable unless this is necessary to improve the starting position. This cervical irritation usually settles without any difficulty, but it is better avoided if possible.

The possibility of irritating the lower thoracic spine, or of creating a thoracic condition, can become a very real problem with strong mobilization and requires watching. Particular care is required with those patients who have, or have had, lower thoracic symptoms as well as the lumbar condition for which they are being treated.

If the rotation is done too vigorously while rotating the pelvis towards the painful side, symptoms of referred pain can be produced in the pain-free leg.

Uses

Rotation is one of the most useful procedures in treating painful conditions arising from the lumbar spine. It is most valuable when used for symptoms which are unilateral in their distribution, whether they are referred to the leg or localized to the lumbar area. In examples where the symptoms are central but the signs are unilateral, these signs can be taken as the guide to the painful side. In such cases the technique is more likely to succeed in relieving the patient's symptoms and signs if it is done with the patient lying on the painless side; that is, with the painful side uppermost so that the pelvis can be rotated away from the painful side.

One further aspect regarding the application of mobilization techniques for distally referred pain requires stating. Frequently a technique performed early in the range results in an exacerbation, even when symptoms are not created during the performance of a technique. In this event the cause of the pain is being excited and nothing is being done to alter the pathology. Under these circumstances the same technique performed at the limit of the available range, in very small amplitudes, will often effect improvement. For example, if lumbar rotation used as Grade I does not produce pain yet causes an exacerbation, the same rotation performed as a very gentle and very small amplitude Grade IV may well effect improvement.

Alternative method of rotation (↻)

When the physiotherapist has difficulty in obtaining sufficient patient relaxation to produce good movement, the following alternative method may give the patient more feeling of security, thus enabling him to relax better.

Starting position

The patient lies on his left side, well forwards on the couch, with his underneath hip and knee flexed slightly and comfortably. He rests his right upper arm on his side and places both forearms, parallel to each other, in front of his abdomen, with his left forearm nearer his chin. The physiotherapist leans across his trunk, facing his pelvis, to place her right forearm along his back. She then holds behind his right femur distally to grasp his inner knee with her right hand. She supports his left leg in approximately 90 degree knee and hip flexion (*Figure 3.31*).

Method

With her trunk and right arm the physiotherapist stabilizes the patient's trunk while rotating his pelvis forwards on the right side through the medium of his right leg. It is important that the technique does not involve any abduction or adduction of the patient's hip; the leg is merely used as a lever to produce the pelvic, and therefore lumbar, rotation.

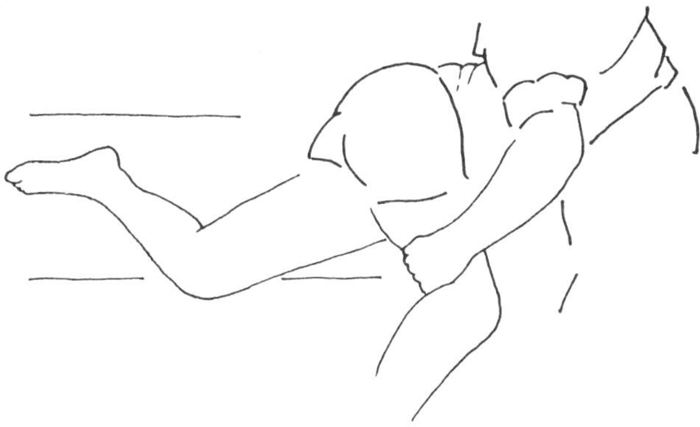

Figure 3.31. – Lumbar region. Alternative rotation method (⟲)

To assist the movement, the physiotherapist can use her right hand on his back:

1. to feel the rotation between adjacent spinous processes;
2. to encourage the rotation at a particular level by lifting the upper spinous process in rhythm with the rotation; or
3. to hold back against the spinous process of the upper vertebra so localizing the movement more to the single appropriate joint.

Rotation with straight leg raising (⟲ ↘)

Lumbar rotation and straight leg raising have been described as separate techniques. However, it is sometimes useful, during a lumbar rotation technique to allow the patient's leg to hang over the side of the couch. One advantage of this is that the weight of the leg assists the rotation being performed by the physiotherapist. However, another important use is that sometimes the effect of the leg hanging over the side acts almost like a straight leg raising technique. Under circumstances when a firm straight leg raising technique is desired the lumbar rotation needs to be done slightly differently so that the physiotherapist can stand in front and use her legs to strengthen the straight leg raising stretch.

Starting position

The patient lies on his right side and the physiotherapist positions him for lumbar rotation as described previously. She allows his leg to hang over the side of the couch with his knee projecting beyond its edge.

She stands in front of the patient and places her right lower leg behind his calf and her left knee in front of his left knee. She leans over

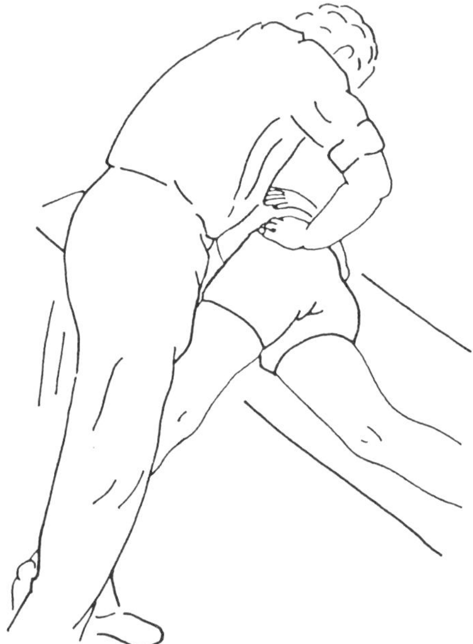

Figure 3.32. – Lumbar region. Rotation with straight leg raising (↷)

the patient to place her left hand cupped over the front of his left shoulder and her right hand cupped over his left hip. She leans far enough across to be able to direct her right forearm back towards herself (*Figure 3.32*).

Method

The physiotherapist provides a holding action with her left hand against his shoulder and performs the rotation with her right hand against his femur. At the same time as she applies rotation to his lumbar spine she also increases the tension in the straight leg raising by pivoting on her feet to both maintain knee extension and to increase the angle of hip flexion.

Precautions

This technique should not be used until other techniques have been tried and it is known that straight leg raising is a necessary part of treatment. It should not be done when pain is reproduced in the lower leg by the technique.

Longitudinal movement (↔)

There are two methods for producing this movement. The operator may use either one or both of the patient's legs.

Using two legs (↔ 2)

Starting position

The patient lies on his back on a low couch with pillows placed under his head, while the physiotherapist stands at the foot end of the couch facing the patient and grasps the patient's heels and ankles from the outside. The patient's legs are lifted, while maintaining some traction, to a height which will allow the lumbar spine to relax in a position midway between flexion and extension. To do this the legs need to be raised approximately 25 degrees from the horizontal plane.

It is advisable for the physiotherapist to stand with one foot in front of the other and crouch forwards over the patient's feet. The physiotherapist's body and arms are then in the position where maximum pull can be given with minimum effort (*Figure 3.33*).

Method

All looseness of contact between the patient and the couch is taken up by gently pulling on the patient's ankles. Longitudinal movement is then produced by the physiotherapist flexing her elbows and extending her shoulders while in the crouched position. With gentle mobilizing there is no movement of the patient along the couch but with stronger grades only three to six tugs can be transmitted because the patient slides a little along the couch. The patient should not make any effort to prevent this movement.

Using one leg (↔ Ⓛ)

Starting position

The patient lies on his back on a low couch with pillows under his head. To mobilize, using the patient's left leg, the physiotherapist stands by the left side of the couch towards the foot end.

The important part of the technique is executed when the patient's leg is straight. It is better, therefore, to take up this position first, so that the physiotherapist can stand comfortably in an efficient position. The physiotherapist grasps the patient's left ankle so that the left hand is placed under the heel grasping it from the outside in the area of the tendo-Achillis, while the right hand is placed in front of the ankle with the thumb lying over the outer aspect of the foot in front of the lateral malleolus with the fingers spreading over the inner aspect of the foot and the medial malleolus. This should give a comfortable encircling grasp of the ankle. The physiotherapist places her feet in a 'walk-standing' position opposite the patient's lower leg, with the feet pointing towards the foot end of the couch and should crouch forwards over the patient's left foot. The angle at which the patient's leg is held should allow the lower lumbar spine to lie comfortably in a neutral position midway between extension and flexion while traction is maintained on the leg, and the knee should be relaxed in extension.

To move from the position described to the true starting position the physiotherapist flexes the patient's hip and knee without moving her own feet. The amount of hip and knee flexion employed is governed by the gentleness of the mobilization desired. If the technique is to be done strongly, a rather full hip and knee flexion position is adopted. If the mobilization starts from a lower position of hip and knee flexion it becomes correspondingly more gentle. As it is necessary for the patient's leg to be relaxed it may be necessary to prevent any lateral rotation of the hip by supporting the lateral aspect of the lower leg with the physiotherapist's right forearm (*Figure 3.33*).

Method

From the flexed position the physiotherapist guides and allows the leg to drop but should be sufficiently ahead of the movement to be in control of the leg position. As the knee drops into the relaxed, fully

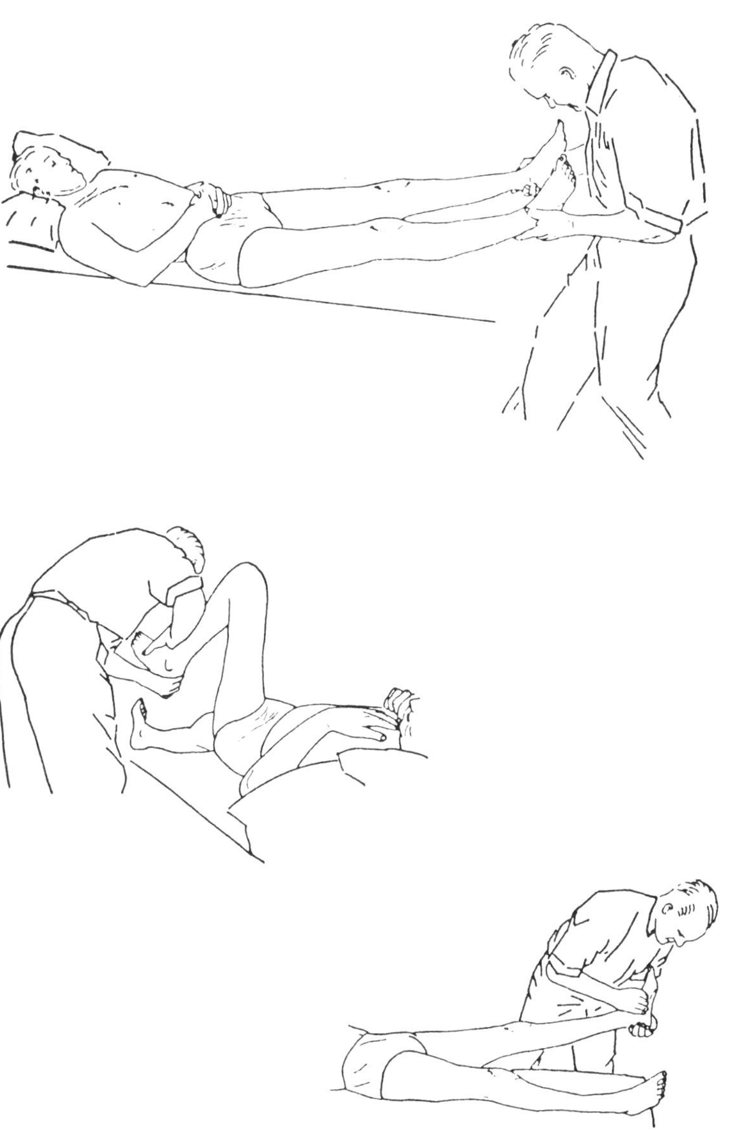

Figure 3.33. – Lumbar region. Longitudinal movement

extended position the physiotherapist applies a gentle, sharp pressure to the patient's ankle so as to continue the elongating action of the leg. The line traversed by the patient's heel must be a straight line from the starting position to the point where the traction is applied, and the line is the position of the straight leg chosen at the outset to place the intervertebral joint being mobilized in its mid-position. *The timing of the physiotherapist's action to coincide with the final dropping of the patient's knee into extension is vital.* The physiotherapist's arms and the patient's foot must at all times be held close to her thorax.

If the patient is unable to allow his knee to drop freely into extension this action can be assisted by asking him to kick gently through his heel. Dorsiflexion of the ankle may assist further.

Once the physiotherapist's action is completed, the patient's leg is returned to the flexed hip and knee position ready for the next movement. A series of three to six movements should be done before reassessing progress. The patient must not hold on to the sides of the couch to prevent sliding, as this may hinder adequate relaxation. As the patient slides along the couch the physiotherapist must move her feet to remain in control of the procedure.

Precautions

When using the single-leg procedure the state of the patient's hip and knee must be checked before and during treatment to avoid injury. If back pain or muscle spasm is produced when the double-leg procedure is being used, the technique should be done gently and changes should be accurately assessed afterwards.

Uses

The double-leg method is used for evenly distributed painful conditions, and the single-leg method (using the painful leg) for symptoms which are unilateral when these symptoms have a lumbar origin below the fourth lumbar vertebra.

This is a very useful technique, particularly when applied as a gentle double-leg procedure for acute pain which is localized to the lumbar spine.

Flexion (F)

Flexion is often considered a movement to be avoided but there are times when it is a necessary part of treatment both with the very gentle and the stronger techniques. Four techniques showing varying strengths are described below.

First starting position

The patient lies prone, arms by his side, his head turned comfortably to one side. The physiotherapist stands to his left side at the level of his thigh, facing his pelvis. She leans across the patient to grasp his right anterosuperior iliac spine in her right hand while holding the left anterosuperior iliac spine in her left hand. She places her right forearm against his lower right buttock (*Figure 3.34*).

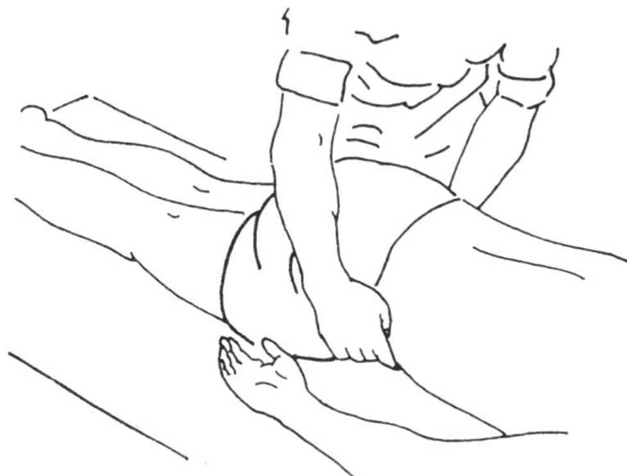

Figure 3.34. – Lumbar region. Flexion: first starting position (F)

Method

Using a very gentle pulling action with her hands, the physiotherapist raises and lowers his upper pelvis slightly. The movement is facilitated by pivoting her right forearm against his buttock.

Second starting position

The patient lies supine with his hips and knees flexed and his feet resting on the table. The physiotherapist stands alongside his trunk, facing across his body, and passes her right arm behind his knees. She reaches across with her left arm in front of his thighs to link her hands together on the outside of his farthest knee. By lifting and pulling with her arms, she flexes his knees towards his chest (*Figure 3.35*).

Method

The physiotherapist uses both arms to flex and return the patient's legs; this gently flexes his lumbar spine and then allows it to unroll. Most of the action is carried out by her right arm but her left arm assists

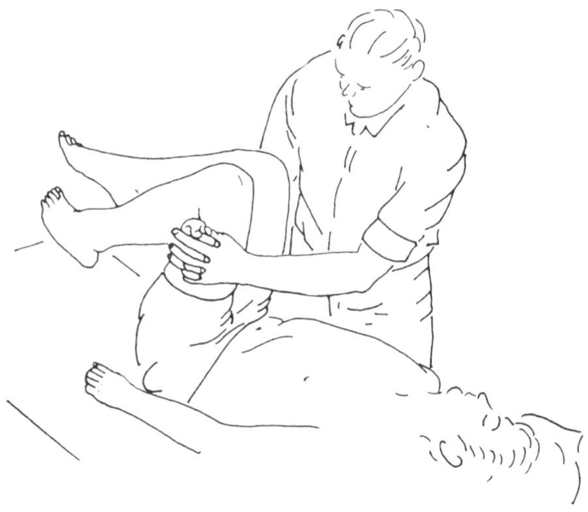

Figure 3.35. – Lumbar region. Flexion: second starting position (F)

the flexing action. By virtue of the position of her right arm behind his knees, she is able to exert a certain amount of traction along the line of his femur, assisting the flexion action on the lumbar spine by raising the pelvis. The oscillatory flexion action can be performed in any part of the flexion range.

Third starting position

The patient sits with his legs extended in front of him with his hands on his shins. The physiotherapist stands closely by his left side with her left hand over his knees and her right hand positioned approximately over his thoracolumbar spine. Her legs are positioned in walk-standing. She crouches forward towards his feet (*Figure 3.36*).

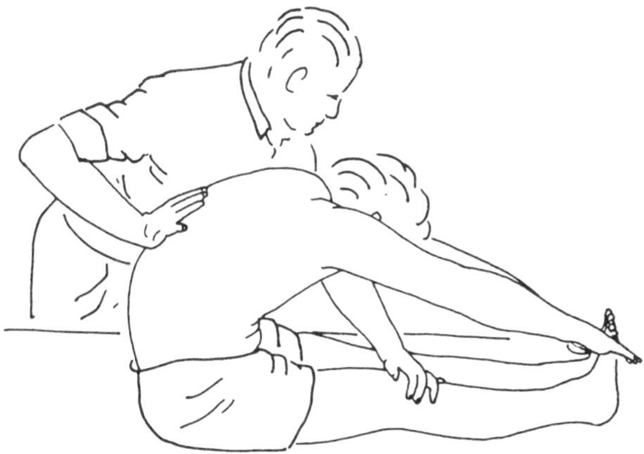

Figure 3.36. – Lumbar region. Flexion: third starting position (F)

Method

The technique has four phases, the first two of which are identical. For the first phase the patient takes his hands off his knees and gently stretches his hands towards or beyond his toes and then returns to hands on knees position. The second phase involves repeating this gentle stretch and return. During both these movements the physiotherapist follows his two gentle stretches, maintaining light pressure with her right hand against his thoracolumbar spine while following his trunk movement with her trunk flexion. The third phase is the actual mobilization which is an exaggeration of the first two phases. In this third phase the patient stretches as far beyond his feet as he can while the physiotherapist, holding his knees down, pushes against the thoracolumbar spine with her hand using her bodyweight to produce an efficient stretch. The fourth phase involves returning to the original starting position where the patient's hands rest on his knees.

Fourth starting position

The patient stands with his feet 10 cm (4 inches) apart. The physiotherapist, standing behind the patient, places her right foot between his feet. She places her right forearm across his middle or lower abdomen and grasps her hands firmly together in the region of his left iliac crest.

The patient then flexes forward and the physiotherapist controls the range to which she allows him to flex by the position of her right forearm through which she exerts pressure (*Figure 3.37*).

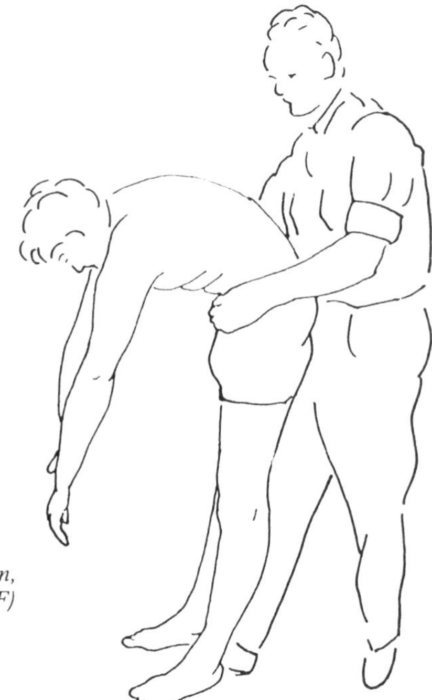

Figure 3.37 – Lumbar region, Flexion: fourth starting position (F)

Method

The patient repeatedly but gently bounces down into flexion. The physiotherapist allows him to go as far as she chooses then returns him some short distance by pulling with her forearm. While pulling with her forearm she leans backwards, levering her right pelvis against his sacrum.

Precautions

The last two methods are not used in the presence of a herniating disc. Flexion is not a technique to use until others which effect movement at the intervertebral joint have been tried without success.

When it is first used it should be performed gently so that its effect can be assessed before progressing to stronger techniques.

Uses

The very gentle technique, described first, is extremely valuable when the patient, on forward flexion, exhibits considerable lordotic muscle spasm. The two stronger techniques cannot be used under these circumstances but are valuable when flexion is limited by stiffness and is not hindered by muscle spasm or pain.

Straight leg raising (SLR,Ⓛ)

This is not a technique to mobilize an intervertebral joint but it is a mobilizing procedure frequently essential in the treatment of lower lumbar conditions.

Starting position

The patient lies supine and rests his left leg on the physiotherapist's left shoulder which is kept as low as is required by the limited range of the patient's straight leg raising. While the physiotherapist kneels alongside the patient she endeavours to keep the patient's right knee extended by resting her left knee lightly just above the patient's knee. The patient's left knee must be kept extended and slightly medially rotated by the physiotherapist's left hand (*Figure 3.38*).

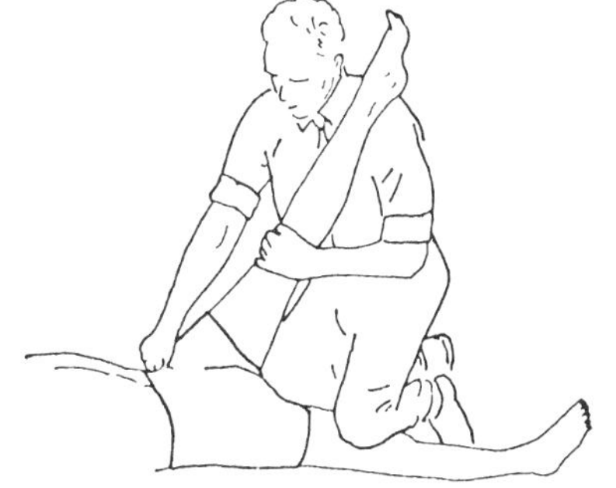

Figure 3.38. – Lumbar region. Straight leg raising (SLR Ⓛ)

Method

Stretch is applied usually as a single fairly rapid stretching movement or as a series of small oscillatory movements, by the physiotherapist raising and lowering her trunk from the squatting position.

As stretch is applied the patient may lift his pelvis on the painful side. If this does occur it can be prevented by thumb pressure in the iliac fossa. Similarly he may abduct and laterally rotate his left leg. This action can be prevented by the physiotherapist's left hand holding the patient's leg medially rotated, and by directing her stretch into flexion and slight adduction of the hip.

Precautions

When lower leg pain is severe or paraesthesiae are present this technique should not be used or should be used extremely gently with careful assessment. Care must also be exercised when neurological changes are present. However, such changes do not necessarily indicate contraindication.

Uses

Straight leg raising can be used when the symptoms or signs indicate pain is arising from the nerve root or its associated investments, whether this is due to nerve root compression or otherwise. The most common indication is unilateral limitation of straight leg raising with minimal pain and when over-pressure produces a pelvic lifting. This sign may be present when the patient has back pain or limb pain. Under some circumstances the range of straight leg raising may be full, then the technique merely mobilizes and stretches the nerve.

It is not the method of choice when the limitation is muscular and it is not a technique which should be used until other techniques which do not move the nerve root so much have been found ineffective.

Lumbar traction (LT)

Traction for the lumbar spine has been described in a variety of ways and using many different types of harness. Some writers have described it with the patient standing (Lehmann and Brunner, 1958) while others have the patient lying; some use a thoracic belt as the means of fixing the upper end of the spine, while others use padded pillars against the axillae (Crisp, 1960); some have described it with the patient in

Crisp, E. J. (1960). *Disc Lesions and other Intervertebral Derangements treated by Manipulation Traction and other Conservative Methods.* London; Livingstone

Lehmann, J. F. and Brunner, G. D. (1958). 'A device for the application of heavy lumbar traction.' *Arch. phys. Med.* 39, 696 the straight position, while others insist on lumbar flexion (Mennell, 1960); some give traction on canvas top couches (Scott, 1955) while others use roller top couches (Judovich and Nobel, 1957); some administer it as constant traction (Cyriax, 1975), and others as intermittent traction (Judovich and Nobel, 1957). Even the application of manual lumbar traction has been described (Crisp, 1960). A useful summary of these and other authors in relation to all forms of traction is given by Licht (1960).

A patient with severe nerve-root pain, if he is to be treated conservatively, should be treated with lumbar traction. However a choice needs to be made between constant traction administered on a 24 hour basis in hospital and traction administered in physiotherapy rooms on a 30 minute per day basis. Provided traction in rooms stands a reasonable chance of success, it is the treatment of choice as it leaves the patient freer than does traction in hospital. When pain is severe it is not easy to make the correct decision from the outset. If constant traction in hospital is to be used the method is as follows.

Hospital traction

The patient lies supine either on a horizontal bed or with the foot of the bed raised 25 cm (10 inches). A comfortable soft pelvic belt is placed on the patient to which ropes are attached and fitted to a spreader. From the spreader a single rope passes over a pulley at the foot of the bed to the weights attached at its end (*Figure 3.39*). It is wisest if the patient remains supine at all times but a change of position may sometimes be permitted. The patient should be allowed commode facilities as the use of a bedpan is too traumatic to the back of a patient with severe pain. Fowler's position (*Figure 3.39*) is only required if the patient has a marked lumbar kyphosis which is not largely reduced when recumbent. If Fowler's position is required, as soon as the kyphosis improves the normal traction position described first should be

Crisp, E. J. (1960). *Disc Lesions and other Intervertebral Derangements treated by Manipulation Traction and other Conservative Methods.* London; Livingstone

Cyriax, J. (1975). *Textbook of Orthopaedic Medicine.* Vol II (6th Edition). London; Ballière Tindall

Judovich, B. and Nobel, G. R. (1957). 'Traction therapy, a study of resistance forces, preliminary report on a new method of lumbar traction.' *Am. J. Surg.* **93,** 108

Licht, S. (1960). *Massage, Manipulation and Traction.* Connecticut, U.S.A.; Licht

Mennell, John McM. (1960). *Back Pain. Diagnosis and Treatment using Manipulative Techniques.* London; Churchill

Scott, B. O. (1955). 'A universal traction frame and lumbar harness.' *Ann. phys. Med.* **2,** 258 adopted. Initially the tractive force should be approximately 5 kg. This weight can be increased on a basis of approximately 1 kg per day up to a maximum of 9–11 kg. Ten days is usually long enough for the traction to be maintained after which the patient should become fully ambulant over the next three days. If there is no improvement after one week on constant traction persistence with the traction will not produce any change.

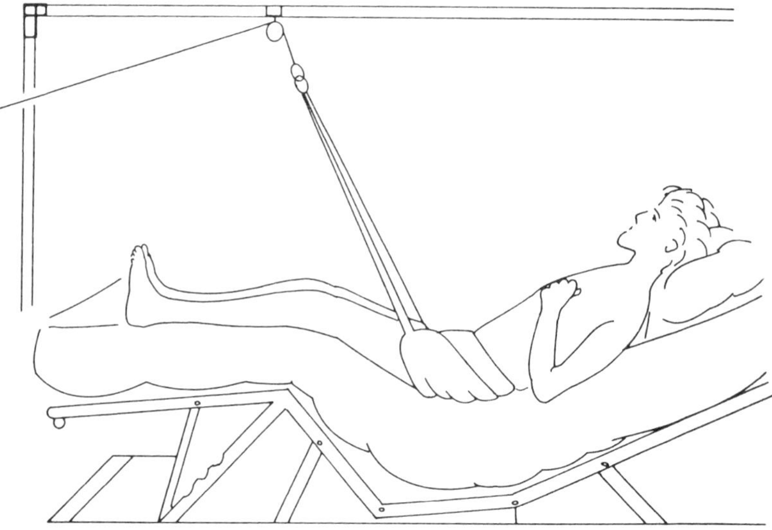

Figure 3.39. – Lumbar region. Traction in flexion (Fowler's position)

Fundamentally the two essentials for lumbar traction administered in treatment rooms are comfortable, adjustable harnesses for attaching the thorax and pelvis to fixed points, and a comfortable position for the patient, to assist relaxation. With these two factors in mind the following method is given as a basis for traction therapy.

Starting position

A belt is firmly fixed around the patient's thorax while he is standing and a second belt around the pelvis while he is lying, making sure that no single garment is caught under both belts.

The patient then lies either face upwards or face downwards on the traction couch. In the supine position it may be necessary for the patient's hips and knees to be flexed. The position of choice is the one which places the intervertebral joint midway between flexion and extension to permit the greatest longitudinal movement.

By means of straps the thoracic belt is then attached to some fixed point beyond the head of the couch and the pelvic belt is attached to a fixed point beyond the foot of the couch. Before the patient is ready for the traction to be applied, these straps must be tightened to remove all looseness from the harness (*Figure 3.40*).

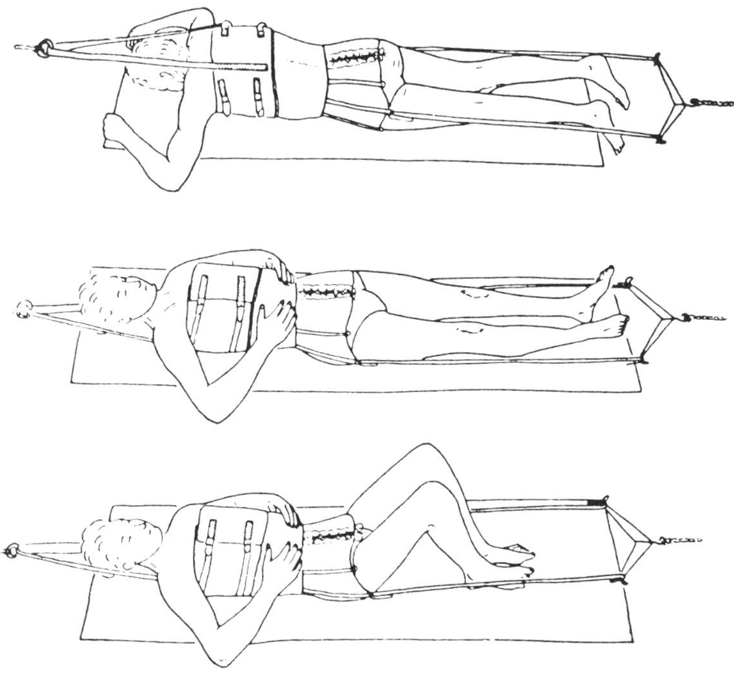

Figure 3.40. – Lumbar traction (LT)

Method

It is necessary to assess accurately the patient's area and degree of pain, while he is lying ready for the traction to be applied.

The traction is then applied from either the head end or the foot end of the apparatus, or from both ends, but care must be taken to eliminate friction between the patient and the couch if a roll-top traction couch is not being used. The physiotherapist does this by raising and lowering the patient's thorax and pelvis alternately to ensure that the stretch is being applied between the belts and that it is not lost in friction between the patient's body and the couch.

Although a friction-free couch is not essential, it is such a tremendous advantage that if it is possible to make up a simple one cheaply the effort is more than rewarded. Most patent roll-top couches consist of a fixed thoracic section and a rolling lumbar section but this arrangement has little to recommend it. An efficient friction-free couch has both sections on rollers. It is also essential to be able to lock the sections together, not only to make it stable for the patient to climb onto but also to make the couch usable for purposes other than traction. Such a couch is described on page 134 and shown in *Figure 3.26*. The cost is minimal.

When a patient is given lumbar traction for the first time a very low strength, not greater than 13 kg, should be used and this should be maintained for a period not exceeding 10 minutes. The patient should not be permitted to have his arms above his head and if he wants to read while on traction this is permissible if, and only if, his elbows are rested on the couch. A careful watch should be kept for low-back symptoms caused by the traction even if these are only felt with movement of the lumbar spine, or coughing. If low-back pain is experienced by the patient, the duration and pressure of this first treatment should be reduced. If 13 kg can be applied, the patient's symptoms, both local back pain and referred limb pain, should be assessed after a waiting period of 10 seconds. One of the following courses of action should then be taken.

1. When severe symptoms are completely relieved (particularly symptoms in the leg), the strength should be reduced by at least half, and the duration should not exceed 5 minutes. If this action is not taken the patient will almost certainly suffer a marked exacerbation of symptoms.
2. The symptoms may be relieved minimally by 13 kg traction and under these circumstances the strength may be increased to approximately 20 kg and the duration can be 10 minutes. However, if 20 kg completely relieves symptoms (especially if they are severe), this strength should be reduced to something less than 18 kg.
3. If the symptoms remain unchanged the traction should be increased to 20 kg and sustained for 10 minutes.
4. If the symptoms are worse the traction should be reduced to a poundage where the patient is the same as before the traction was applied and the duration should be reduced to 5 minutes.

While the traction is being released slowly, the patient should move his pelvis gently by rolling from side to side or tilting it. If pain is experienced with this pelvic movement the traction should be held at that point until the pain disappears. When the traction has been removed the patient should rest for a few minutes before standing. This is not always necessary, but should be insisted upon at the first treatment. The patient should be warned that it is normal for his back to feel strange for approximately 2 hours.

Method of progression

On the day following the first stretch the patient's symptoms and signs are assessed and compared with those present before traction. From these facts one can determine whether traction should be repeated and how it should be graduated. Signs can be assessed immediately following the traction but flexion frequently does not provide any useful information and certainly it is not the main criterion on which to base further treatment as it is nearly always more limited immediately after traction. In the absence of other signs one factor which will show whether traction is being successful is if it is known that at a certain strength pain is produced, and if this poundage can be increased at a subsequent treatment without producing the discomfort the patient's condition must be improving.

If, during the first treatment, the symptoms were made worse initially and the strength had to be reduced considerably and if the symptoms remain increased and the signs have also deteriorated, traction must be discontinued. If, however, the symptoms do not remain worse and the signs do not deteriorate the traction can be repeated. During the second treatment an assessment should be made of the strength which can be applied without increase of symptoms, to be able to compare this with the previous treatment. If a higher strength is possible then favourable progress has been made.

When the strength on the first day was reduced because symptoms were completely relieved while the patient was on traction, the progression is guided as much by changes in the severity of any temporary exacerbation which followed the treatment, as by the changes in signs. Over the period of the first three or four stretches the improvement in signs will probably be small. When signs indicate that traction should continue, any increase in the treatment should be in the length of time and not by an increase in the strength. When there is no exacerbation following treatment or after the duration of 15 minutes, the poundage can be gradually increased.

Under circumstances other than the two just discussed, strength and time can be increased together. Generally the average strength is reached between 30 and 45 kg but occasionally when the rate of progress seems too slow with lower strength, stretches of up to 65 kg are necessary. Duration does not need to exceed 15 minutes, as longer periods do not produce any further progress except when treating disc pathology causing nerve root symptoms.

Although strengths have been suggested, the scale should not be the controlling guide during treatment. In fact it should only be referred to when traction has been applied to the level required by the patient's symptoms and signs. The main value of a scale measurement is for recording purposes.

As in other areas of the vertebral column, intermittent variable traction can be used for the lumbar spine. The duration and strength of such treatment falls within the same limitation as set out above. Timing for the hold and rest periods varies as discussed on page 118.

Precautions

With the exception of discomfort from the harness used, there is no natural soreness to be felt with low strengths of traction. With this in mind great care should be taken when any low-back discomfort is felt while the traction is being given. It is advisable, once the traction has been applied, to ask the patient to attempt alternate flattening and lordosing of the lumbar spine as well as coughing to see if this causes any back discomfort.

It is wise to consider the first session of traction as a 'dummy run' so that the embarrassing harmless situation of a patient having difficulty getting onto his feet is avoided. Following carelessly strong traction, particularly the first time, a patient may be unable to get to his feet because of sharp pains in the lower back. This is unpredictable but can be avoided if care is exercised with every first treatment.

Uses

Traction has three primary uses in the treatment of pain arising from the lumbar spine.

1. Any symptoms, whether they are localized to the lumbar area or referred into the leg, which have gradually appeared over a period of days or longer, and which have not been preceded by any known trauma, may be treated successfully by traction.

2. An ache arising from the lumbar spine in the presence of marked bony changes, whether these have been brought about by excessive degeneration, old trauma or postural deformities, usually responds well to gentle traction, or intermittent variable traction.
3. Pain arising from the lumbar spine in the absence of any obvious loss of active range of movement in the lumbar spine usually responds better to traction than manipulation.

Traction should always be tried when no further progress can be obtained by mobilization.

It is often necessary for traction to be preceded by manipulation, particularly when traction is given in the presence of painless limitation of movement at an intervertebral joint. When traction of a particular patient has reached a stage when it is not producing any further progress, it is advisable to return to mobilization as it is then often successful where it had not been before traction.

GENERAL

The techniques can be performed in general or very specific ways. For example if cervical rotation is being used to treat C4/5 the physiotherapist's 'head' hand can be moved down from the occiput so as to grasp C4. Similarly, if we again take C4/5 as the level but treatment is by postero-anterior unilateral vertebral pressure on the left side, the technique may be used generally by employing the technique from C3 to C6 or it may be used only on C3 or C4 on the apophyseal joint line between C3/4. Also C4 articular pillar can be held in one hand and the C3 articular pillar in the opposite hand. While C3 is moved postero-anteriorly, C4 can be either moved in the opposite direction to C3, or just stabilized. When transverse pressures are being used similar accuracy to one level can be achieved by pushing adjacent spinous processes in opposite directions.

4 Application of Mobilization

Many people believe that to use manipulation as a form of treatment requires only the learning of techniques. This is a dangerous mistake and could not be further from the truth. This same thought is also, unfortunately, carried into some of the courses on manipulation and this is deplorable. Obviously it is important that the techniques must administer movement properly but even a technique performed well may do harm or may fail completely if the wrong movement is selected or if it is done at the wrong depth. The choice of a technique and the changing from one technique to another is determined by repeated accurate assessment of the patient's symptoms and signs before and after each application of a technique and from treatment to treatment. This routine must be rigidly adhered to if the treatment is to be objective and safe at all times. However, safety and guidance for changing from one technique to another are not the only reasons for continually assessing symptoms and signs; it is by this means that the manipulator gains experience in predicting the possible outcome of treatment.

When a particular technique does not produce any change it should be repeated perhaps more firmly, and if it still fails to produce any change then the technique should be discarded. Traction is usually slower in producing changes and should not be discarded until up to four daily applications have failed to produce any change. When a patient says his symptoms have improved, or if any of the signs show improvement, the same technique should be repeated. Repetition would be indicated if only one of the signs had shown improvement, provided of course that the remainder had not been made worse. When the symptoms or signs are made worse by a technique, it should not be repeated. However, it may be attempted again at a later stage of treatment when, provided there has been an alteration in joint signs, it may be useful. Care needs to be taken in assessing symptoms because a patient may say that his symptoms are worse when in fact the pain may be of a different nature, being rather a response to stretching than a worsening of the existing symptoms. In such cases it is unlikely that the symptoms have been made worse if there is no associated deterioration in the signs.

TREATMENT ASSESSMENT

Although it has been suggested that two applications of a mobilizing technique or four daily applications of traction are sufficient to show the value of a technique, this is not always so. The whole point of

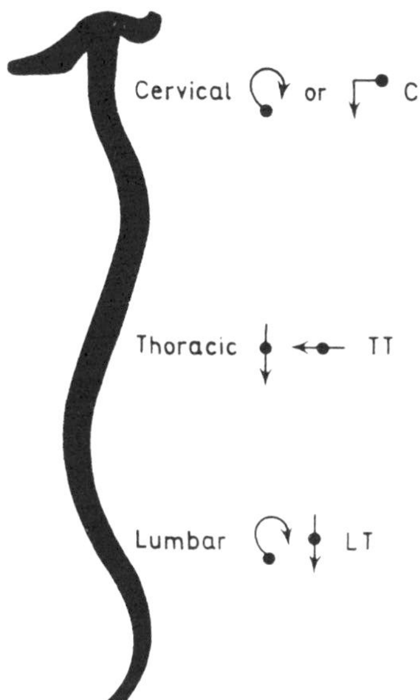

Figure 4.1. – Spinal techniques in order of efficacy

assessing between techniques is to have a means whereby their effect can be measured. Before treatment, during the initial examination of a patient, the physiotherapist should assess whether it will be possible to bring about quick improvement in the patient's condition or whether the progress is likely to be slow. If quick progress is possible, changes from one technique to another can be made more rapidly (*Figure 4.1*).

For example, when a technique is producing improvement, if it is thought that the rate of improvement is slower than might be possible, a change of technique may increase the rate of progress. When it is known that improvement will be slow, it may be wrong to change from a technique until it has been used for two or more days.

How much improvement in a patient's signs is enough to justify continuing to use a particular mobilizing technique? This is difficult to learn except through practical experience based on continual assessment of changes produced by the technique under various conditions. Obviously some patients will show a greater rate of change than others. It has been found (Maitland, 1957) that as pain is referred further and further from the source, treatment takes longer and is less likely to be successful (Table 4.1). As the survey consisted of 220 patients pre-selected by medical practitioners it cannot be expected to be precise, and it is not the author's wish that it should be accepted as anything more than an approximate guide. Because the results from treatment of cervical syndromes follow a somewhat similar pattern, the survey can help the student to know how much treatment a particular patient may need.

TABLE 4.1

Results of Treatment

Symptoms	*Patients relieved (percentage)*	*Average length of successful treatments (days)*
Back pain		
without protective scoliosis	96	4.5
with protective scoliosis	91	6
Back to buttock pain		
without protective scoliosis	95	4
with protective scoliosis	95	4
Back to knee pain		
without protective scoliosis	96	5.7
with protective scoliosis	60	11
Back to foot pain		
without protective scoliosis	91	7
with protective scoliosis	50	9
Pain with neurological changes*	54	9

*Pains with neurological changes referrable to the third lumbar nerve root were more difficult to relieve than those from the sacral nerve roots and both of these were more difficult to relieve than were all others of lumbar origin

Maitland, G. D. (1957). 'Low back pain and allied symptoms, and treatment results.' *Med. J. Aust.* **2,** 851

The routine of treatment is as follows. The patient is first assessed for his response to the previous day's treatment. This questioning is not as easy to carry out effectively as some may think. Great care must be taken to avoid misinterpreting the patient's words and it is essential to be critical of one's interpretations. The second assessment consists of comparing the important movement signs with those which were evident before. These findings are recorded as set out in Chapter 8 (*see* page 245).

Following the assessment a technique is chosen and this is performed for approximately a minute before the patient is reassessed. The reassessment of the patient's symptoms and his signs must be made in a way which will endeavour to prove the value of the technique which has just been used. If the improvement is adequate the technique is repeated but if there is not adequate improvement then a change in technique is made. The new technique is applied for the required time and another assessment made. Unless the patient's symptoms are minimal the number of mobilizations between assessments is limited to approximately four per session.

It is important to remember that there is an optimum amount of improvement which can be achieved in any one day. It is therefore necessary to realize that the amount of treatment which can be given at any one session is limited. The treatment must therefore be balanced if the optimum advantage is to be gained from changes in technique.

Although it is possible to have some idea of whether a quick or slow progress with treatment might be achieved, it is necessary to give some examples of what can constitute adequate improvement of signs with the successful application of a technique. The following figures are not intended to be taken too literally and are offered only as a guide. With a patient who can be helped quickly these changes should be expected after each technique but with slower examples the same changes should not be expected in under two or three days. The minimum improvements which justify repeating a technique are increases of 2.5 cm (1 inch) of forward flexion in the standing position, 5 degrees of straight leg raising or 5–10 degrees of trunk or cervical rotation.

There are many pointers which may be found on examination to indicate that a slow rate of progress can be anticipated. These may appear singly or in combination. The pointers can be thought of under the headings deformity, movements, and pathology.

Deformity

1. A patient whose pain radiates to one leg and who also has a scoliosis displacing his shoulders towards the side of pain

(ipsilateral tilt) is certain to be much slower in his response to conservative treatment than if he had a contralateral tilt.

2. A patient who has a protective type scoliosis which alternates from side to side is always difficult to help. However, the more easily the scoliosis can be changed, the harder it is to help him.
3. When a patient on forward flexion exhibits marked spasm of the extensor muscles to limit the movement, his condition can be expected to be difficult to help. This lordotic type of muscle spasm can be bilateral or unilateral. Occasionally a patient is seen who has an ipsilateral tilt combined with a unilateral lordotic type of muscle spasm. When these two factors are combined the response to treatment is likely to be even more difficult.
4. A patient who has a lumbar kyphosis is usually fairly easy to help with mobilization unless the degree of kyphosis is in excess of 30 degrees. Under these circumstances it is almost impossible to help him conservatively unless rest is a part of the treatment.

Movements

1. When a patient with pain in his back and leg has a marked restriction of forward flexion and straight leg raising on the painful side he is likely to be difficult to help (Charnley, 1951).
2. A patient may have limb pain and extension of his neck or back may reproduce some of this limb pain. However, if the range of extension is markedly limited and this movement reproduces the distal area of the pain then the patient is likely to be very difficult to help.
3. When a patient's movements in all directions are very limited and these movements produce sharp pain then the degree of severity and restriction indicates the slowness with which the patient can be expected to respond to treatment.
4. A patient with thoracic or lumbar pain may have the tension sign where passive neck flexion is very limited while reproducing the symptoms. The more the movement is restricted by pain the more difficult it is to relieve him of his symptoms.
5. It is common for patients with gross arthritic or spondylitic changes to have localized aching. Their movements, though generally stiff, are not painfully restricted by this aching. These

Charnley, J. (1951). 'Orthopaedic signs in the diagnosis of disc protrusion.' *Lancet* **1**, 186 patients are reasonably easy to help. However, if the patient with these radiological changes has a localized joint lesion then he is certain to be slow in his response to treatment (*see* example page 291).

6. A patient having bilaterally distributed pain from his lower back into both legs of symmetrical distribution and equal severity is certain to be difficult to assist.

Pathology

1. Severe nerve root pain is always a concern in its response to treatment. Initially it may be seven to ten days before any lessening of the pain is noticeable to the patient. However, the total treatment time is likely to be longer than that for referred pain from other sources. There are three nerve roots which seem to respond less readily to conservative measures than others: L3, which is harder to help than S2; in the cervical area, C8.
2. A primary posterolateral protrusion is always slower in its results though it can usually be helped (Cyriax, 1975).
3. Patients whose symptoms arise from an unstable spondylolysis or spondylolisthesis are always difficult to help with mobilization. Also their response to treatment is not as complete as would be that of patients with similar symptoms from other sources.
4. Patients whose symptoms arise directly from trauma are always more difficult to help and presumably this is because the extent of damage is greater. A particular form of trauma which should also be included in this category is the post-surgical patient who has not responded as well to surgery as was anticipated.
5. One particular group of patients is always difficult to help and this difficulty must be due to the type of pathology or the extent of pathology involved. Any young patient, that is somebody in his teens for example, who has not recovered from his symptoms without requiring treatment, will always be difficult to help. Young people have extremely good powers of recovery and therefore almost without exception any junior who has pain which lasts long enough for him to have been through medical channels to the physiotherapist is likely to be far slower in his response to treatment than his adult contemporary with similar signs.

Cyriax, J. (1975). *Textbook of Orthopaedic Medicine* Vol. 1 6th edn. London; Baillière Tindall

TABLE 4.2

Sequence of Selection of Techniques

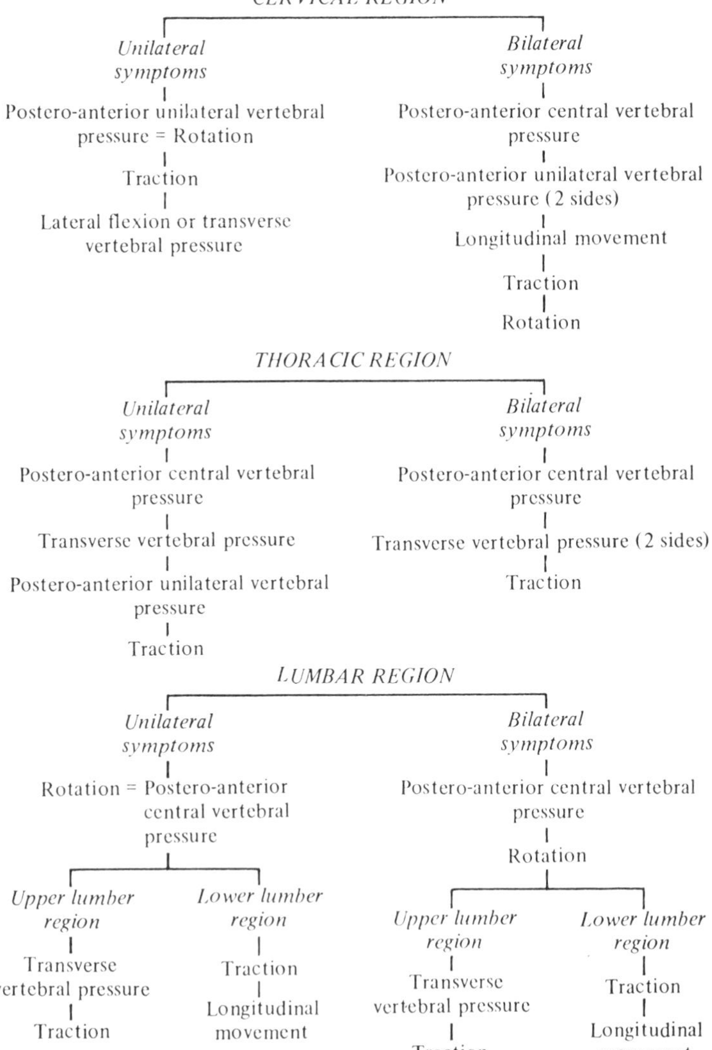

In each region the order may be changed by removing traction from its designated position and placing it anywhere in sequence. The remaining techniques are then used in the same order as shown in this table

SELECTION OF TECHNIQUES

For physiotherapists who are new to this work Table 4.2 is given to assist in the selection of techniques. It lists those techniques for each area of the vertebral column which are most likely to produce some improvement.

This table has been divided into three regions of the spine, and these have been further divided into two groups depending upon whether the symptoms have a unilateral distribution or a bilateral distribution. Under each heading the techniques are listed in what has been found to be the best order. A condition causing bilaterally distributed symptoms must also have signs which can be elicited bilaterally to fit into the 'bilateral symptoms' group. For example, a patient who has pain over the spinous process of the seventh cervical vertebra which can be reproduced by rotation of the head to the left should be considered in the 'unilateral symptoms' section of the table and not under the bilateral symptoms.

Each technique listed in Table 4.2 is used in the direction indicated in Table 4.3; however, if this sequence of selection fails to produce the anticipated result, the techniques can then be tried in the opposite direction.

Because assessment of the value of traction as compared with mobilization can take longer, the feeling can easily develop that the two are not readily interchangeable during treatment. However, it is just as correct to change from one mobilizing technique to traction and thence to another mobilizing technique (when attempting to assess the relative values of each), as it is to make changes which do not include traction. The only difficulty lies in interpreting the relative value of the different procedures. For example, a mobilizing technique takes a minute to do and can be discarded if it proves ineffective after two applications, whereas traction may need to be used for four days before being sure that it is ineffective.

The statement that manipulation is an empirical form of treatment is still perhaps largely true, and must necessarily remain so until every abnormality of the intervertebral joint can be completely understood in terms of clinical signs, and diagnosed. However, when manipulation is used to restore movement to a stiff intervertebral joint the treatment is not empirical. The mobilizing techniques described in Chapter 3 have been listed as having special uses. These uses have been found by keeping careful statistics of some hundreds of patients treated and are not based on pathology. There are many factors which guide in the selection of techniques and these factors are now described separately.

Area of pain

A patient's symptoms may be completely unilateral in which case the type of technique used must be one which affects the joint in a unilateral manner. That is, it should effect the movement of the whole intervertebral joint which moves in such a way that it is a different movement on the right hand side from that on the left.

A patient's symptoms may be bilateral in their distribution from the vertebral column, whether near to the vertebral column or referred does not matter. The technique chosen would be one which affects the joint similarly on both sides. This refers to techniques such as postero-anterior central vertebral pressure, longitudinal movement or traction. However, patient's symptoms do not always fit neatly into one of these two categories and frequently they have symptoms on both sides of the body, with the symptoms on one side being either much greater than the other or are referred much further from the vertebral column than the other. The choice of technique then is more difficult, but the more unilateral in distribution or intensity the symptoms, the more the tendency is to choose a unilaterally effecting technique.

Techniques

As has already been pointed out the techniques of postero-anterior central vertebral pressure, longitudinal movement and traction are all techniques which effect the same movement on one side of the intervertebral joint as on the other. All of the other techniques have a different effect on one side as compared with the other. Whenever these techniques are used they should initially be done in a way which opens the intervertebral space on the side of pain. This thus avoids any narrowing of the intervertebral foramen. To produce this opening on the side of pain the techniques should be performed as follows.

Cervical rotation

The intervertebral foramen on the painful side is widened with the head turned away from the side of pain. Although it is possible to treat occipito-atlantal and atlanto-axial joint pain by rotating the head towards the side of pain, great care should be taken if this is to be done on lesions below this level. Rotation of the head to one side below C2 produces considerable narrowing of the intervertebral foramen on that side. However, above this level such narrowing does not occur.

Lumbar rotation

This technique should initially be performed rotating the patient's pelvis away from his painful side. The amount of foraminal narrowing which takes place during lumbar rotation is very small and it is not unrealistic to endeavour to use rotation in the opposite direction. However, it is wise for the initial movement to be attempted away from the pain.

Cervical lateral flexion

This technique is initially performed tilting the patient's head and neck away from the side of pain to open the foramen on the painful side. Similar care to that described for cervical rotation should be exercised if cervical lateral flexion is to be used towards the side of pain.

Transverse vertebral pressure

This should be performed pushing the spinous process towards the side of pain so that the intervertebral space is open on the painful side.

Postero-anterior unilateral vertebral pressure

This technique should be performed with the pressure being applied on the side of pain. In this way the foramen is open on the painful side. These techniques are set out in Table 4.3.

Section of spine

Many techniques have been described for each section of the vertebral column but some of these are much more useful and effective than others. It can be reasonably said that a quick run-through of two or three techniques will give a fair indication of the value of those techniques, and others, which may be applied to that section of the vertebral column. There are possibly two reasons for these particular techniques being most useful. The first is that they are techniques which are more easily applied to the spine and are therefore more readily controlled during treatment. The other reason is that they involve the main movements of the spine. In the cervical and lumbar spines the two main techniques are rotation and pressures. The next major technique in each of these areas is traction. In the thoracic spine the main technique whether the symptoms are unilateral or bilateral is postero-anterior central vertebral pressure. The second most useful technique is transverse pressure, and the third technique is traction. It should be said at this point that the upper lumbar spine behaves more like the thoracic spine than the lumbar spine (*Figure 4.1*).

TABLE 4.3

Mobilizing Techniques and Their Uses

Technique	*Primary uses*
CERVICAL REGION	
Longitudinal movement	Frequently of value in presence of a spasm deformity
Postero-anterior central vertebral pressure	Bilaterally distributed symptoms. Bony changes from all causes; muscle spasm. Not for severe symptoms
Postero-anterior unilateral vertebral pressure	Unilaterally distributed symptoms particularly if middle or upper cervical in origin. (Direct the push downwards on the side of pain)
Transverse vertebral pressure	Unilaterally distributed symptoms. Bony changes from all causes. (Direct the push towards the side of pain)
Anteroposterior unilateral vertebral pressure	Unilaterally distributed symptoms. (Direct the push on the side of pain)
Rotation	Most valuable–usually the first technique used. Unilaterally distributed symptoms. (Rotate the head away from the side of pain)
Lateral flexion	Unilaterally distributed symptoms. Often used to restore rotation. (Flex away from the side of pain)
Flexion	Minor symptoms in the presence of intervertebral flexion restriction.
Traction	Any cervical condition–severe arm pain with markedly limited neck movements
Traction in neurtal	Upper cervical conditions
Traction in flexion	Lower cervical conditions
Intermittent variable traction	Gross radiological degenerative changes

TABLE 4.3 (cont.)

Technique	*Primary uses*
THORACIC REGION	
Postero-anterior central vertebral pressure	Usually the first technique used. Bilaterally distributed symptoms; unilaterally distributed symptoms if poorly defined or widespread
Transverse vertebral pressure	Unilaterally distributed symptoms. (Direct the push towards the side of pain and mobilize adjacent rib)
Postero-anterior unilateral vertebral pressure	Unilaterally distributed symptoms. (Direct the push downwards on the side of pain and mobilize adjacent rib)
Traction	Widely distributed symptoms especially if radiological degenerative changes are present; when pain is not aggravated by active movements
LUMBAR REGION	
Postero-anterior central vertebral pressure	Bilaterally distributed symptoms. (Equal in usefulness with rotation.) Bony changes from all causes
Postero-anterior unilateral vertebral pressure	Unilaterally distributed symptoms particularly if middle or upper lumbar in origin. (Direct the push downwards on the side of pain)
Transverse vertebral pressure	Unilaterally distributed symptoms. More useful for upper lumbar spine than lower. (Direct the push towards the side of pain)
Rotation	Often the first technique used. Unilaterally distributed symptoms. (Rotate the pelvis forwards on the side of pain)
Longitudinal movement 2 legs	Bilaterally distributed symptoms of lower lumbar origin
1 leg	Unilaterally distributed symptoms of lower lumbar origin
Flexion	Bilaterally distributed symptoms of a chronic nature in the presence of flexion restriction

TABLE 4.3 (cont.)

Technique	*Primary uses*
	LUMBAR REGION
Traction	Gradual onset of symptoms. When pain is not aggravated by active movements
Intermittent variable traction	Gross radiological degenerative changes
Straight leg raising	Unilateral limitation of straight leg raising without extreme pain.
	For symptoms of a chronic or stable nature arising from the nerve root. (The technique is not used as a first technique)

Pain on movements

The point often discussed by writers is whether a technique should be used into a painful range or into a painless range (Maigne, 1964). It is necessary to point out that when using mobilizing techniques it is quite reasonable to use the patient's most painfully restricted movement as the treatment movement but it should be emphasized that the movement is not done into the painful range. If this fact is accepted the choice when selecting techniques sometimes needs to be made between choosing the most painfully restricted movement or the least painfully restricted movement. It does not matter which of these techniques is chosen provided the value of the technique is carefully proven by continuing assessment. If, having chosen the least painful movement, this technique is found to be ineffective, the most painful movement should be chosen though this movement should be performed in a pain-free part of the range. To choose the most painful movement has one distinct advantage. This advantage is based on the fact that, while performing the technique, a small percentage improvement becomes immediately appreciated by the physiotherapist. It is easy to see that a very small percentage of improvement is far more easily discerned in a movement which is markedly limited as compared with a movement which is not very limited. Such information is not available during mobilization if the least painful movement is chosen.

Maigne, R. (1964). 'The concept of painless and opposite motion in spinal manipulation'. *Am. J. Phys. Med.* **44**, 55

Pathology

Diagnosis plays a very important part in the selection of techniques though rarely it is clear that with certain disorders only certain techniques *will* produce improvement. Not only is this so but a pathology may produce different symptoms during its various stages of development. However the following points are helpful in the selection of techniques.

Severe nerve-root pain

As has already been discussed in the chapter on Techniques, with particular reference to the use of traction, the only treatment which should be given during the stages when nerve-root pain is severe is traction. When pain is severe and neurological changes are present this rule must not be altered.

Locked joint

When a patient has carried out a movement and become stuck, and on examination a joint is found to be so limited as to prevent the normal movements of that joint, the joint can be considered locked. Past history and response to previous treatment will indicate how easily this joint is likely to become free. Gentle techniques of longitudinal movement or rotation may easily free the joint. However if these techniques do not produce the desired change then the technique required is a localized manipulation which fully opens the joint on the restricted side. For example, if a patient has quickly turned his head to the left and become stuck in this position, unable to rotate to the right, laterally flex to the right or extend his head, the initial treatment should be longitudinal movement and failing this, rotation to the left. If both of these techniques fail, then the localized manipulation such as described on pages 198 and 199 should be used to open the joint on the right hand side. The important thing is that the joint should be able to be unlocked on the day of treatment.

General stiffness

A patient may have symptoms of a general nature resulting from stiffness of a section of the spine. These symptoms, usually aching in nature, are not severe and usually result from either arthritic changes in the apophyseal joints or spondylosis. The loss of range does not alter significantly with the onset of symptoms.

These patients respond well to general mobilizing techniques applied in a very general manner to the section of spine involved. The techniques should include localized pressures in all directions, rotation and lateral flexion to both sides, and longitudinal movement or intermittent variable traction. Obviously it would be incorrect to apply all of these procedures during the first treatment. The pressures could be applied on the first day, the rotation and perhaps lateral flexion added on the second day, and if there is no unfavourable reaction, the longitudinal movement or intermittent variable traction could then be added. The sequence does not matter greatly but assessment should be made carefully so that the most effective of the groups of techniques can be determined. In subsequent treatments the most effective of the groups of techniques should be used last so that advantage can be taken of the gain made by the other techniques.

Discogenic pain

This aspect of pathology is raised for one purpose only. If it is possible to know certainly that a patient's pain has its source in the disc and that there is no indication of herniation, and if rotation is the technique chosen to be used, it must be performed in a particular way. Rotation can be performed in two basic ways. In the lumbar spine either the pelvis or femur may be used as the medium through which the intervertebral rotation is produced or the rotation may be produced by pulling on one spinous process while pushing on the adjacent spinous process. In the cervical spine pressure against the articular pillar may produce the rotation. When the localized pressures are used to produce the rotation the main effect of the movement is centred on the apophyseal joints. If the indirect techniques are used, once the rotation reaches the limit of the range, any further pressure to increase the rotation applies a strong torsion strain on the disc pivoting about fixed apophyseal joints. Therefore, when wishing to centre the main effect of rotary techniques on the disc the general indirect techniques should be used.

Spondylolysis and spondylolysthesis

Asymptomatic conditions are common, but examination may show clearly that either of these conditions may be causing a patient pain. When this is the case, mobilization may be used as treatment to relieve the pain. The extent to which such treatment can effect improvement is limited by the pathology, as also is the strength with which the techniques may be performed. However the two techniques most likely to produce improvement are rotation and traction but neither can be performed strongly at any stage.

Tension signs

This title refers to those signs found on examination which indicate a loss of pain-free movement of the pain-sensitive structures in the vertebral canal or intervertebral foramen. The obvious signs are straight leg raising, prone knee flexion and supine neck flexion.

These signs clearly indicate signs of tension in the canal or foramen. However, tension signs may show in other ways. For example, on standing, a patient may have a protective scoliosis and he may list, say, towards the right. His lateral flexion to the left would obviously be restricted. The protective scoliosis may be an example of a tension sign or it may be a mechanical block to intervertebral movement. In either case the movement of lateral flexion to the left will be restricted. In other words it is sometimes impossible to know whether certain restrictions of joint movement are joint signs or tension signs. Moreover, if techniques which mobilize the joints produce improvement in some movements and not in others then it may be that the movements not improved are tension signs requiring special techniques.

Tension techniques are ones which effect movement of structures in the vertebral canal and foramen, for example, supine neck flexion (page 108), straight leg raising (page 159) or prone knee flexion. It is sometimes useful to perform lumbar rotation with the leg hanging or held in a position of straight leg raising (page 149).

DEPTH OF MOBILIZATIONS

At first it is difficult to know how firmly mobilizations should be done. Any technique used for the first time should be performed gently, so that the movement produced at the intervertebral joint seems too small to cause any change in the patient's symptoms or signs. Gentle technique is particularly important in the presence of severe pain, neurological changes or muscle spasm. The factors which guide the depth at which a technique is performed are pain, muscle spasm and any other type of physical resistance which may limit the movement. The severity and relative position of these factors in the range of movement are the important guides.

Pain

Pain on movement is perhaps the most important guide to how deeply a technique should be performed and pain which is localized to the vicinity of the joint must be considered separately from referred pain. When the pain is localized to the joint the mobilization should be done in the range which is pain free but the movement should be carried up to the point where pain begins. When pain is felt at the beginning of the range the mobilization must be performed with very small rhythmical movements (Grade I, *see* page 85). As this technique increases the range of pain-free movement the mobilization can be performed further into the range (Grade II). A stage may be reached when it is necessary to carry the movement into the pain to reach the resistance. This is necessary when progress with this technique has slowed down and changes of technique have not effected progress.

Greater care is necessary when a mobilizing technique produces pain which is referred into a distal segment. To begin with the movement must be performed in the painless part of the range and a very careful assessment should be made of its effect immediately following the technique and 24 hours later. Provided the symptoms or signs have not been made worse the technique can be repeated. It may even be necessary to increase the movement minimally to the point where discomfort in the referred area can be felt. Assessment must be meticulously repeated. While performing a mobilization which does cause distal discomfort, the physiotherapist must continue the technique at a fixed amplitude and position in the range whilst assessing any change in discomfort. If referred symptoms increase without any increase in technique the amplitude and position in the range of the mobilization must be reduced. Assessment over 24 hours, or on the day following a further gentle mobilization in the same range, will clearly show whether the technique should be continued or not. Frequently it is necessary to provoke discomfort very gently to produce an improvement in movements and subsequent lessening of symptoms.

When pain is found to begin in the last quarter of the range of the mobilization, it is likely that the technique can be taken through pain, whether it is a local pain or a referred pain, up to the limit of the range or up to any physical resistance which may be restricting movement. When a resistance can be felt the choice will be between a large and a small amplitude movement (Grade III and IV, *see* page 85). The small amplitude stronger movements tend to produce more local soreness, even though this grade of movement may be necessary, but the larger amplitude movements will lessen soreness though they may not increase the range as quickly.

When a patient has pain in an arc of movement or if it is a catching pain, the mobilization chosen should be performed in a large amplitude (Grade II or III).

Severe pain must be handled gently and movements must be small, usually Grade I. When there is very little pain but there is restriction of movement, Grade IV movements can be used and in fact are frequently the only movements which will help. Gentler Grade III movements will relieve any local soreness produced by the Grade IV movements.

Spasm

There are many varieties of muscle spasm but the one referred to here comes into effect in response to pain. When a mobilization produces a quick muscle contraction, the technique must be performed more slowly and at a depth which avoids the spasm. If pain is used as the guide to the depth for performing the technique, spasm will be avoided because pain starts earlier in the range than the spasm. As the signs improve, the depth at which the mobilization is performed may need to be increased to a point in the range which fails to provoke spasm. Because mobilization can effect prompt improvement an occasional oscillation should be taken further to elicit spasm to ensure that the technique is being performed deeply enough. Careful technique in this way can be expected to produce quite rapid increases in the range of spasm-free movement. The presence of such spasm in a patient is not a contraindication to mobilization. In fact, the opposite is true, the technique to choose is the one which would cause the protective spasm if done too strongly.

Muscle spasm which limits a range of movement, and is always present at that point in the range no matter how gently or slowly the technique is performed, is spasm of another kind from that described above. Techniques in treatment can be done as described above, up to the point where spasm begins. Naturally all spasm must be respected but this variety, which is so strong that further movement is prevented, must never be forced. The spasm described in the foregoing paragraph, however, can be avoided if the technique is done more slowly or gently. No attempt should ever be made with any technique to force a way through spasm.

DURATION AND FREQUENCY OF TREATMENT

The amount of treatment which can be given on the first day should be considered separately from that of subsequent treatments because it involves a full examination of the patient before any treatment can be given, and this adds to the movements being exerted upon what is presumably a faulty joint. Also the first stretching of a joint appears to cause more reaction than subsequent stretchings. The first day's treatment therefore should be less in regard to the number of mobilizations given. At the end of this first treatment the patient should be given adequate warning of the temporary increase of symptoms which may follow, to allay fears which can arise from an unexpected increase in pain. The number of mobilizations which can be given in subsequent treatments depends entirely on the reaction to previous sessions. If there is no undue reaction and the patient's symptoms and signs are not severe, much more can be done than if the reverse is the case. It should be remembered, however, that there is an optimum which can be achieved at any one treatment period and to continue mobilizing a joint beyond a certain length of time will cause increased soreness and regression. Obviously this optimum will vary with different joint conditions but the amount of treatment is approximately three or four mobilizations of a joint lasting approximately 30 seconds each. With extremely painful joint conditions this should be halved, and when symptoms and signs are minimal it can be increased.

Treatment should be carried out daily, at least initially if not throughout. If the patient asks, 'Should I continue taking my tablets?' or, 'Should I cut down on my activities?' the physiotherapist should say, 'In the initial stages of treatment I want to assess, as exactly as I can, the effect of my treatment. With this thought in mind continue doing whatever you have been doing so that I will have a better chance of telling whether changes which do take place are due to what I am doing and not to what you have changed to doing or not doing as the case may be.' Frequently a stage may be reached in treatment when it is difficult to tell whether it should be continued or stopped. The difficulty of assessment may be because treatment is perpetuating joint soreness, or it may be because a stage has been reached when the condition may continue to improve without treatment. Under either of these circumstances treatment might well be discontinued temporarily and a reassessment made in 7–14 days. Depending on whether the signs have shown further improvement or not, treatment may or may not need to be reinstituted.

There is one final point which occurs quite commonly and should not be forgotten. A patient may be treated over a period of 10–14 days without producing any noticeable change in symptoms or signs. A two week break from treatment is advisable in the hope that over the break, as a result of the treatment, the symptoms go. The patient should therefore be asked to telephone and report any changes so that assessment and advice can be formulated. With this thought in mind, it is a good policy for referring doctors to review patients two weeks after treatment ends. Such timing gives a more accurate assessment of the effect of the treatment.

5 Techniques of Manipulation

The point has already been made that a mobilization, even though it may be done firmly, does not consist of a sudden movement. A sudden movement or thrust constitutes a manipulation. There are two types of manipulative technique, namely those which are the same as the mobilizations already described but performed much more rapidly, and those which localize the manipulation as much as is possible to one intervertebral joint to free its range of movement. Whatever type is used it is always a quick movement of very small amplitude. Strong traction is unnecessary and, in some instances, it is a distinct disadvantage. If it is applied strongly, it lessens the range available for the manipulation. Some manipulators believe it provides a safety factor. This is false, the safety being provided by gradual progression of the strength of the technique coupled with continual assessment.

TYPE 1

During treatment by mobilization, the improvement rate may slow down even though the early mobilizations were methodically increased in depth and produced adequate progress. Under these circumstances it may be necessary to alter the technique to include a sudden movement near the limit of the range. Such an over-pressure is usually only necessary in the mobilizing techniques of postero-anterior unilateral vertebral pressure in the thoracic region, postero-anterior central vertebral pressure in the thoracic and lumbar regions, and rotation in the cervical and lumbar regions.

Postero-anterior central vertebral pressure (thoracic and lumbar regions) and postero-anterior unilateral vertebral pressure (thoracic region)

When increasing the strength of the thoracic mobilizations mentioned above, it becomes necessary to use the hands to produce the pressure localizing with the pisiform bone as described on page 137, instead of the thumbs. Conversion of these mobilizations to manipulations necessitates a sudden increase of pressure, given from the position where the joint is stretched to its limit, to produce a sudden movement of very small range. The pressure required to produce this small movement is considerably greater for the lumbar region than for the thoracic region. To increase the effectiveness of the manipulation on the lumbar spine the patient's trunk or legs can be supported in extension, thereby increasing the lumbar lordosis (*Figure 5.1*).

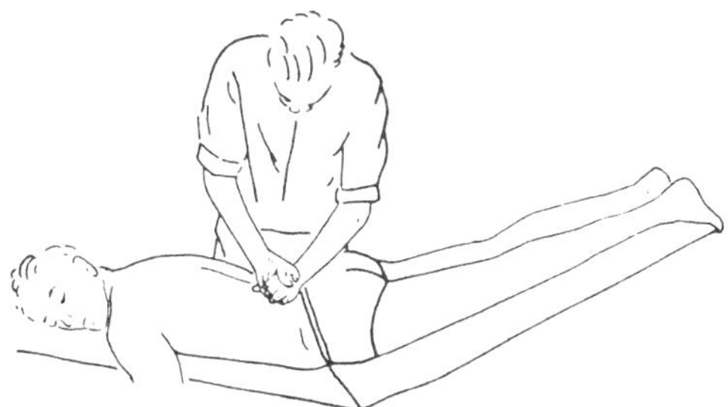

Figure 5.1. – Postero-anterior central vertebral pressure (lumbar)

Cervical rotation (↻)

The symbol indicates the direction of the rotation of the patient's head.

This mobilization can be converted to a manipulation by applying a sudden movement of tiny amplitude to the neck. Manipulation in this instance presupposes that treatment has progressed through stages from gentle mobilization to the stage when manipulation has become necessary.

The position used to manipulate is the same as that described for the mobilization (*see* page 102); the head and neck are rotated as far as possible, and then a quick rotary movement through 3–4 degrees is given. This movement should never be a large movement through a full range from the central position.

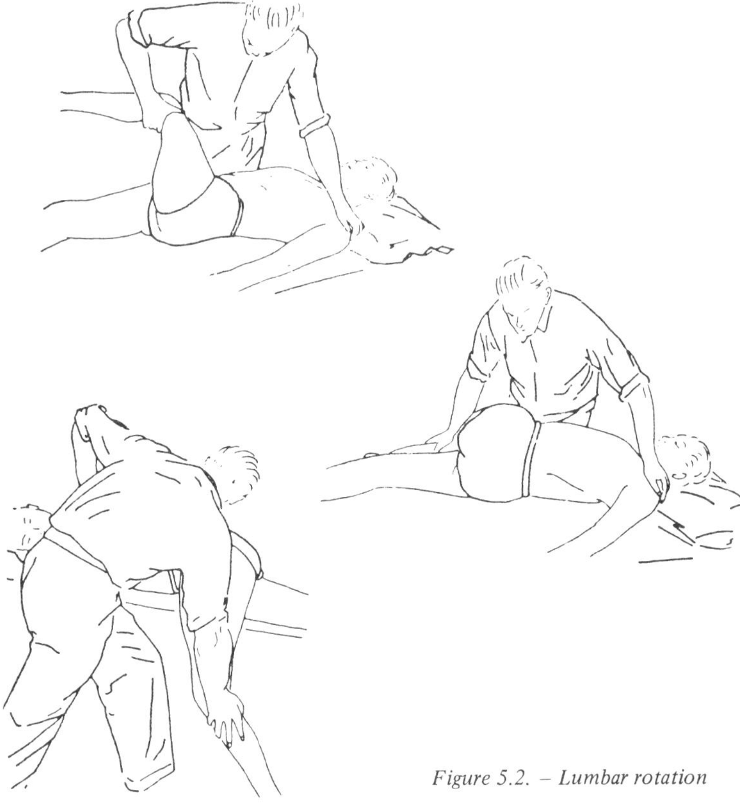

Figure 5.2. – Lumbar rotation

Lumbar rotation (↻)

The symbol indicates the direction of the rotation of the pelvis.

Although the mobilization described on page 144 can be converted to a manipulation by a sudden increase of the operator's effort, the starting position described below is easier to perform.

Starting position

The patient lies on his back with his head supported on a pillow while the physiotherapist stands by the right side of the couch facing the patient. She abducts the patient's right arm out of the way. The physiotherapist cups her left hand over the patient's left shoulder, grasps behind the patient's left knee from the outside with her right hand and flexes the hip and knee to a right angle. Then, by adducting the patient's left hip to pull the knee across the body and downwards towards the floor, the pelvis will be rotated to the right. Careful positioning of the patient at the beginning will prevent squeezing his left leg against the edge of the couch (*Figure 5.2*).

Method

When the position of full rotation has been reached, the physiotherapist changes her right hand to grasp the posterolateral aspect of the upper calf; the heel of the hand lies behind the head of the fibula and the fingers extend down the calf. Rotation is stretched further by increasing the pressure against the patient's shoulder and leg, then a sudden downward and rotary thrust is applied to the leg and strong counter-pressure at the shoulder. The all-important factor is that the direction of movement of the patient's left leg must produce rotation of the pelvis and not adduction of the hip. This rotation can be done with the lumbar spine in flexion or extension by positioning the underneath leg and altering the angle of hip flexion used for the leg which acts as the lever.

TYPE 2

Where an almost painless limitation of movement, which is presumed to be the cause of a patient's symptoms, cannot be sufficiently improved by mobilization or the manipulative techniques described above, the manipulation must be localized to the one joint. This manipulation aims at directly restoring movement to the faulty intervertebral joint.

Occipito-atlantal joint (rotation ↻)

Starting position

The patient lies supine and the physiotherapist stands at the head end towards the patient's left shoulder. By reaching around the right side of the patient's head, the physiotherapist grasps the chin in her right hand. She then places her left hand under the patient's head so that her middle finger is against the posterior margin of the right arch of the atlas with the pad of the tip of the finger pressed firmly against the posterior margin of the transverse process. A firm grip of this vertebra is then achieved by hooking the thumb round the left transverse process of the atlas to reach its anterior surface. Rotation of the patient's head to the right is then carried out until the occipito-atlantal joint is felt to be stretched (approximately 10 degrees short of full rotation), from which position the head is rotated back approximately 10 degrees. In this position the grasp of the atlas is tightened (*Figure 5.3*).

Method

Sudden rotation of the patient's head to the right through 10–15 degrees should be effected by the physiotherapist's right hand while the left hand attempts to prevent any movement of the atlas. There is no danger attached to this procedure since, although a maximum range of occipito-atlantal movement is achieved, the range of head movement is still short of the patient's full range of active rotation.

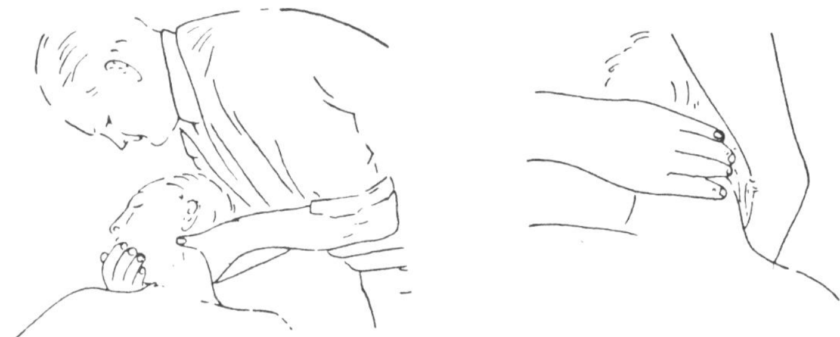

Figure 5.3. – Occipito-atlantal joint. Rotation

Occipito-atlantal joint (unilateral PA thrust ↴)

Starting position

The patient lies supine with his head beyond the end of the couch. If the technique is to be performed on the right side the physiotherapist stands by the right side of the patient's head. She supports his chin and head in her left arm and holds his right occipital area in her right hand. She places her right hand in such a position that the contact point of her right hand is placed behind the right occipito-atlantal joint. *The position she adopts with her right hand is one which is used in many techniques. The contact point is the anterolateral surface at the junction of the proximal and middle thirds of the proximal phalanx of the index finger. If the contact is made too far laterally it becomes very painful. The position of the rest of the hand is also important. The fingers are comfortably flexed at the interphalangeal joints while also supporting the patient's head. The thumb is brought forwards to hold the occiput more laterally. The wrist is ulnar-deviated and held in a position midway between flexion and extension. This description of the thrusting hand position (Figure 5.4) will be referred to when adopted in other techniques.*

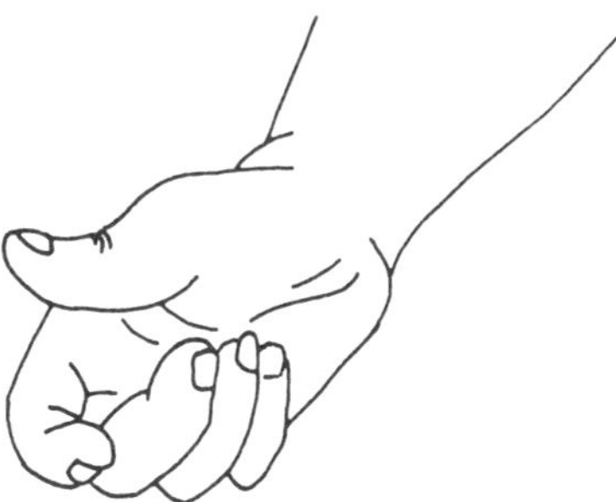

Figure 5.4. – Thrusting hand position

The patient's head is now rotated to the left through approximately 30 degrees for convenience. His head is then firmly stabilized between her left arm and her shoulder. While she palpates behind the occipito-atlantal joint with the proximal phalanx of her index finger she adjusts the position of the occipito-atlantal joint with her left arm as follows. Firstly, she adjusts the flexion/extension position of the patient's head on his upper cervical spine until the occipito-atlantal joint is positioned midway between these two movements. Secondly, she adjusts the lateral flexion position for the joint. This she does by tipping his head sideways in an oscillatory fashion on the upper cervical spine. Once this neutral position has been adopted the head should be held stably so that the position is not lost (*Figure 5.5*).

Method

The physiotherapist hugs the patient's head firmly in her left arm and tightens her contact against the right occipito-atlantal joint. She then directs her forearm pointing towards his right eye. Small preparatory oscillatory movements are produced by pushing through her right hand

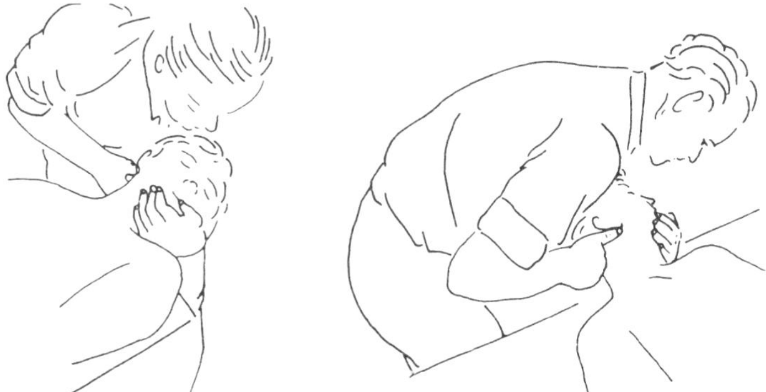

Figure 5.5. – Occipito-atlantal joint. Unilateral postero-anterior thrust

plus very tiny movements of his head with her left arm. These movements allow the head to be tipped by the right handed push but do not allow it to move far.

The manipulative thrust is then executed with a short, sharp stabbing type movement through her right hand countered by a controlling and guiding movement with her left arm.

Occipito-atlantal joint (longitudinal movement ←•→ R)

Starting position

The starting position for this technique performed on the right side varies in only one aspect from that described for the postero-anterior thrust. The thrusting hand makes contact with the occiput immediately adjacent to the right occipito-atlantal joint and the physiotherapist adjusts her right forearm to thrust through the crown of the head. The neutral extension, and lateral flexion, positions are adopted in the same manner as that described above (*Figure 5.6*).

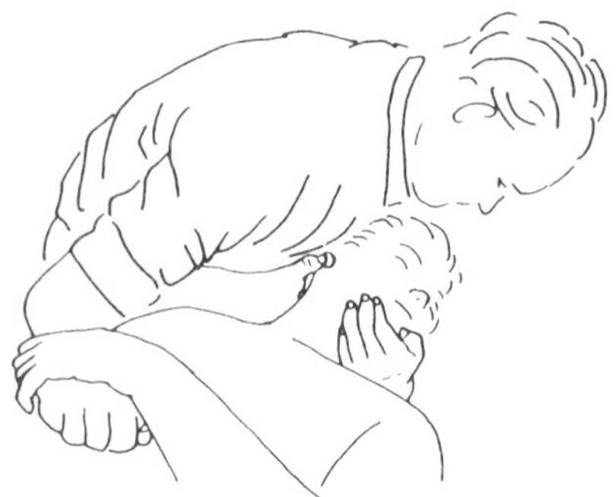

Figure 5.6. – Occipito-atlantal joint. Longitudinal movement

Method

The physiotherapist hugs the patient's head to hold it firmly and by pressure, directed through the crown of his head with her thrusting hand, she takes up the slack of longitudinal movement in his neck. The manipulative thrust is one of very small amplitude performed at maximum speed and without force.

Atlanto-axial joint (rotation ↻)

Starting position

The technique will be described for rotation to the left. The patient lies supine with his head well clear of the end of the couch. The physiotherapist holds his chin and head in her left arm and rotates his head through 40 degrees. With this degree of rotation there has been no movement of the second cervical vertebra. She palpates for the tip of the spinous process of C2 with her index finger and then slides her index finger beyond the spinous process keeping firm contact between the spinous process and the index finger's lateral surface. This firm contact must be maintained with the skin and the spinous process throughout so that the tissue can be held tightly. This sliding movement is continued, her arm at right angles to the skin of his neck, until the spinous process of C2 is cradled in the first interosseous space. She is then in a position to hold C2 firmly cradled between the metacarpo-phalangeal joint of her index finger behind the left articular pillar of C2 and her thumb which holds the transverse process of C2 on the right hand side almost from in front. Her forearm is by this time well underneath the patient with the elbow pointing towards the floor. This hand position is vital if the technique is to be a success. The physiotherapist's hand remains at right angles to the skin throughout the technique and the fingers of her right hand pass the back of the left hand during the manipulation. The physiotherapist needs to stand behind the patient's head to be in the most efficient position (*Figure 5.7*).

Method

Before carrying out the manipulation the position is checked by two movements. Firstly, the physiotherapist rotates his head back and forth through a small amplitude to ensure that all slack has been taken up between the two hands. This is done by rotating the patient's head with the left arm to see if the right hand is forced to follow. This is followed immediately by a de-rotation movement with her right hand to see if the left hand is forced to return to its original position because in fact the head is being turned back by the right hand's contact against C2. The second exploratory movement is a counterclockwise movement

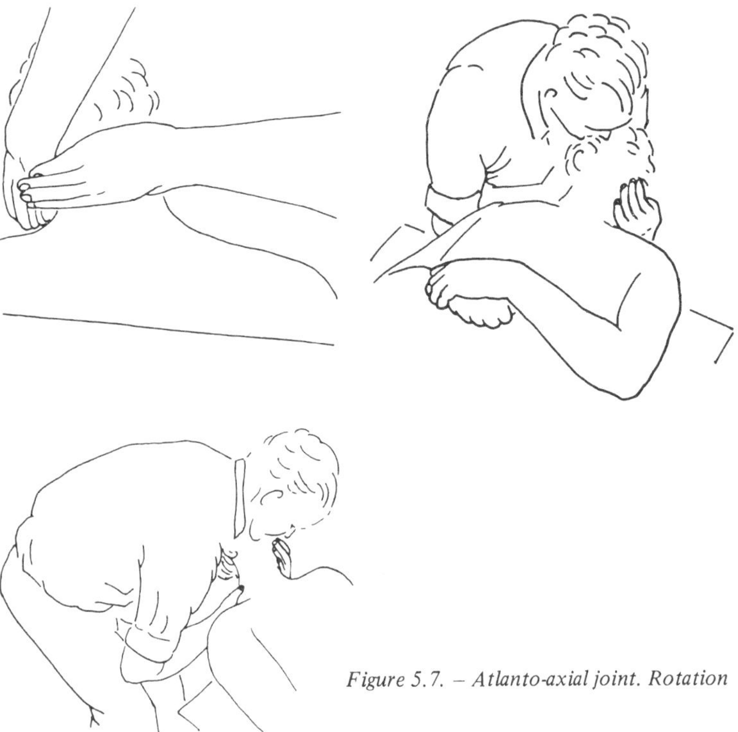

Figure 5.7. – Atlanto-axial joint. Rotation

with both hands. These are done as small jabbing movements with both arms and are the forerunner of the manipulative thrusts. These exploratory movements will give a good guide to the strength of the movement required to manipulate the joint. The manipulation consists of a tiny rotary movement with the left hand and a small amplitude sharp thrust with the right hand. The movement of the right hand consists of a unilateral postero-anterior thrust on the left side of C2 while her whole contact with that vertebra with her right hand effects a rotary movement of C2.

Intervertebral joints C2–C7 (rotation ↻)

Starting position

The technique is described for rotation left of the C3/4 joint.

The patient lies supine with his head beyond the end of the couch. The physiotherapist stands by the right side of his head, supporting his head in the crook of her left arm and holding his chin in her hand. She flexes his neck to place the C3/4 joint midway between flexion and extension. With the tip of her right index finger the physiotherapist finds the C3/4 interspinous space and then moves her hand laterally to bring the anterolateral surface of the proximal phalanx of the index finger behind the C3/4 apophyseal joint. She places her fingers on the back of his neck and head to provide support and her thumb lightly on his jaw. While holding this proximal phalanx stationary against the articular pillar of C3/4, she oscillates the head in a rotary movement, starting from the straight head position and gradually turning the head further until rotation is felt by the phalanx at the C3/4 joint. She then tightens her right hand grip with the fingers and thumb so that if the head is turned further and the right hand follows the turn, C3 also follows the turn. This unifying of the spine above C3 with the head is vital (*Figure 5.8*).

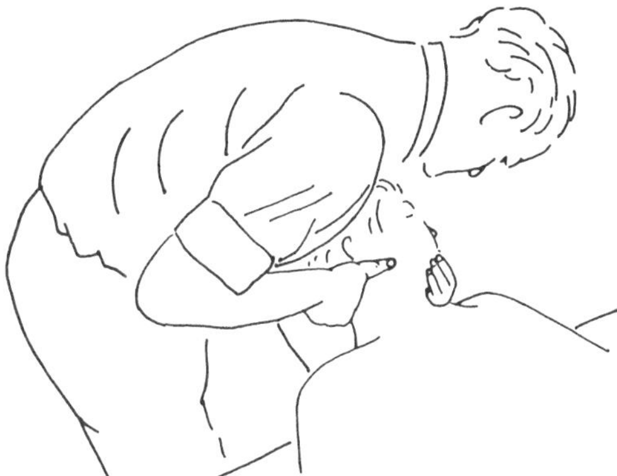

Figure 5.8. – Intervertebral joints. C2–C7 (rotation)

Method

The manipulation consists of a small amplitude sharp rotation of the unit, head to C3, with a thrust being exerted behind the articular pillar of C3.

Intervertebral joints C2–C7 (lateral flexion)

Starting position

The patient lies supine with his head beyond the end of the couch and the physiotherapist, standing at the head of the couch, grasps the patient's chin in her left hand while her left forearm lies against the left side of the patient's head. With the palm of the right hand at right angles to the neck and the fingers supporting under the head and neck, the patient's head is laterally flexed to the right through a few degrees while the physiotherapist moves her body and feet until she is standing by the patient's right shoulder facing his head.

To localize the level of the manipulation, the physiotherapist uses the tip of the right index finger to palpate for the desired interspinous space, and when the level has been ascertained the anterolateral surface of the base of the proximal phalanx of the right index finger is placed against the articular pillar on the right at that level. The physiotherapist

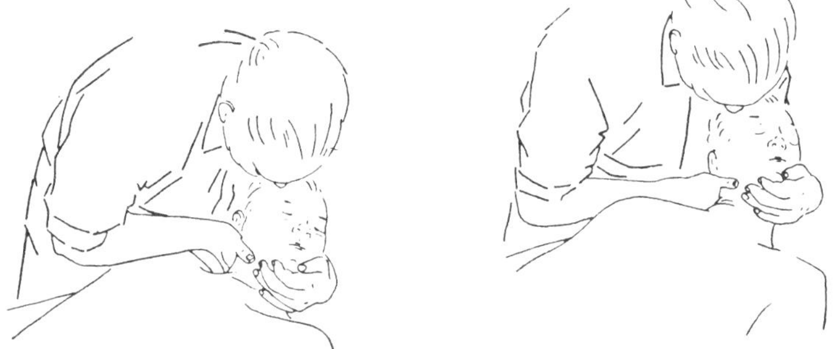

Figure 5.9. – Intervertebral joints. C2–C7 (lateral flexion)

then combines a push against the articular pillar with the right hand (thus displacing the neck to the left), with a lateral flexion of the patient's head to the right by the left hand and forearm. In this way a position can be reached where the intervertebral joint opposite the base of the physiotherapist's right index finger can be felt to be fully stretched. To complete the tension at this joint the head must be passively rotated to the left by the physiotherapist's left hand until this stretch can also be felt under the finger. The right wrist is held flexed to the mid-position to keep the heel of the hand away from the patient's right ear, thereby keeping the more lateral aspect of the proximal phalanx to bear against the articular pillar. At the same time the physiotherapist directs her forearm in line with the plane of the apophyseal joint under the base of the index finger. To perform this manipulation with minimum effort the physiotherapist should crouch over the patient's head to hug it and hold both arms firmly against her sides (*Figure 5.9*).

Method

When the physiotherapist is sure that she has the joint fully stretched she gives a sudden thrust through the base of the right index finger along the line of the right forearm, at the same time applying an equal counter-pressure with her left arm at the head and neck. The aim is to produce a sudden stretch at the apophyseal joint opposite the fulcrum. This stretch may result in a crack-like sound.

Intervertebral joints C2–C7 (transverse thrust ←•−)

Starting position

This technique will be described to open the joints on the left hand side. The patient lies supine with his head extended beyond the head of the couch and his right shoulder near the right hand edge of the couch. The physiotherapist supports his head in her left arm holding his chin with her hand and stands by the right side of his head. With her right index finger she finds the interspinous space between the two vertebrae which she plans to manipulate. She then places the anterolateral border of her thrusting proximal index finger phalanx against the articular pillar at that level on the right hand side. She then rotates his head to the left in a series of small amplitude oscillations increasing the range until the movement can be felt to take place at the joint to be manipulated. This rotation will vary between 45 and 55 degrees depending on the level being manipulated; the higher the level the smaller the rotation. The right palm is at all times kept at right angles to the skin surface. The physiotherapist, with firm contact held against the articular pillar, tilts his head back towards his right shoulder with her left arm. This movement is a combination of slight extension with lateral flexion. The movement is continued until the joint can be felt to be tight under the physiotherapist's right hand. At the same time that she tilts back the patient's head and neck, the physiotherapist displaces the mid-cervical area away from her towards his left shoulder (*Figure 5.10*).

Method

Small oscillatory thrusting movements are employed by the physiotherapist through her right hand to ensure that the right degree of slack has been taken up. These small amplitude thrusting movements are countered by tiny tipping movements of the patient's head, held in her left arm. A small amplitude manipulative thrust with the body transmitted through the right hand effects the technique.

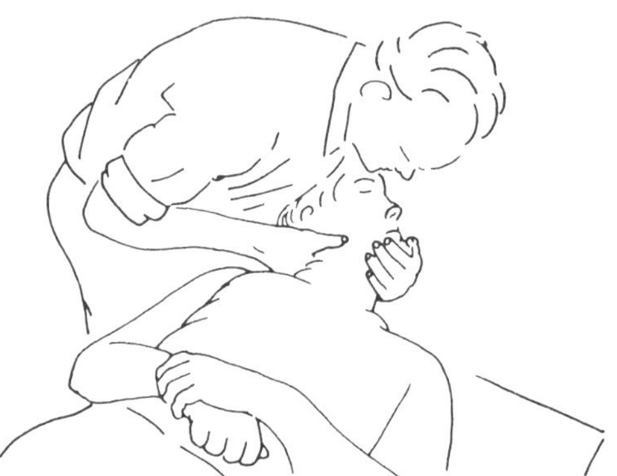

Figure 5.10. – Intervertebral joints. C2–C7 (transverse thrust)

Intervertebral joints C7–T3 ( )

Starting position

The patient sits well back on a medium height couch while the physiotherapist stands behind. To provide the patient with comfortable support the physiotherapist places her left foot on the couch next to the patient's left buttock, rests the patient's left arm over her left thigh, and asks the patient to relax back against her. Localization of the manipulation is achieved by firmly placing the tip of the right thumb against the right side of the spinous process of the lower vertebra of the intervertebral joint. Pressure is applied horizontally in the frontal plane by this thumb while the fingers spread forward over the patient's right clavicular area. These fingers also hold to stabilize the vertebra. The next step is to flex laterally the patient's head to the right until the tension can be felt at the thumb. While maintaining the lateral flexion tension the middle position between flexion and extension is found by rocking the neck back and forth on the trunk. After determining this position, rotation (face upwards) is added in small oscillatory movements until the limit of the rotary range is found. She then positions both forearms to work opposite each other (*Figure 5.11*).

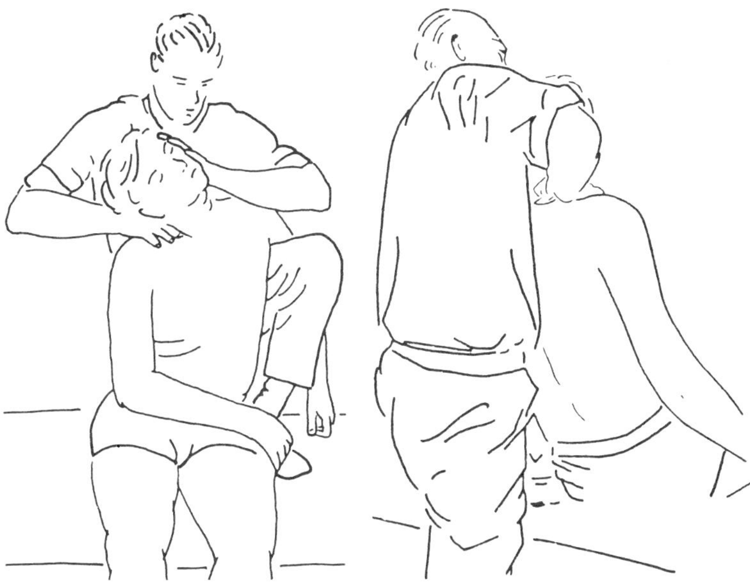

Figure 5.11. – Intervertebral joints. C7–T3

Method

The manipulation consists of a sudden short range thrust through the right thumb transversely across the body, while a counter-thrust is given by the operator's left hand against the left side of the patient's head.

Intervertebral joints T3–T10 (↕)

Starting position

The patient lies supine without a pillow and links his hands behind his neck while the physiotherapist stands by his right side. By grasping the patient's left shoulder in her right hand and both elbows in her left hand, the physiotherapist flexes the patient's head, neck and trunk and twists them towards herself. While the physiotherapist holds the patient in this position, she releases her hold on the shoulder and leans over the patient to palpate for the spinous process of the lower vertebra forming the intervertebral joint being manipulated. Still holding the patient in this position, the physiotherapist makes a fist with the right hand by flexing the middle, ring and little fingers into the palm but leaving the thumb and index finger extended. A small

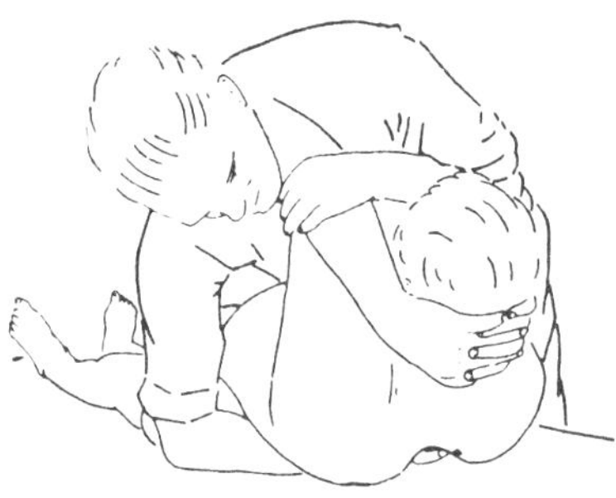

Figure 5.12. – Intervertebral joints. T3–T10

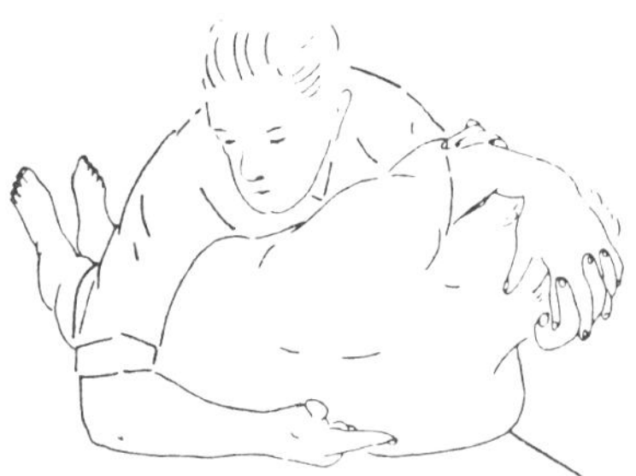

pad of material grasped in the fingers will give added support. This fist is then applied to the patient's spine (the thumb points towards the head) so that the lower spinous process is grasped between the terminal phalanx of the middle finger and the palmar surface of the head of the opposed first metacarpal. The patient is then lowered back until the physiotherapist's right hand is wedged between the patient and the couch. The weight of the patient's trunk is taken on the flat of the dorsum of the hand (not on the knuckles) and the forearm should project laterally to avoid interference with movement of the patient's trunk. If the surface of the couch is too hard, it will be difficult for the physiotherapist to maintain her grip of the spinous process. To achieve firm control of the patient's trunk, his elbows should be held firmly and pressed against the physiotherapist's sternum. However, when a patient has excessively mobile joints it may be necessary for him to grasp his shoulders with opposite hands while keeping the elbows in close apposition rather than clasping the hands behind the neck. The patient's upper trunk is then gently moved back and forth from flexion to extension in decreasing ranges until the stage is reached where the only movement taking place is felt by the underneath hand to be at the intervertebral joint to be manipulated (*Figure 5.12*).

Method

Pressure is increased through the patient's elbows causing stretch at the intervertebral joint, and the manipulation is then carried out by a downward thrust through his elbows in the direction of his upper arms. This thrust is transmitted to the patient's trunk above the underneath hand. The thrust may be given as the patient fully exhales.

Intervertebral joints T3–T10 (longitudinal movement ↔)

Starting position

The patient sits well back on the couch and grasps his hands behind his neck allowing his elbows to drop forwards. The physiotherapist stands behind the patient and threads her arms in front of his axilli to grasp over the dorsum of his wrists. When grasping his wrists she encourages his elbows to drop forwards while at the same time holding his ribs firmly from each side with her forearms. She then turns her trunk slightly to one side to place her lower ribs against his spine at the level requiring manipulation. While feeling for movement with her rib cage she flexes and extends his thoracic spine above the level to be manipulated until the neutral position between flexion and extension is found for the joint to be treated (*Figure 5.13*).

Method

The physiotherapist lifts his trunk in the direction of the long axis of the joint being treated and makes a final adjustment of the flexion/ extension position to ensure that the mid-position has been retained. The manipulation then consists of a short amplitude sharp lift.

Some degree of extension may be added into this technique. This extra movement is achieved by a very small movement with her ribs against the spine performed at the same time as the lift is executed through the arms.

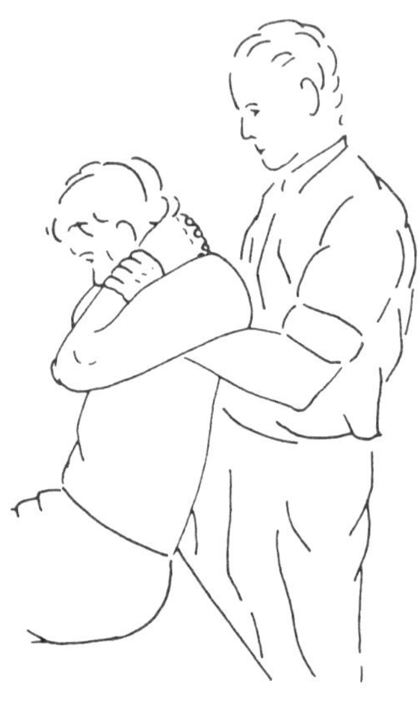

Figure 5.13. – Intervertebral joints. T3–T10 (longitudinal movement)

Intervertebral joints T3–T10 (rotation ↻)

Starting position

If rotation to the left is to be performed the patient sits on the edge of the couch near his right hand end while the physiotherapist stands behind his right side. The patient hugs his chest with his arms and turns his trunk to the left. For the mid-thoracic area the physiotherapist reaches with her left arm around his arms to grasp his right shoulder while placing the heel of her right hand along the line of the right rib above the joint to be manipulated. She cradles his left shoulder in her left axilla (*Figure 5.14a*). For the lower thoracic levels she grasps around his chest under his arms to reach his scapula. This time she places the ulnar border of her right hand along the line of the ribs (*Figure 5.14b*). With both techniques she then takes the movement to the limit of the range taking up all slack.

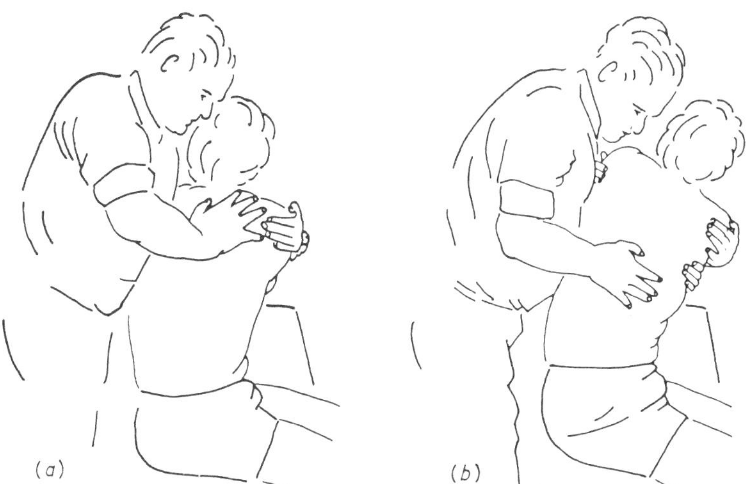

Figure 5.14. – Intervertebral joints. T3–T10 (rotation): (a) mid-thoracic area; (b) lower thoracic area

Method

The manipulation consists of a synchronous movement of the physiotherapist's trunk and an extra pressure through her right hand. With her trunk she carries out an oscillatory rotation back and forth at the limit of the rotary range. At the same time she maintains constant pressure with either the heel of her right hand or its ulnar border exerting an extra rotary push at the limit of the rotation. The manipulation consists of an over-pressure at the limit of the range being done in a very small amplitude and very sharply.

Intervertebral joints T10–S1 (rotation ↻)

Starting position

The patient is asked to lie on his right side while the physiotherapist stands at the side of the couch facing the front of the patient. From this position it is advisable to tell the patient to relax, explaining that he will be put into the required position. The first step is to flex the patient's left hip and knee until the dorsum of the foot can lie behind his right knee. Then the straight right leg is put into slight hip flexion sufficient to place the particular intervertebral joint midway between flexion and extension. The patient's left arm is extended at the shoulder and flexed at the elbow to allow the forearm to rest on his side. To achieve the next step involving rotation at the intervertebral joint, the patient's right arm is pulled towards the ceiling to twist his thorax until his left knee lifts from the table. Care must be exercised to see that the joint is still in the mid flexion–extension position. The arm is then allowed to relax in an abducted and laterally rotated position out of the way. The physiotherapist leans over the patient, threads her left forearm through the triangle made by the patient's left arm and trunk, and places her left upper forearm against the patient's left shoulder. At the same time she places her right upper forearm behind the patient's left hip. This position leaves both hands free to add to the rotation at the intervertebral joint. The left thumb presses downwards against the left side of the spinous process of the upper vertebra, and the right middle finger (usually the strongest) pulls upwards against the right side of the spinous process of the lower vertebra (*Figure 5.15*).

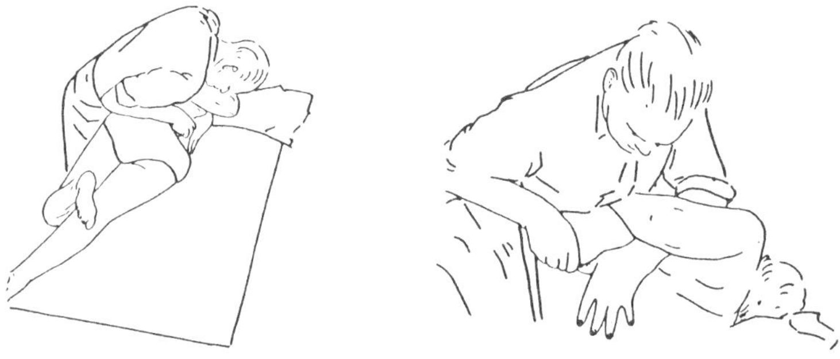

Figure 5.15. – Intervertebral joints. T10–S1 (rotation)

Method

Maximum rotary stretch is applied by rocking the patient back and forth with the forearms, altering the position of the right forearm on the buttock if the lumbar spine position needs to be adjusted. Gradually as more and more stretch is achieved, the pressure against the spinous process is increased until the joint is tight. The manipulation then consists of increasing the push through both forearms and sharply increasing the pressure against the adjacent spinous process.

MANIPULATION UNDER ANAESTHESIA (MUA)

A very constructive review of the third edition of *Vertebral Manipulation* was published. In it, and in subsequent correspondence with the author, the reviewer advocated acknowledgement in the text of the existence of 'manipulation under anaesthesia' (MUA) as it is used widely by doctors and by some physiotherapists, and with this view the author heartily concurs.

Mr R. A. Bremner (1958) provides evidence of the effectiveness of MUA in the treatment of lumbosacral strain. Probably the same applies to any local pain and stiffness of spinal origin; it certainly does in the cervical spine. Dr J. Cyriax (1975) sets out clearly the indications and contraindications for MUA.

A patient's condition may be improved initially by mobilization and manipulation but a stage may be reached where the rate of progress slows down; MUA may then be indicated. The build of the patient, or a degree of voluntary muscle contraction which prevents manipulation while a patient is conscious may well make MUA the treatment of choice. The reviewer so rightly asserts that in 'determining management of difficult and unresponsive cases it proves very profitable for the doctor and physiotherapist to confer'.

If a patient can relax completely, the end-feel of the range of movement being manipulated is the same whether he be manipulated consciously or under anaesthesia.

Care must be taken not to manipulate under anaesthesia too vigorously. Rather than trying to achieve a full range of movement in one manipulation it is often better to manipulate more gently on two or more occasions. In a second article Mr Bremner (Bremner and Simpson, 1959) relates 'follow-up' physiotherapy after an MUA has been carried out.

The degree of success of an MUA will be known within two or three days. If the patient gains complete relief of his symptoms, follow-up treatment is unnecessary. However, if the symptoms do not improve sufficiently, passive mobilization will be required. When radiological evidence of joint changes (which account for some of the stiffness) is present, the patient should be taught to perform daily mobilizing exercises. When there is instability, stabilizing exercises should be performed daily.

It is important to bear in mind that follow-up treatment should only be given selectively and not routinely for all patients.

Where manipulation of the conscious patient has failed, MUA may be successful. The converse is also true. Sometimes, as evidenced by the reviewer, patients may require a balance of both.

Bremner, R. A. (1958). 'Manipulation in the management of chronic low backache due to lumbosacral strain.' *Lancet* **1**, 20

Cyriax, J. (1975). *Textbook of Orthopaedic Medicine.* Vol. II (6th Edition). London; Baillière Tindall

Bremner, R. A. and Simpson, M. (1959). 'Management of lumbosacral strain.' *Lancet* **2**, 949

6 Application of Manipulation

The question now arises as to when mobilization is used and when manipulation is used. Manipulation is rarely chosen at the beginning of treatment and certainly never in the presence of a very painful joint or a joint whose movement is protected by muscle spasm. One of the cardinal rules of treatment of passive movement is that a movement must never be forcibly thrust through protective spasm. Manipulations are usually progressions from mobilizations which have increased in strength and shown clearly that further increase is necessary. Grades of mobilizations have been discussed (*see* page 85) and a manipulation is similar to a Grade IV mobilization in amplitude and position in the range; it differs only in speed. A Grade IV mobilization is an oscillatory movement which the patient can prevent if he chooses to do so, whereas the movement of the manipulation is so quick it cannot be prevented by the patient. Because there is this link between the two procedures it is perhaps an advantage to consider manipulation as a Grade V movement.

One of the occasions when manipulation might be used early in treatment is when a stiff and almost painless joint is responsible for minor symptoms. However, whether manipulation is used or not will depend partly on whether it is believed that an attempt must be made to forcibly increase the range of movement of the joint. In most circumstances the symptoms can be relieved by mobilization without having to resort to manipulation.

It is not always possible, nor is it necessarily advisable, to aim for restoration of a full range of movement. For example, in the presence of degenerative or arthritic changes, or when adaptive shortening has taken place in response to postural deformities, it will be impossible to regain the full range of movement which would exist in an unaffected spine. Also a limitation of movement may be present to protect an otherwise unstable intervertebral joint. It is not always in the best interests of the patient to continue manipulative treatment in an effort to produce a full range of movement beyond the stage where symptoms have been relieved. In practice approximately 85 per cent of patients successfully treated will respond to mobilization, leaving 15 per cent requiring the stronger techniques.

If mobilization is being used successfully in treatment the patient should show marked improvement within four or five days. However if there has been progress yet the progress is not as great as expected then it is probable that manipulation should form part of the treatment. Under these circumstances the treatment would commence with mobilization which would be followed by manipulation and then completed by more mobilization. Similarly, manipulation might be used as a forerunner prior to the administration of traction. Under these circumstances it is intended that the increased movement obtained by the manipulation would assist the effectiveness of the traction. So it can be seen that manipulation may be used separately or in conjunction with mobilization.

Manipulation differs from mobilization in its effect on a joint. If it is done vigorously it must have some traumatic effect. The tissue reaction from the trauma influences the treatment plan, which normally aims at producing the quickest result possible with the minimum discomfort to the patient. As a joint should not be manipulated until all soreness from previous manipulations has gone, it may not be possible to manipulate until 2–3 days after the first manipulation. This soreness tends to increase, and can result in a break of 4–5 days before the third manipulation and 5–7 days before a fourth manipulation can be given. However, it should not take more than 4–5 manipulations to gain the maximum possible improvement in the range of movement of a joint. By allowing the soreness to subside, progress may be more accurately assessed. Although symptoms should be the ultimate guide to treatment, intervertebral movement should be checked each time for improvement.

Crack-like sounds coming from joints of the spine may be heard during manipulation, but they are only of significance in treatment when the joint is being manipulated to restore its movement. When there is almost no movement in an intervertebral joint, early attempts to manipulate it will possibly produce little more than a forcible stretch of the joint. However, when the movement has improved a little, the manipulation is more likely to produce a 'crack', which indicates an increased range of movement. This crack is different from the tearing sound associated with rupturing adhesions.

CONTRAINDICATIONS

The possibility of serious damage resulting from manipulation, particularly cervical manipulation, is often emphasized when this form of treatment is discussed. Although deaths have occurred (Smith and Estridge, 1962) it must be realized that if the number of manipulations carried out daily by lay manipulators is compared with the mortality rate, the danger is extremely small (Brewerton, 1964). Coupled with this fact is the record (Liss, 1965) that similar damage resulting in death can occur with daily activities. With care of application and the continual assessment of the patient's symptoms and signs advocated in this book, serious damage is almost impossible especially if it is realized that patients with serious pathological conditions are excluded from manipulative treatments by the medical practitioner.

There are many considerations influencing contraindications to manipulative therapy. For example, some medical conditions may be considered contraindications because manipulation is potentially harmful, while other conditions may be considered contraindications in the sense that the conditions are unsuited or unlikely to be affected by the treatment. On these grounds the doctor will exclude such conditions as Paget's disease, rheumatoid arthritis, osteomyelitis, ankylosing spondylitis, malignancy, cord and cauda equina syndromes and vertebral artery involvement.

Another consideration is that some conditions may be contraindications to the more forceful manipulations yet they may not be contraindications to the mobilizations described in this book. In fact, one of the important facets of mobilization is that by its gentleness with careful assessment most of the possible dangers are eliminated and the treatment can be applied more widely. Neurological and radiological changes cover two groups of conditions which may be contraindications to any but the gentle techniques.

Neurological changes

Pain associated with disturbances of reflex activity, muscle power or sensation due to nerve-root compression are frequently cited as

Brewerton, D. A. (1964). 'Conservative treatment of the painful neck.' *Proc. R. Soc. Med.* **57**, 163

Liss, L. (1965). 'Fatal cervical cord injury in a swimmer.' *Neurol. Minneap.* **15**, 675

Smith, R. A. and Estridge, M. N. (1962). 'Neurological complications of head and neck manipulation.' *J. Am. med. Ass.* **182**, 528 contraindications to manipulation. Patients having these signs certainly should not be manipulated vigorously at the commencement of treatment. However, provided the proper care is taken and the nature of the complaint is appreciated, the gentler mobilizing techniques can be used from the beginning. It may even prove necessary, as treatment progresses, to strengthen the techniques and eventually manipulation may be indicated.

Herniated disc material at one intervertebral level in the lumbar spine can cause compressive signs in two nerve roots but in the cervical spine only one nerve root can be involved. Therefore, a patient with arm pain and neurological signs attributed to two nerve roots has a pathology which is a contraindication to manipulative therapy. Disturbances of bladder or bowel function or perineal anaesthesia are similar signs of contraindications.

Cord signs are also a contraindication to any form of forceful manipulation. Very gentle mobilizing may be quite safe but it is unlikely to be of any value. Cervical traction is quite safe also, and although it is occasionally ordered it is difficult to see how it can effect a favourable change in the cord signs. Gentle techniques may be used to treat joint pain when this exists with cord signs but if gentle techniques fail, forceful measures must not be employed.

Radiological changes

Osteoporosis and rheumatoid arthritis are two conditions which should preclude forceful manipulation yet both conditions can be present in a patient who has pain which can be relieved by mobilization. Both conditions present situations where the safety measures detailed in this book are not enough to prevent fracture or serious damage if forceful procedures are used. There are no signs to warn the physiotherapist that an osteoporotic bone or diseased ligament is about to give way under the strain until it actually does. Therefore, forcible manipulation must never be used. However, it is wrong to preclude gentle mobilization.

Two techniques require particular care. Cervical rotation in the presence of marked rheumatoid arthritic changes can rupture the transverse and alar ligaments and cause atlanto-axial dislocation. Rib pressures used to manipulate the costovertebral joints may fracture an osteoporotic rib.

Differential diagnosis can be difficult and in the early stages of a disease a patient may have symptoms and signs which are believed to be skeletal in origin. This patient may be referred for manipulative therapy. However, if the signs do not follow the usual patterns or if the patient does not improve during treatment he should be referred back to the doctor. Treatment must not be continued for prolonged periods when only minimal improvement is being gained. Occipital headaches and neck stiffness, even wry neck, can be the first sign of subarachnoid haemorrhage or of a cerebellar tumour. If such a patient is referred for manipulation before a correct diagnosis is possible the physiotherapist should send the patient back to the doctor as soon as it becomes clear that the pain and signs do not improve with mobilization.

Vertigo

Vertigo is another condition which requires close observation when manipulative treatment is requested. Although vertigo can have a cervical origin (Cope and Ryan, 1959) it is usually only when it is secondary to headache that mobilization techniques will help (Ryan and Cope, 1955). It has already been mentioned (page 28) that exploratory movements should be made with cervical techniques before they are used and that a technique which causes any feeling of giddiness must not be used.

Hypermobility

Hypermobility and instability are two words which are frequently used loosely thus causing considerable misunderstanding. When dealing with spinal problems the term 'hypermobility' can be interpreted in two distinctly different ways.

The first is illustrated by the patient who has general laxity of ligaments, allowing excessive ranges of movement of all or most joints of the body. This hypermobility is easily detected. Although patients may have hypermobile joints they do not necessarily have pain from them.

The second kind of hypermobility is particularly evident, and of importance, in spinal problems. Under the circumstances being referred to here, the patient is not generally hypermobile as described above but rather has one (or more) intervertebral joint which is excessively mobile in relation to the neighbouring joints. When such a patient presents for treatment of pain arising from this area the passive intervertebral movement tests described on pages 44 to 64 are used to assess which joints are stiff and which are hypermobile. When it comes to treating such a

Cope, S. and Ryan, G. M. S. (1959). 'Cervical and otolith vertigo.' *J. Lar. Otol.* **73,** 113

Ryan, G. M. S. and Cope, S. (1955). 'Cervical vertigo.' *Lancet* **2,** 1355 patient it is firstly necessary to decide whether the pain is coming from the stiff joint or the hypermobile joint. If the stiff joint requires treatment then reasonable care should be taken to avoid putting excessive strain on the hypermobile joint. However, when the hypermobile joint becomes painful and requires treatment then the considerations are quite different, as will now be explained.

It is a generally held opinion that hypermobility is a contraindication to manipulation. This statement, however, requires clarification. A clinical or radiologically hypermobile joint may become painful in just the same way as a stiff joint or a joint with an average range of movement. There is usually some loss of movement when a hypermobile joint becomes painful. However, its loss of range may be small enough for the joint to still appear hypermobile on examination (*Figure 6.1*).

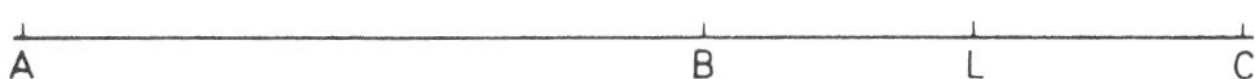

Figure 6.1. The hypermobile joint movement has become stiff (limited to point L in the range) yet it still appears to be hypermobile because the limited range AL is still greater than the normal average range AB: that is the range is still hypermobile whilst still being stiff for that joint. A = beginning of a range of movement; B = end of the normal average range for that movement; C = end of the normal range of the movement when it is hypermobile; L = limit of range of movement when the hypermobile movement AC is painful.

Mobilization is not contraindicated under these circumstances and, in fact, it would be the treatment of first choice. Forcible manipulation of a full range hypermobile joint is another matter. Although there may be occasional circumstances when a further increase of range is advisable, the general rule is that hypermobile joints should not be forcibly manipulated.

The above description identifies two kinds of hypermobility. It needs to be pointed out that under neither circumstances is the joint necessarily 'unstable', the movements still being within the patient's muscular control. Instability refers to the joint which has laxity of supportive ligaments permitting the joint to move abnormally in a manner which makes the joint unstable. The joint does not have to be generally hypermobile for it to be unstable in any one particular direction. Reference to the testing of flexion/extension on page 62 indicates how the lumbar spine can be tested in such a manner as to reveal instability in a particular intervertebral joint.

Any patient having symptoms arising from either a hypermobile joint or an unstable joint can be treated by mobilizing techniques and the effect of such treatment assessed as described in the chapter on assessment. Once the joint has been made symptom free it is essential that the patient be shown exercise to strengthen the muscular support around the hypermobile or unstable joint in an endeavour to add greater support for that joint. If pain is not relieved readily, then stabilizing exercises should be added or substituted early in treatment. If pain is aggravated by mobilizing exercises they should be discontinued and stabilizing exercises substituted. The addition of supports to make the area more stable should also be considered. It should also be pointed out here that hypermobility does not directly relate to the orthopaedic diagnosis of 'instability'.

Clearly, the dangers of manipulation increase as the strength of the technique increases. Safety measures taken with manipulative treatment must be emphasized if the medical profession is to have confidence in its use. Every effort has been made in this book to emphasize the importance placed on gentleness with techniques which are only increased in strength as the continual assessment of signs indicates the need for increase. Even then, no attempt is ever made to forcibly thrust through muscle spasm.

Some people believe that maintaining strong traction while performing cervical and thoracic manipulations is essential for safety but this can give the physiotherapist a false sense of security. If pain and spasm are ignored because traction is being used, dangers will still exist. Care and assessment together with knowledge of pathology provide the safety.

7 Assessment

Over the years various diagnoses have been put forward by manipulators to explain what they are doing with the many spinal pain syndromes they treat successfully. Many of the suggested causes of the patient's problems are not wholly accepted by the medical profession and consequently treatment by passive movement is not used to its fullest advantage. How much better off we and our patients would be if passive movement treatment were used and controlled by proper assessment so that its role in the overall management of musculoskeletal problems could be learned.

During the last few years passive movement has gained greater recognition as an effective mode of treatment. Furthermore, its use as a source of information regarding the behaviour of the joint disorder has been realized by some doctors to be of great value if the joint movements are assessed accurately throughout treatment. Without assessment, treatment is merely an application of techniques lacking guidelines.

'Examination' has been described in Chapter 2. However, for the purpose of this chapter on 'Assessment' it is necessary to elaborate certain points because without accuracy and detail in examination the proper assessments cannot be made.

In the opening chapter Dr Brewerton has given information regarding diagnosis, indications and contraindications for manipulative therapy and it is obvious that diagnosis is vital before manipulative treatment is undertaken. This diagnosis may only disclose that the patient has a musculoskeletal disorder, signifying that mobilization or manipulation could be a treatment of choice. If a physiotherapist is asked to treat by passive movement it is then necessary for her to examine individual movements in detail.

It is universally accepted that medical diagnosis of spinal conditions is extremely difficult. However, a diagnosis indicating that no disease process is involved is usually possible. From the manipulative therapist's point of view the main concern, once the patient is referred, lies in appreciating the mechanical factors related to each patient's symptoms. Many difficulties and complications are associated with this examination.

Firstly, and most importantly, examination of the patient should reveal which particular intervertebral joint is responsible for his symptoms and the effect the disorder has on his spinal movements. It is by restoring these movements to normal that his symptoms will be relieved.

Secondly, abnormality of the movement of the faulty joint should be determined by passive movement tests, testing each intervertebral joint separately, and the examination must divulge:

the presence and behaviour of pain through the available range;
the movements which are restricted or hypermobile;
the extent and behaviour of stiffness during movement or at the limit of range; and
the extent and behaviour of muscle spasm during movement or at the limit of range.

Behaviour of pain is the most important aspect.

The 'behaviour' of the aspects listed above relates to movements of the faulty intervertebral joint. In relation to the pain-sensitive structures in the vertebral canal and the intervertebral foramen (i.e. the dura, the nerve-root sleeves and the nerve roots) their movements must also be examined for range and the behaviour of any resulting pain. Also, in the day-to-day management of the vertebral disorders, it is essential to know the state of conduction of the nerves in those patients whose symptoms indicate involvement of the nerve root.

Many tests can be used to assess the joint movements mentioned above: among the principal ones are the movement tests produced by pressures on the palpable parts of the vertebrae. These have been described in detail in Chapter 2, pages 34 to 42.

The importance of 'Assessment' has been referred to in Chapter 3 but, because of its extreme importance in the management of intervertebral joint disorders, greater detail of the mechanics of assessments made during treatment needs to be given.

An important part in assessment is the ability to recognize patterns of syndromes. Also it is necessary to be aware of the extent of improvement which it is possible to achieve with treatment. The only way to gain this proficiency is by clinical experience based on accurate critical assessment. Armed with this competency, and as a member of a team, the physiotherapist can offer constructive suggestions to the referring doctor regarding the physical side of the management of the patient. Achieving this competency is a slow process not to be rushed. Miss Jennifer Hickling (1967), a physiotherapist of note in this field in England, once said to me:

> Manipulation depends upon clarity of thought and critical thought. People have to be trained at it in a most detailed way. It is easier to achieve this with undergraduate students than with postgraduate people because the latter have got into the habit of thinking in other ways, and it is difficult to undo these habits.
>
> This business of methodical, critical thinking resulting in adding brick to brick is terribly important. Novices must expect to get fewer results more slowly than the experienced person, and they must resist the temptation to try short-cuts.
>
> Novices need to clearly understand that every little bit of clinical knowledge they get out of a patient, provided they are certain about what it is and what the results are, adds up to a brick which is clear-cut; a fact that is not only useful for *that* patient but also for other patients they must meet.
>
> For example, an experienced person who is prepared to take a calculated chance, not in an unscrupulous or unprofessional way but mentally, may go straight for a particular technique and say, do rotation to the left as a V, right at the beginning of treatment, and she may get a quick result. Others who feel their way into it, might finally come to the conclusion that this V is necessary but it might take them six or seven treatments to get there. [*Author* – A grade V movement is a manipulation that is a small-amplitude movement performed at a speed which gives the patient no time to prevent it. It is a general procedure compared with the IV shown in *Figure 3.2.*]
>
> It is much better to have taken six or seven treatments to get there and to have proved all the way along the line that rotation is the right choice, and that the dosage is the right one. To arrive at the result by guesswork does nothing for the novice's future good management of manipulation generally, whereas arriving at the right result more slowly, having proved to her satisfaction the correctness of every step along the way, will pay hands down in the future.
>
> Unless novices are prepared to sort out their knowledge as far as possible into these clear-cut proven facts they will end up with a welter of rather wishy-washy knowledge which is of little use in the different situations which come along.

Hickling, Jennifer (1967). Personal communication

Even with present-day knowledge it is impossible to relate directly the techniques of passive movement treatment to a diagnosis given by the referring doctor, so how does the manipulative physiotherapist plan and carry out treatment? The diagnosis and pathology must of course be understood by the physiotherapist, but it is not this information which will direct the technique to be used, at what strength it should be used and also when to change from one technique to another. The physiotherapist bases the selection and change of treatment techniques on the assessment of changes in the symptoms and signs which take place during treatment. Judgements regarding management and changes are so intricate and need to be so exact that, though manipulation is still empirical, it can be very precisely applied and assessed.

Diagnosis is very important, or where diagnosis is not possible the recognition of the different syndromes is important, and so too are the patient's symptoms and signs. When discussing diagnoses of patients suitable for treatment by manipulation, doctors have differing opinions which lead to disagreements as to the use of manipulation. However, the patient's symptoms and signs consist of clear-cut indisputable facts so there can be no disagreement in this area. Therefore, while not ignoring diagnosis and pathology, passive movement treatment can be used on the basis of the musculoskeletal and neurological symptoms and signs and the changes which take place in these symptoms and signs.

To make manipulative treatment an acceptable part of routine medical care, physiotherapists need to split their thinking into two compartments. One part comes under a general heading of 'history, symptoms and signs' and the other under a general heading of 'anatomy, biomechanics, pathology and diagnosis' (*Figure 7.1*).

LEFT COMPARTMENT	RIGHT COMPARTMENT
History, symptoms and signs	Anatomy, biomechanics, pathology and diagnosis
S & S	D

Figure 7.1. – Mode of planning treatment

On examination, a patient will have certain symptoms and signs which both the doctor and the physiotherapist can determine and agree upon. (These findings fit into the first compartment described above and they clearly indicate the state of the disorder.) Doctors may vary in their opinions regarding the diagnostic title for this particular disorder and may differ as to which structures are causing it. Such discrepancies emphasize the importance of the first compartment which is free of disputable components.

Figure 7.2 is intended to show two examples which further add to the need for the physiotherapist's 'two-compartment' thinking. A particular patient may have a history and set of symptoms and signs (S_1 & S_1) indicating to the referring doctor one of two diagnoses (D_1 or D_2). However, one of the conditions (say D_1) could have different symptoms and signs if the disorder were at a different stage. Diagrammatically these symptoms and signs could be referred to as S_2 & S_2; that is D_1 may have symptoms and signs represented by 'S_1 & S_1' or by 'S_2 & S_2'. Furthermore, one of these groupings of symptoms and signs (let us say S_2 & S_2) may indicate the possibility of another diagnosis, D_3 (*Figure 7.2*), and so the discussion and confusion centred around diagnosis can continue and sometimes a conclusion may not be possible.

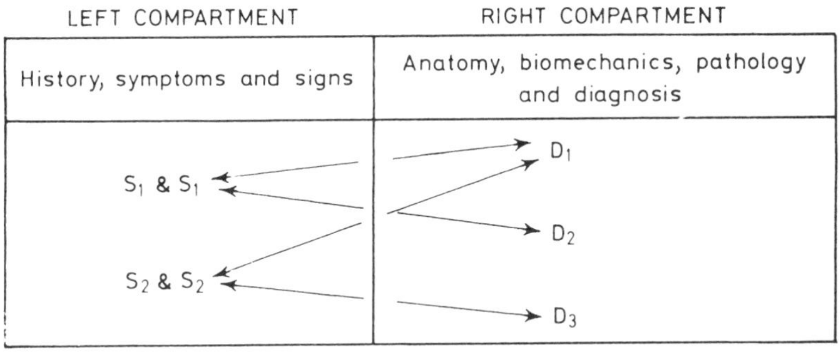

Figure 7.2. – Varying relationships between diagnosis and symptoms and signs

It can be clearly seen that there would be many difficulties if passive movement treatment were to be directed by the diagnosis alone. Even when a clear diagnosis can be given, treatment cannot be directed by the diagnosis because different techniques have to be used at different stages of such disorders.

A patient with nerve-root pain and compression signs arising from a disc prolapse may have any one of a number of combinations of symptoms and signs, particularly in regard to the behaviour of his pain with movement. Some of these combinations of symptoms and signs would indicate very gentle treatment with great emphasis on assessments, while another patient with a combination of symptoms and signs may have a chronic condition requiring vigorous treatment to gain improvement. It is not therefore the diagnosis which indicates the kind of passive movement treatment required; it is the behaviour of the symptoms and signs during movement. This means that the symptoms and signs (the left compartment referred to in *Figure 7.2*) combined with the knowledge of anatomy, biomechanics, pathology and the diagnosis (the right-hand side of the compartments in *Figure 7.2*) guide the selection of the initial treatment. *Subsequent* treatments are directed by the changes which take place in the symptoms and signs. This is where assessment is so very important.

The suggestion of the 'two-compartment' thinking for the physiotherapist does not conflict with Dr Brewerton's opening chapter. It is assumed that the referring doctor has been able to diagnose the patient's disability to a degree where contraindications have been excluded and passive movement treatment is indicated. This present text is rather a refining of the examination by the physiotherapist of the patient's joint movements in such detail as is required for accurate assessment during passive movement treatment.

It can be seen from the above that the examination of the range of movements and the behaviour of resistance, pain and muscle spasm within the available range (i.e. the first compartment of the 'two-compartment' thinking) is fundamental to effective and informative treatment. The treatment is empirical yet it is very precise if based on full and proper assessments throughout treatment.

There is another good reason for this 'two-compartment' thinking. Frequently a manipulator is asked: 'What are you doing when you use "such and such" a technique on Mr X?' To answer by relating treatment to pathology is to tread on dangerous ground. Obviously, any conscientious manipulative physiotherapist will have some idea of what she thinks she might be effecting but to express these 'thoughts' as 'facts' leaves her wide open to justifiable criticism. In answer to the above question the physiotherapist should say that 'no-one really knows what is happening' but she can say that she is endeavouring to restore as much range of movement to the intervertebral joint as is possible and by doing so she expects the patient's symptoms to be relieved. She may be prepared to go further and say, 'If you will allow me to stand in the right-hand compartment of *Figure 7.2*, i.e. on the diagnosis side, there is a possibility that I may be moving "such and such" so that the relationship between structure A and structure B is altered, permitting the movement to return to its normal state and so relieve the pain.'

All of this chapter's preamble is necessary to emphasize and make understood the need for assessment, with all its complications and implications.

To what do we refer when we speak of 'assessment'?

Dictionaries give many shades of meaning but in the context of manipulative treatment 'assessment' means judging the changes in the patient's symptoms and signs effected by passive movement treatment. This means comparing the symptoms and signs at set times during treatment and also by comparing the symptoms and signs with the initial examination findings.

There are four times when Assessments are used:

1. At the initial examination and treatment session
2. During a treatment session and also over a period of treatment
3. At the end of treatment
4. To assist in differential diagnosis

ASSESSMENT AT THE INITIAL EXAMINATION

A patient may have symptoms for which a doctor, following examination, may not be able to give the diagnosis. It is possible for a patient to have what seem to be musculoskeletal symptoms and signs as the first presenting indications of a diagnosis of more sinister origin. It is very important therefore that a physiotherapist should not carry out passive movement treatment on patients who have not been referred by a medical practitioner. If they were to do so they would be undertaking the responsibility for the diagnosis. Such practice is to be condemned. Physiotherapy, particularly passive movement treatment for the spine, should only be carried out under circumstances where there is the closest liaison between the physiotherapist and the referring doctor. This is without doubt in the best interests of the patient.

For the physiotherapist treating musculoskeletal disorders by passive movement, two important assessments are made at the initial examination.

The first is related to diagnosis.

The second is related to movement of both the intervertebral joints and the pain-sensitive structures in the vertebral canal.

The examination of these movements must take into account the behaviour of the patient's related pain, stiffness and muscle spasm.

Assessment related to diagnosis at the initial examination

Even though the referring doctor has examined and diagnosed the patient's condition before referral, at the initial interview with the physiotherapist, the patient is questioned and examination tests are repeated by her. By bringing together all the findings, an assessment is made of the present stage of the disorder.

Even if the doctor has been able to make a diagnosis of (say) irritation or compression of a nerve root, this does not give all the information regarding the cause of the compression.

Macnab (1971) has shown that the nerve root can be irritated or compressed by mechanical means other than disc prolapse. Therefore, thinking must not be limited to the intervertebral disc when seeking causes of nerve-root pain. Also it is wrong to believe that in all patients who have nerve-root symptoms and signs manipulation is contraindicated for many will respond to passive movement treatment even when they have neurological changes.

The behaviour of a patient's nerve-root pain, spreading from the back posteriorly to the heel can vary widely when lumbar movements are examined. For example, one patient may have a full range of forward flexion of the lumbar spine which causes back pain only. Another patient, with identical symptoms, may be able to flex only 20 degrees before his calf pain is reproduced. Both patients may have the same diagnosis but the treatment for each would need to be different.

Diagnosis is a coadjutant factor linked with a patient's presenting symptoms and signs. In fact, an initial diagnosis may need to be changed in retrospect when it is seen how the patient's symptoms and signs alter with passive movement treatment. An example will clarify this.

A woman was referred from an orthopaedic surgeon who requested manipulative treatment for 'disc prolapse causing C7 nerve-root symptoms and compressive signs'. On examination, the three cervical movements of extension, lateral flexion to the left, and rotation to the left, were all markedly restricted and all reproduced tingling in the patient's forearm and hand. She had diminished sensation in the pad of the terminal phalanx of the index finger, marked weakness of triceps, and diminished triceps reflex. She was in considerable pain. Traction was the treatment chosen, and by continual assessment over the first four days noticeable improvement was apparent in pain, cervical movements and neurological changes. She only required 10 treatments, with mobilization and gentle manipulation being added for the last sessions. At the conclusion of treatment there was complete recovery of cervical movements and all neurological changes had returned to normal.

After re-examining the patient, the orthopaedist appreciated that she could not have responded so quickly if the original diagnosis of disc

Macnab Ian, (1971). 'Negative disc exploration. An analysis of the causes of nerve root involvement in sixty-eight patients.' *J. Bone Jt. Surg.* **53A**, 891 prolapse had been correct. In retrospect, he considered the symptoms were caused by synovitis or inflammation of the synovial joint reducing the diameter of the intervertebral foramen thus compressing the nerve.

A further problem related to making a diagnosis is the fact that some doctors consider that a patient can have one diagnosis only. There are instances, however, where careful assessment and skillful planning of passive movement treatment will show that a patient having pain (say) arising at the base of the neck and radiating to the shoulder and mid upper arm may have a shoulder disorder causing the shoulder and arm pain, coupled with a cervical joint disorder causing the neck and scapular pain. Examination of the joint signs for both the cervical spine and the glenohumeral joint should be accurately assessed at the initial examination. If joint signs are found in both the shoulder and in the appropriate intervertebral joint, then ideally treatment should be applied only to the cervical spine at first. The joint signs in the spine may improve, resulting in the patient losing his neck and scapular pain but retaining the shoulder and arm pain. Re-examination of the glenohumeral joint may reveal that the glenohumeral joint's signs have remained unchanged. Under these circumstances treatment should then be applied to the glenohumeral joint in an effort to clear its joint signs, so gaining an improvement in the shoulder and arm pain. There are many such examples of combined joint involvement to explain the different pain patterns and syndromes which occur from patient to patient.

Another example of multiple causes for a patient's pain is seen frequently with patients having pain in their back which radiates down the full length of the leg. In relation to this area of pain physiotherapy students may find themselves in a dilemma when learning dermatomes. Confusion is understandable when one textbook (e.g. *Figure 2.4* in this book) shows the L4 dermatome as starting in the low back area and spreading throughout the buttock and leg to the top of the foot, while another text (Cyriax, 1975) shows the L4 dermatome starting below the knee and radiating down the shin into the foot. There is good reason for each of these presentations. There are various causes of referred pain from pressure or irritation of a nerve root. For example, there may be a prolapse of the nucleous pulposus, or the prolapsed material may be in direct contact with the nerve root (and not the dura or nerve-root sleeve). Under these circumstances the pain will only be felt below the knee, as shown by Dr Cyriax. An important point is that if the pain is felt only from the knee downwards, and if it can be

Cyriax, J. (1975). *Textbook of Orthopaedic Medicine.* 6th edn, Vol 1. London; Baillière, Tindall shown that this pain is arising from the back, then the pain must be due to irritation or compression of the nerve root alone.

Another example, which is far more common, is the patient who has a diagnosis of L4 referred pain extending from the centre back area through the buttock and leg to the top of the foot. The reason for this *may* be that the extruded disc material is irritating other pain-sensitive structures in the vertebral canal, such as the posterior longitudinal ligament, the dura and the nerve-root sleeve, as well as the nerve root. Under these circumstances we may have four contributary causes for the patient's pain.

If a patient has pain radiating from the buttock down the leg to the top of the foot, and he complains that the worst part of the pain is in the lower leg, then one can confidently assume that the nerve root is involved, particularly if spinal movements reproduce all of this pain, and in particular the distal pain. When pain is felt from the lower spine to the foot, the disc and adjacent posterior longitudinal ligament may be causing some of the proximal pain and the nerve root and its sleeve may be the source of the distal symptoms. Therefore more than one factor is causing the patient's pain.

From the foregoing it is easy to see that there are many problems associated with diagnosis, and there is still much more that medicine has yet to unravel. However, the problem must be tackled, and in the meantime when a diagnosis is incomplete the ability to make the proper use of the 'two-compartment' thinking makes it possible to use manipulation within routine medical care, and the treatment is made safe and informative by virtue of good assessment.

Assessment related to abnormal movements at the initial examination

The manipulative therapist bases most of her selection of techniques on the patient's history, symptoms and signs. As has already been said, this does not infer that diagnosis is unimportant. Changes of treatment techniques are guided by changes in the 'behaviour' of the pain and the 'behaviour' of the joint stiffness and muscle spasm. In this context the word behaviour has a special meaning. Behaviour of pain during joint movement is one of the most important aspects of examination and also the most important aspect to assess continually during treatment. The following examples will provide clarification.

Let us assume two patients present for treatment. They both have constant pain in their lower lumbar area which radiates into the buttock, posterior thigh and calf and then runs along the lateral border of the foot to the little toe; an area of pain indicating an S1 nerve-root problem. Both patients have been referred with a diagnosis of 'disc prolapse causing nerve-root compression'.

The first of the patients, standing with his back towards the physiotherapist, is asked to bend forward until his pain changes in any way. This he does, stopping when his fingers reach the top of his patellae. He returns to the upright position and states that at that point in the movement the pain in his back started to increase in intensity. He is asked to repeat the movement and on reaching his knees the physiotherapist gently encourages him to move a little further into the range and then returns him to the upright position. On questioning, the patient reports that on flexing beyond his patellae he experienced further increase in his back pain while his leg pain remained unchanged. Again he is asked to bend forward and is encouraged to gradually move further and further into the range, at the same time describing any changes in his pain. The end-result of testing forward flexion for this patient is that a full range of flexion is possible and only the pain in his back is increased. The movement has no effect on his leg pain.

Now let us consider the second patient with the same distribution of pain. On forward flexion he too can only reach the top of his patellae before pain starts to increase. He is returned to the upright position and asked what happened to his pain. This patient reports that the pain in his buttock and posterior thigh started to increase. This fact is noted and then, as with the previous patient, he is encouraged to flex a little further into the painful range. The physiotherapist carefully guides and controls the extent of this movement, asking the patient to signify changes in his symptoms as he flexes further. It is found that after moving only a few inches further into the range the pain in the calf increases. The patient is immediately returned to the upright position and is asked to inform the physiotherapist when increased symptoms, especially the calf pain, have subsided to the original state, and a note is made of the time taken for the pain to subside.

Both patients have the same distribution of pain and the same diagnosis, yet on testing their movements the 'behaviour' of their pain is quite different. Each patient will require different management by passive movement treatment. For example, as the second patient has referred pain provoked by movement tests, the initial treatment techniques must be very gentle so as not to provoke this pain. The first patient may need more vigorous treatment because the examination movements do not provoke his referred pain.

The above examples have been related to referred pain whether it is of nerve-root origin or not.

Some doctors consider that nerve-root involvement contraindicates manipulation. Of the two examples of nerve-root compression given above it may be reasonable to state that in the second patient, whose distally referred pain is easily provoked, manipulation is contra-indicated for the novice, but not necessarily for the experienced manipulator. However, the first example should not be classed as a contraindication to manipulation because the behaviour of the pain on movement does not increase referred pain. Neither patient should be classed as a contraindication *provided* the rules of continual assessment and gentleness with initial techniques are adhered to.

The above patients are perfect examples of the advantage of having the 'two compartments' of thinking, enabling treatment to be applied to the faulty area by assessment of the patient's history, symptoms and signs while full awareness of possible pathology is still retained.

What makes the pain pattern in these two patients differ? We do not know. Endeavouring to understand the differences in pathology is an interesting and important exercise facilitated by an in-depth appreciation of the history, symptoms and signs while endeavouring to relate the two compartments! The above examples also depict the care with which the examination of movements should be undertaken and continually reassessed during treatment.

There are other variations of referred pain which it is important to appreciate. These can be described as:

1. Recovery pain
2. Referred pain which can only be reproduced by sustained positional tests
3. Latent pain

Recovery pain

In this category the patient feels pain as he brings his body back to the upright starting position following test movements. For example, during examination of the trunk movements of a patient with central low back pain his trunk flexion is tested. The range may be full and painless, yet as he returns to the upright position from the fully flexed position he experiences low back pain during an arc of the return movement. From an assessment point of view, if, following treatment, the pain felt on the return movement to the upright position after flexion is less severe, or if the arc becomes smaller, this indicates improvement.

Referred pain which can only be reproduced by sustained positional tests

An example will explain this phenomenon. A patient presents with pain in his scapula and triceps area. On examination, the routine cervical test movements are found to be full range and painless. However, if cervical extension is sustained (for say 10 seconds) while some over-pressure is also maintained at the limit of its range, the pain may only be reproduced at the end of the 10 seconds. Also, when the patient's head is returned to the upright position it may take some seconds for that pain to subside. This kind of behaviour is a very accurate measuring-stick. If treatment is successful, the sustaining time required to reproduce the pain will increase, or the time taken for the symptoms to subside will decrease. The goal of treatment is to achieve symptom-free movement no matter how long the extension position is sustained, even if it is sustained while applying very strong overpressure.

Latent pain

This is a reasonably frequent finding and an example will help to explain it. A patient may have pain in his left scapula radiating into the back of the upper arm. During the examination of his cervical movements all are full range and painless. However, during, or immediately following, the examination of his movements, the patient may have a surge of pain into the scapula and arm. When this occurs the first time, it will not be possible to know which of the test movements has stimulated this latent pain. The examiner should see this phenomenon as a warning to be gentle with examination movements and take longer to do them. If the patient sits quietly without moving his head this latent surge of pain will subside. The length of time taken for the exacerbation to settle will vary from patient to patient but will be consistent with any one patient. (This is another example when the time taken for the symptoms to subside is a valuable measuring-stick.) When these test movements are repeated, they should be examined in a slightly different manner to elicit the exact behaviour of the pain with each direction of movement. Let us take examination of cervical lateral flexion first. This movement should be tested towards the side of pain and if no pain is found at the limit of the range, over-pressure should be applied. If the movement is still painless the position should be sustained for a short time (say 10 seconds). The patient's head should then be returned to the upright position. The patient is then asked to remain sitting for 10 or more seconds to determine whether there is any resulting surge of pain (i.e. latent pain) from that movement. If there is no pain from this test then rotation towards the side of pain should be tested in the same manner, with care being taken to allow enough time for latent pain to show up. If these test movements prove negative all other movements should be tested, with sufficient time for accurate assessment between each test movement being allowed each time. When the particular movement producing the latent pain is determined, the next step is to discover *how much* movement is needed to produce *how much* latent pain, i.e. the intensity and area of the pain. The time taken for the latent pain to subside after return to the upright starting position should also be noted.

These fine assessments of the behaviour of pain on movement may seem tedious and time consuming. They are important, however, and familiarity with the different ways pain can behave with movement makes the examiner dextrous in carrying them out.

Assessment by re-examination

Examination of movements of the spine must be done with care to allow assessment by re-examination to show if there has been improvement following a treatment technique, even if this improvement is only in the order of one per cent. An example of the depth of detail required is exemplified in a patient who feels pain on the left side of his neck at the mid-cervical level. During the examination he is asked to turn his head to the left until the symptoms are first felt. This range is estimated and recorded to be, say, 70 degrees. The physiotherapist then applies a small degree of controlled over-pressing through a further 5 degrees approximately and he judges how the pain behaves with this further movement. If the patient reports that the pain has not changed, firmer over-pressure is then applied. This further movement may result in a marked increase in the left neck pain. Some readers may doubt that such detail in examination is necessary. The answer to this statement is that these findings give the physiotherapist a guide as to the treatment technique to use, while also providing a very fine measure by which the effectiveness of the chosen treatment technique can be assessed. For example, having made the initial assessment of rotation as detailed above, the physiotherapist carries out a selected treatment technique, then sits the patient to reassess the rotation, taking note of the three facets of the rotation test.

Favourable changes would be indicated by any of the following findings:

1. As the patient turns his head to the left he feels the same pain as he did at the initial test. Over-pressure is applied with the result that the movement can be pushed further without increasing the pain.
2. If the patient's active *range* of rotation to the left is unchanged though it becomes symptom free, and the response to over-pressure is as it was at the initial examination, the fact that he can turn actively without pain indicates improvement.
3. When the patient turns his head to the left he feels no pain, nor does the first gentle over-pressure provoke any pain. With firmer over-pressure, however, pain increases as it did in the initial test. These findings indicate greater improvement than (2) above, even though the patient still feels the same degree of neck pain with the stronger over-pressure.
4. If the patient can turn his head without pain and the over-pressures also do not cause any pain, the patient's disorder is obviously improving favourably.

If the treatment technique is of no help the signs found on re-examination will not have altered.

Should the treatment technique have made the condition worse, then either

1. the patient's cervical rotation to the left will be slightly more limited and pain will start earlier in the range; or
2. the active range of rotation and its associated pain may be unchanged, but with even the slightest over-pressure applied to the movement, his pain will increase more than at the initial test.

As the first use of the technique is very gentle, any worsening of the signs will be minimal and not harmful, and the changes will be informative.

Two or more pains

There is yet another problem associated with careful assessment of a patient's movement and his pain. A patient may have two or more pains. One movement, or a group of combined movements, may be found to reproduce one particular part of the patient's symptoms while a different movement reproduces a second and different part of the patient's pain. This is particularly important if we can accept that it is *not uncommon* for a patient to have more than one kind of pain—either in the same area or in a closely linked area. It is important for the physiotherapist to be fully aware of these possibilities lest differences be missed during examination. For example it is common for a patient to complain of two distinctly different kinds of headache. The patient must be adequately questioned to determine the differences, and each pain should be examined, treated and assessed independently.

Joint stiffness

Let us now consider differences in the behaviour of joint stiffness. In the normal person the movement of one joint surface on its companion is a completely friction-free movement. However, examination of a patient's joint may show that while the range is full yet on oscillatory movements, through range, it lacks this feel of friction-free movement. With experience it is possible to feel a slight resistance to movement as described above even though the range is full. This resistance may be accompanied by crepitus though this is by no means always the case. It is important that physiotherapists develop the skill of feeling this lack of friction-free smoothness.

When a joint is limited by stiffness there are two ways in which this resistance may behave.

1. In the first part of the joint's movement slight restriction to the friction-free movement may be felt through a large part of the range and it only increases markedly in strength at the limit of the range.
2. Resistance may be felt early in the range and the further the movement is carried into the range the stronger the resistance becomes until a point is reached where the physiotherapist is not prepared to stretch the joint further. In other words, the rate of increase of strength of the resistance is proportional to the movement through range.

The physiotherapist must be aware that these variations in joint stiffness can and do exist; proficiency in assessment of their differences will only come with clinical experience.

Recording findings

At the initial examination it is behaviour of pain, of resistance, and of muscle spasm that form the basis for selecting treatment techniques and assessing the effect of treatment techniques. On rechecking (i.e. assessing) the patient's original abnormal movements it should also be possible to interpret the value of that technique as applied to that particular joint, at that particular state of the disorder. This is the whole purpose of assessment: PROVING THE VALUE OF EACH TREATMENT TECHNIQUE.

When recording the examination findings in the case notes, the important findings, which on reassessment will clearly and objectively reveal changes resulting from treatment, should be highlighted by marking them with asterisks. This procedure makes the main joint signs easy to find in the case notes.

ASSESSMENT DURING TREATMENT

Assessing changes in the patient's symptoms and signs which occur as a result of treatment is made at the following times:

1. At the beginning of each treatment session
2. During the performance of a treatment technique
3. Between each treatment technique used during a treatment session
4. As a retrospective assessment after a period of say five sessions

Assessment at the beginning of each treatment session

Assessment of changes in symptoms and signs at each treatment session needs to be carried out in a particular manner. There are three times when the patient's interpretation of the effect of treatment (i.e. the symptoms he feels) are most valuable.

(*a*) Immediately following treatment
(*b*) During the evening of the day of treatment and that night
(*c*) On first getting out of bed the following morning

It is better not to ask the patient initially for this information: questioning should be so planned that the physiotherapist can evoke spontaneous remarks which then prove to be very informative.

When assessing at the beginning of a treatment session, the first question should be, 'How have you been?' The answer will be valueless if the patient takes it as a general remark and answers, 'Fine thanks, how are you?' If this happens, the advantage of an initial, spontaneous, informative reply is lost. However, if the patient says, 'Much better, thank you,' then useful information has been expressed.

If the first question produced a valueless answer, the next question should be, 'What do you feel was the effect of yesterday's treatment?' The reply, 'Better' or 'Worse', needs further clarification. For example a patient may, in wishing to emphasize the degree of his present pain, give the impression that he is worse, whereas on closer questioning, it may be proved that he was better after his treatment until he performed some activity which aggravated his pain. Under these circumstances treatment helped rather than made him worse. This kind of information may be gained through the following questions:

> 'In what way is the pain worse' (is it more severe, sharper, changed to a throbbing pain, or has it increased in area, etc. etc.?)
> 'When did it start to become worse?'
> 'What do you think made it worse?'
> 'Was it related to treatment or did you do something which may have aggravated it?'

The physiotherapist must be prepared to accept the possibility that she has performed a technique too strongly. If a patient comes in feeling cross, saying 'What you did to me yesterday made me a lot worse', the beginner is going to feel disconcerted and disheartened. She will find it easier to accept the blame if she can reply, 'Good – not that I wanted to make you worse but it shows me exactly what to do and how to do it'; or she may say, 'If I can make you worse by too much or too heavy mobilizing of your spine then I should stand a good chance of being able to improve it.'

If the vital spontaneous information sought is not forthcoming it may be necessary to ask the direct questions:

> 'How did you feel when you got up first thing the next morning compared with how you felt when you came in for the last treatment?'
> 'How did you feel for the rest of that day and that night?'
> 'How did you feel when you got up first thing the next morning?'

Should the answers still not give a clear assessment, the physiotherapist may need to ask, 'Has your pain altered at all as a result of treatment?' If the patient has to hesitate before answering, then it is fairly clear that the symptoms could not have changed much, if at all.

If the patient reports feeling better from the treatment it is equally important to clarify what it is that has improved and in what way it has improved. This is particularly relevant when a patient has referred pain.

The above is the *subjective* assessment of the effect of the previous day's treatment. This is followed by retesting the previously abnormal movements and assessing the quality of any change resulting from treatment. Changes in these signs will, hopefully, agree with the findings of the subjective assessment, so reinforcing each other. This will then make the total assessment more reliable.

Assessment during the performing of a treatment technique

When the physiotherapist is carrying out a passive movement technique on a patient, she should first ascertain whether the patient has any pain while positioned for the treatment technique to be carried out. The movement is then performed at a chosen grade and the patient is asked whether the technique is causing any alteration to the symptoms. This information is necessary from three points of view.

1. The patient may have referred pain while positioned for treatment. As the treatment technique is carried out this pain may gradually lessen and go, it may remain at the same level throughout, or it may worsen. Assessment during the technique will guide the decision as to whether to continue with the technique, to perform it more gently, or whether a change of technique is indicated.

   (*a*) For example, in the early stages of treatment of a patient who has pain radiating throughout his leg, if treatment initially causes slight calf pain, and especially if this calf pain increases as the technique is continued, then the physiotherapist should discontinue that technique. She should stand the patient and reassess the other movement signs before going on to the next technique.

   (*b*) On the other hand, if the condition is more chronic in nature, it may be necessary to provoke this calf pain with the treatment technique to gain improvement. On reassessment it would be hoped that the provocation had brought about a definite improvement in pain-free range of active movement.

   (*c*) While performing the treatment technique, only the back pain, and not the referred pain, may be reproduced. If this occurs the technique should be continued. Whether it should be repeated or not would depend on the assessment of its effect.

2. The patient may have no pain while positioned prior to performing the technique but during the performing of a technique he may feel centre back pain. The physiotherapist may choose to continue with the same technique, at the same grade and ask the patient three, four, five or six times during the performance whether the centre back pain remains the same, improves, or worsens. If pain increases she may lessen the grade of the technique, or she may stop. If there is no change in the symptoms or should they improve she may need to do the technique more firmly.
3. There is one other response which can be determined during treatment. It is a difficult assessment to make because misunderstandings between physiotherapist and patient occur easily. It is useful to know when performing a technique whether pain is provoked at the limit of the oscillation only. The easiest way for the physiotherapist to make this assessment is to say to the patient, while performing the technique, *'Does–it–hurt–each–time–I–push?'* The words in italics are said in rhythm with the strongest part of the treatment technique. The patient then easily understands this question and has no hesitation in answering clearly.

These assessments should be recorded on the treatment record as is discussed in Chapter 8.

Assessment between each treatment technique used during a treatment session

The main points to be considered under this heading have already been covered in the section on Assessment at the beginning of each treatment session (*see* page 231). Care must be taken firstly, in the manner of questioning and secondly, in the accuracy of testing movements which form the basis of comparison.

Having carried out a treatment technique at a chosen grade long enough to expect some change in the symptoms and signs, the physiotherapist asks the patient to sit up (or stand up) for the assessment. She then asks, 'How does that feel now?' If there is no immediate spontaneous response she asks 'Is there any change?' Again, accuracy in questioning and interpretation are important to subjective assessment.

The patient's movements are then retested and a comparison made with those present before the treatment technique was used.

When reassessing the movement signs the same sequence of test movements must be used each time. The reason for this is that one movement which provokes pain may alter the signs for the next movement tested. Similarly, if cervical movements were tested in standing at the beginning, they should be reassessed in standing. It is inconsistent to test movements one time in standing, another while sitting in a chair and a third time with the patient sitting on the treatment couch without foot support.

It is hoped that the subjective and objective assessments will agree.

In principle, when a physiotherapist is in the learning stages of treatment by passive movement, this assessment should be made following each use of every technique. As experience is gained she learns to expect a certain improvement when particular techniques are applied to particular disorders. For example, if she is treating an elderly patient with general neck pain which can be reproduced at the limit of all movements, all of which are stiff, she can assume that there will not be much change during one treatment session though there may be considerable improvement over two treatment sessions. In these circumstances it would not be necessary to assess after each technique but the assessment should be made by comparing the symptoms and signs at the end of the second treatment session with those at the beginning of the first treatment session.

If the physiotherapist is able to judge that changes in symptoms and signs may be expected to take place quickly, she should assess them after each application of a technique and if the *rate* of change is not as much as desired, then a change in technique should be made. This procedure should be continued throughout the treatment, changing from technique to technique to find the one which produces the quickest and best improvement.

Retrospective assessment

Even when it is possible to make confidently an objective assessment that progress has been made, it is still of value to know how the patient feels he is progressing.

When questioned regarding his symptoms, a patient's answer may well be influenced by factors related to his work, his home problems, compensation, his ethnic group, his desire to please the physiotherapist, etc., etc. Therefore the physiotherapist must be sure the patient is giving accurate answers to her questions, and that she interprets them as he means them. In the context of 'question and answer' she must *never assume anything*. At the beginning of treatment it is not uncommon for a patient to reply day after day that he is feeling much better. Then, when asked, after say four treatments, 'How do you feel now compared with before we started treatment?', he may say cautiously, and after a long period of thought, 'I'm sure it's a little better; at least it certainly isn't any worse.' Such a retrospective answer alerts the physiotherapist from falling into the trap of believing she is making as much daily progress as she thought she was.

It can be of help to ask the patient, 'What percentage of progress do you think you have made compared with when we began treatment?' Often the patient finds it difficult to use percentages but he may answer by some other comparison which is equally useful. The physiotherapist should make her own percentage assessment before putting the question to him. If there is agreement in judgement then obviously communication and assessment are good.

Sometimes the subjective and objective assessments do not agree. For example, a patient's pleasure at improvement in his symptoms may not be equally reflected by improvement in his signs. The converse may also occur. However, these are exceptions to the general rule and usually at a slightly later stage of treatment they will agree.

Even when a patient has clear objective signs on which assessments can be made, it is still important to find out how he considers he is progressing. It is poor policy to just continue treatment time after time without making this 'retrospective assessment'. It is very easy to continue treatment unnecessarily, leading to perpetuating the joint disorder.

ASSESSMENT AT THE END OF TREATMENT

Assessment at the end of treatment is similar in many ways to the retrospective assessment discussed above. However, two other aspects should be taken into account when deciding whether or not treatment should be discontinued. The first of these is related to the stage of the pathology, and the second is related to 'what is normal in the way of pain and range of movement for this patient?' In other words, perhaps the goal of treatment may have to be a compromise rather than a 'cure'.

Pathology

When it is possible to be sure of the diagnosis then it is also possible to have a good idea of what treatment can achieve and whether a recurrence is likely.

Two examples of assessment related to pathology are worthy of consideration.

Example 1

The first relates to a patient who presents with symptoms arising from a low grade active arthritis where it is known that to regain a full painless range of joint movement is impossible. The question is when does one discontinue treatment.

In the early stages of passive movement treatment for such patients a gratifying improvement in movement and pain can be expected. Later during treatment a point will be reached when the patient's symptoms remain static and it is difficult to be sure whether the range of movement is improving ever so slightly or not at all. The physiotherapist should know that a stage can be reached when, in fact, the mobilizing is perpetuating the complaint. At this point the patient can be asked the direct question, 'Do you feel you have continued to improve over the last three or four treatments?' If the answer is 'No', then the treatment should be discontinued for a period of approximately two weeks, after which the patient's signs and symptoms should be reassessed.

1. If the symptoms have improved, then the patient should be left for a further two or three weeks and then reassessed. If then there is additional improvement, the patient can be discharged on the assumption that the symptoms will continue to improve without treatment.

2. If the symptoms and signs have remained the same, the patient should be given four or five more treatments and then taken off treatment again for two weeks. At the end of this period it will be possible to determine whether the extra treatment produced any improvement and whether a further few treatments should be administered.

This pattern of management must be very accurately assessed if it is to be used constructively.

It may be of interest to mention here that when these patients have recurrences, and they always do have recurrences, usually:

1. they seek treatment at an earlier stage of the exacerbation,
2. they respond more readily to treatment,
3. they have progressively longer periods between exacerbations, and
4. many of their exacerbations recover quite quickly without treatment.

Example 2

The second type of pathology problem, though uncommon, is a good example of the mental processes the physiotherapist has to exercise in formulating her assessment.

A patient has pain in his left buttock spreading down the posterior thigh to a point in his calf just distal to the knee. On examination he is found to have two sets of movement signs associated with his symptoms. One set is due to movement of the joint while the other is due to movement of pain-sensitive structures in the vertebral canal. The physiotherapist finds *marked* limitations due to pain in the following movements, all of which reproduce his pain.

Forward flexion
Extension
Left lateral flexion
Left straight leg raising

As treatment progresses a stage is reached when the assessment of the movements shows the following.

Extension has become full range and painless.
Forward flexion has improved 50 per cent.
Lateral flexion to the left remains unchanged.
Straight leg raising remains unchanged.

Interpreting these assessments and taking advantage of the 'two compartments' method of assessment, it is reasonable to assume in retrospect that the marked limitations found at the initial examination were due to two factors.

1. Restricted movement of one vertebra on another.

2. Restricted movement of the pain-sensitive structures in the vertebral canal.

If this reasoning can be accepted it is possible to assess the amount each factor played in the initial limitations of movement. It is reasonable to assume that the marked limitation of straight leg raising was not caused by mechanical lack of movement of the interbody joint or the apophyseal joints, and therefore the restricted straight leg raising was due to loss of movement of the pain-sensitive structures in the vertebral canal or intervertebral foramen. The treatment techniques used have not improved this part of the movement signs.

The range of extension improved with treatment from being markedly limited to being full range and painless. Therefore it is reasonable to assume that the limitation of extension bore no relationship to movement of the pain-sensitive structures in the vertebral canal. Therefore it must have been due to an intervertebral joint disorder.

Forward flexion improved 50 per cent with treatment. The assumption that can be made under these circumstances is that part of the limitation of forward flexion proved to be due to faulty intervertebral joint movement and the remainder of the limited range was due to restriction of movement of the pain-sensitive structures in the vertebral canal.

As lateral flexion to the left did not improve at all it can reasonably be assumed that the limitation was entirely due to the loss of movement of the pain-sensitive structures in the vertebral canal. Also, as it did not improve, the marked limitation bore no relationship to the faulty intervertebral joint movement. If it had been due to joint mechanics, it too would have become full range and painless as did extension.

This example may seem complex but if repeated assessment is carried out carefully enough, it is possible to change one's techniques and so relate them to the right structures. In other words, in this example, techniques should now be used in an endeavour to move the vertebral canal structures to see if improvement here can be achieved.

However there are many other factors which can arise to confuse assessments as seen in the above example where all movements caused pain throughout the leg. If back pain and not leg pain were produced by one or more of the test movements, different interpretations would need to be made. Also, on examination a particular intervertebral movement may be stiff and on testing its movements it may be painless or cause only slight local back pain.

The above example is a clear instance of why treatment techniques should be related to symptoms and signs rather than to diagnostic titles. It would have been impossible at the initial examination of the above example to give an exact diagnosis, yet with careful assessment the physiotherapist is able to relate accurately her treatment techniques to the signs found on examination.

The example also shows that loss of movement of pain-sensitive structures in the vertebral canal can limit trunk movements. Limited forward flexion as a result of disc prolapse is a common and accepted example. If the change of techniques does not improve the canal signs then manipulation would be discontinued and perhaps surgery would need to be considered.

Determination of 'normality'

The second consideration in relation to assessment at the end of treatment is 'What is normal in the way of pain and movement for this patient?'

People have widely differing norms. For example, forward flexion of the trunk in standing can vary between one person being able only to reach just beyond the knees, to someone else being able to put flat hands on the floor. Such variations occur in other movements also. It is necessary to bear in mind these ordinary variations if an accurate assessment is to be achieved.

Example 1

Consider a patient who presents for treatment of low back pain. On examining forward flexion it is found that he can only reach his knees and at this point his back pain is reproduced. On first seeing this it might be considered that flexion is markedly limited and painful and therefore the patient's condition is assessed as being quite bad. However if this patient had been asked, 'How far could you bend before the onset of your pain?' he might have replied 'I've never been able to bend much further than my knees.' This information puts the interpretation of the flexion disability into a different perspective.

Example 2

An elderly patient with neck pain also shows radiological evidence of gross degenerative change. Passive movement treatment is very helpful for a patient such as this but the assessment must take into consideration the fact that rotation to either side will never reach a stage of being 90 degrees. The same will apply to all his other cervical movements. Therefore the assessment must take into account the range of movement which is likely to be normal for this patient. The role of treatment will be to eliminate the painful aspect of joint movement. The end-result will be slightly improved movement though movements will remain stiff in all directions. Importantly the neck pain will have gone.

When assessing progress the physiotherapist should be alert to situations where improvement in symptoms and signs do not occur synchronously. There are times, particularly if the patient has severe pain, when the signs may show improvement without the patient being able to appreciate any change in symptoms. Severe nerve-root pain fits into this category. In these situations the slight improvements in the movement signs indicate that the same treatment should be repeated; improvement in the symptoms will soon be noticeable. Conversely, circumstances may arise where the symptoms improve quite dramatically but progress in the joint signs is not so rapid. The adolescent disc lesion is a good example of this phenomenon. If either the subjective or the objective assessment shows improvement then it can be considered, with one very important exception, that the disorder is improving.

The important exception to this rule concerns patients who have severe nerve-root pain and neurological changes. These patients should be examined neurologically daily by the physiotherapist and any worsening of neurological changes, or the appearance of neurological changes which were not apparent before, should be reported immediately to the doctor. It is common for such patients to report dramatic improvement in symptoms over a period of one or two days, even to the extent of becoming symptom-free, or almost symptom-free. In these cases pain does markedly and rapidly lessen while the neurological changes either appear or worsen considerably. As has already been stated, the referring doctor should be notified at once as the patient may require immediate surgery.

ASSESSMENT ASSISTING IN DIFFERENTIAL DIAGNOSIS

At the initial examination of a patient the doctor may not be able to make a definitive diagnosis. If the problem is a musculoskeletal disorder then under some circumstances passive movement treatment can be applied in such a way as to assist in making the diagnosis.

For example, a patient may have pain in the region of his shoulder and the referring doctor may not be certain whether the pain is emanating from the patient's shoulder or from his neck. The patient can be referred to a manipulative physiotherapist with a request that he be treated in such a manner as to assist in forming the diagnosis.

To do this successfully the physiotherapist needs to examine both the neck and the shoulder in the kind of detail mentioned earlier in this chapter so that all joint signs, both cervical and glenohumeral, are revealed in detail. She should then treat the cervical area first and assess the effect of this treatment on both the cervical and shoulder signs. If treatment to the cervical spine produces favourable changes in both the cervical and the shoulder signs then the cervical treatment should be continued. However, if there is no improvement in the shoulder signs within three treatment sessions, despite trying all techniques applicable to the cervical spine, treatment to this area should be discontinued. The shoulder should then be treated and its response assessed. In this way the response to treatment will give the answer as to whether or not the cervical spine is involved, thus assisting the diagnosis.

IN CONCLUSION

Just as there are communication difficulties in normal conversation, arising out of misinterpretation of the meanings of things said or not said, so there are difficulties in assessing the patient's subjective response to treatment. Because of these difficulties the physiotherapist should be *most* careful in questioning to assess any variations in the patient's symptoms.

None of the patient's feelings about his pain should ever be assumed. For example, if a patient is asked to bend forward, and as he does so, says 'Ouch!', the physiotherapist should immediately follow up with 'Did that hurt?' 'Yes.' 'Where did you feel it?' As the examination continues and the patient repeatedly feels pain with each movement, it can be irritating to him to be continually asked 'Where did it hurt?' Under such circumstances, when the patient cringes while testing movements, the physiotherapist can ask, 'In the same spot?' This avoids reiteration while still getting the correct message. Assume nothing. If the pain alters in its area he will say where it is, even if only asked, 'In the same spot?' It is this close communication between physiotherapist and patient which makes assessment so informative and valuable and thereby makes treatment more specific and effective.

Although some will say this is too time consuming to be of value, successful treatment compels this degree of accuracy; it is essential if the physiotherapist is to remain in control of the treatment situation. Given practice and experience, it is not a lengthy procedure.

8 Principles Applied

Manipulative techniques and the indications for their use can be taught, but this is not enough. Experience teaches the finer points of treatment so that the best result is produced in the shortest possible time. The best way to learn from manipulative treatment is to record accurately the cause and effect of all that occurs during treatment. This written record should begin with a summary of the patient's account of changes which have resulted from the previous treatment. Perceptive questioning by the examiner may be required to obtain the relevant information. The record should then indicate changes in the important signs being checked throughout treatment (*see* Table 8.2).

The advantages of a written planning stage in relation to the examination of a patient have been discussed (*see* page 16) but it is even more valuable when recording treatment. Once the changes which have resulted from previous treatment have been assessed, the physiotherapist must choose whether to continue with the same techniques or not and she must know clearly why she makes such a decision. If she chooses to change to a particular technique she must know why she has chosen that particular technique. Writing this plan down facilitates clearer thinking and encourages consideration of the next day's treatment.

Treatment is recorded by naming the technique used, stating the grade in which it was used, and noting any effect it had on the patient's symptoms while it was being carried out. Following the record of the technique and separated by a clear and thick vertical line a record must be made of both the assessment of what the patient feels has happened as a result of the last treatment, and also the physiotherapist's assessment of the changes which have taken place in his joint signs. One of the main complaints made about recording treatment in this way is that it is too time consuming; this is quite wrong. Abbreviations will make the task quicker and encourage the omission of unnecessary words. Table 8.1 offers descriptive symbols which might be used to describe each of the techniques. (Full credit for the origin of these symbols must be given to Miss Margaret Jenkinson, MCSP, of King's College Hospital, London, and agreement as to their identification was reached by a group of physiotherapists in England in 1966.) If the number of times a technique is used is written in numbers, and grades are recorded in Roman numerals the whole procedure can be very quickly recorded once the habit is established.

TABLE 8.1

Technique	Symbol	Description
Postero-anterior central vertebral pressure		
Postero-anterior unilateral vertebral pressure		(on the right side of a vertebra)
		(on the left side of a vertebra)
Transverse pressure		(pushing the spinous process towards the right)
		(pushing the spinous process towards the left)
Anteroposterior unilateral vertebral pressure		(on the left side of a vertebra)
Rotation		(head or pelvic rotation to the left)
		(head or pelvic rotation to the right)
Lateral flexion		(lateral flexion of the vertebrae to the left)
		(lateral flexion of the vertebrae to the right)
Longitudinal movement		

To enable easy reference to previous treatments it is suggested that each treatment should be written up as shown in Table 8.2.

Only by this means can a methodical treatment be given and the steps taken be clearly understood. It will also avoid unnecessary waste of treatment time resulting from false impressions.

The foregoing part of this book has been concerned with teaching techniques and the principles involved in their application. Now this knowledge must be put into practice. Supervised treatment of patients is of course the best way to do this, but selected case histories have been given in some detail as a guide. These will indicate the reasons for each step taken, and the results which followed.

TABLE 8.2

C/O	Assessment of what the patient feels has happened as a result of the last treatment	
O/E	Operator's assessment of changes in any of the signs resulting from the last treatment	
Plan	Which technique is to be used and why	
Treatment	Title of technique How it was used (Grade) Number of times it was used Effect on symptoms during application	C/O O/E
Plan	State what you will do next time if certain changes occur	

EXAMPLE

	3x ↓ L4 and L5 III slight spasm and slight local deep pain	'Feels freer' F. imp. 2in.
Plan	May need IV+ to hasten progress.	

In the case histories which follow, there will be aspects of the examinations which have not been mentioned, but it can be assumed that all relevant abnormalities known at the time of treatment have been included. These case histories have been set out so that they can be readily used for quick reference. With each history there is a quick reference diagram showing the area of pain of which the patient complained, and a title showing the particular reason for its inclusion.

Examination

The examination deals with the appropriate aspects of the patient's history and the associated signs, and is divided into the following.

1. Brief statements setting out the history of the condition as it stood at the time of treatment.

2. The relative physical findings on examining the patient at the first visit.

Treatment

Treatment is divided into the following.

1. A list of the general principles involved in the manipulative treatment.
2. A record of the treatment given and its effect, and the factors involved in any alteration.

It is hoped that the following section will guide the student through the early stages of making decisions on treatment, and also guide the medical practitioner in assessing the treatment results his physiotherapist should be getting when he refers patients for such treatment. These cases are intended not as reading material but as references and guides to the student.

The basis for this book has been to relate treatment to the symptoms and signs found on examination. This concept is unacceptable to many medical practitioners and it is reasonable to consider that manipulation should not be undertaken unless a diagnosis is possible. However two sets of circumstances apply. Sometimes it is not possible to make a diagnosis, and mobilization can be administered diagnostically. Secondly, although a diagnosis may be possible, this does not necessarily give enough indication to guide the type of treatment necessary. This is so because under one diagnostic title the patient may have any one of a number of related symptoms and signs each of which may indicate a different approach to treatment. Hence, although diagnosis is important, a clear appreciation of the symptoms and signs present on examination is the vital issue. Stoddard's manual (1969) clearly relates treatment to the diagnosis but the divisions can be carried even further.

As an example in the first four case histories the patients all had a diagnosis of 'disc lesion with nerve-root compression'. However on examination their signs were markedly different and each was treated in a different manner. It is for these reasons that symptoms and signs play such an important part, and it is essential that they must be given much consideration.

Stoddard, A. (1969). *Manual of Osteopathic Practice.* London; Hutchinson Medical Publications

CASE HISTORIES

The case histories that will be dealt with are listed in Table 8.3.

TABLE 8.3

NERVE ROOT

SEVERE CERVICAL NERVE-ROOT PAIN

Examination

History

A man aged 42 years developed aching in his right scapula in November for no apparent reason. Over a period of two weeks these symptoms subsided but did not completely go. In January the symptoms recurred but settled over a period of three weeks. The symptoms recurred again in April and gradually, over a period of four days, spread into his right arm. Treatment began three weeks after the April onset. When first seen, he was obviously in distress because of pain. The two main areas of pain were the right scapula and right forearm. He also complained of a general puffy numb feeling through his whole hand (*Figure 8.1*).

Physical findings

All cervical and arm movements were full range while cervical extension, lateral flexion to the right and rotation to the right all produced right scapular pain. If these three movements were sustained at the limit of the range, right forearm symptoms developed and a general tingling appeared in the right hand. Following examination of his cervical movements there was a marked exacerbation of his symptoms which took five minutes to subside. Moderate weakness of the right triceps was the only definite neurological change.

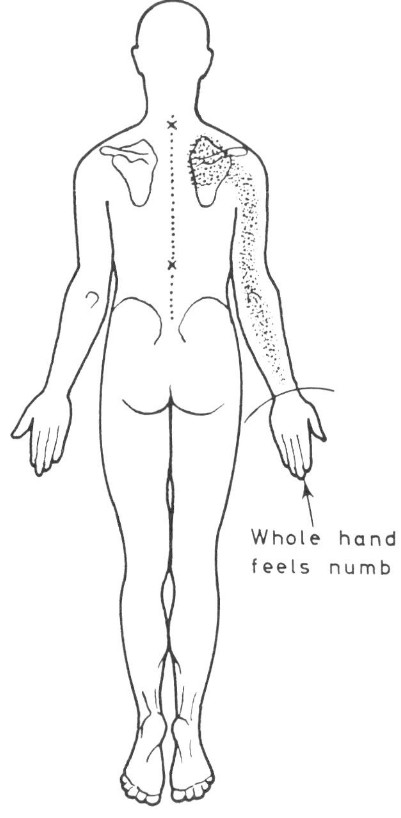

Figure 8.1. – Severe cervical nerve-root pain

Treatment

Guiding factors

1. As an example of severe cervical nerve-root pain traction is the only form of conservative treatment which should be considered from the physiotherapist's point of view.
2. With an exacerbation so easy to produce, initial treatment must be very gentle.

3. Mobilization of any form is not considered appropriate at this stage.
4. The patient should be advised that he may not notice much improvement in his symptoms for the first seven days. Despite this, we should be able to assess that progress is forthcoming by the signs.
5. The patient should also be warned of the possibility of some exacerbation following the first treatment.

First day

Very gentle cervical traction in flexion in lying was administered for 15 minutes. This treatment was continued daily for five days and over the last two days the duration of each stretch was increased. By the fifth day he was having 25 minutes' traction. At this stage he was unaware of any improvement, though on examination his extension was slightly less painful in the scapula area and the position required sustaining longer before arm symptoms developed.

Sixth day

By the sixth day the patient was able to say he was feeling better and traction was then increased to 30 minutes.

Eleventh day

By the eleventh day he was feeling 70 per cent better and at this stage sustained extension did not produce any symptoms.

On the fifteenth day he was able to say the arm was the best it had been and his movements were then almost symptom free. Treatment was discontinued and he was reviewed two weeks later. His symptoms were then 90 per cent better and were not worrying him. Movements were painless and the triceps muscle power was unchanged.

SEVERE LUMBAR NERVE-ROOT PAIN

Examination

History

This man aged 45 years had had a sudden onset of back pain six weeks previously while lifting. Over a three week period he developed lower

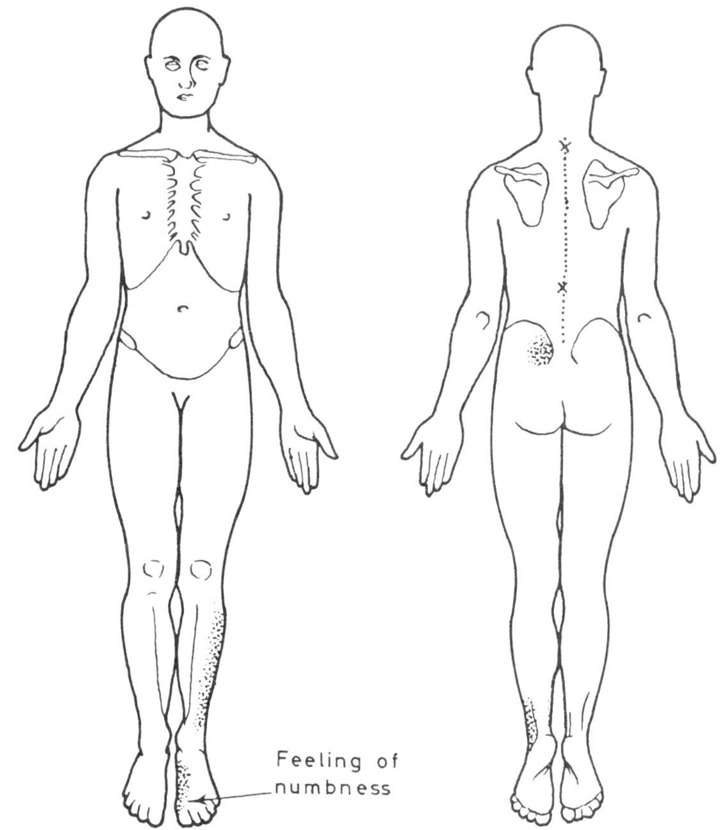

Figure 8.2. – Severe lumbar nerve-root pain

leg and foot symptoms and muscle weakness. He was admitted to hospital and given constant traction for 12 days. He was then referred for continuing physiotherapy (*Figure 8.2*).

Physical findings

In forward flexion the patient was only able to reach his knees and at this position he had pain only in his back. Extension was full range and painless. Lateral flexion to the left was limited and caused pain in his back at 40 degrees, and at 45 degrees the pain increased in his back and appeared also in his foot. His tibialis anterior was 1, extensor hallucis longus 2, and toe extensors 2+.

Treatment

Guiding factors

1. Traction would probably be the first treatment which should be considered. However, as he has had traction in hospital and been considerably relieved of his symptoms, the last improvement in his movements may come more rapidly with mobilization.
2. If mobilization is to be used, general rotation would be the treatment of choice because symptoms are unilateral and the cause of the pain is likely to be the disc.
3. In the presence of marked neurological changes treatment must be gentle and cautious and assessment of the neurological changes made daily.

First day

Lumbar rotation, pelvis rotated to right, was performed very gently as a Grade IV. Following two uses of this technique the assessment was as follows. Symptomatically his lower leg felt better, and his left lateral flexion seemed a little improved. Left straight leg raising was unaltered.

Second day

On assessment his movements were unchanged but he thought his leg might have been better at times. The same technique was repeated, this time for three times. The technique improved his flexion and straight leg raising by 5 cm (2 inches) but his symptoms were unchanged.

Third day

The patient's symptoms and signs were unchanged so it was decided to make a change in treatment. Traction was chosen and it was decided to use intermittent variable traction instead of constant traction because the oscillatory movement of the lumbar rotations did seem to produce some change. Twelve kg was given for 10 minutes with a 5 second hold and no rest period.

Fourth day

He reported feeling definitely a little better so the treatment was repeated for a duration of 12 minutes.

Fifth day

He still felt a little improved and both flexion and straight leg raising had maintained the 5 cm (2 inches) improvement in range. It was then decided that perhaps rotation could be added to the traction to see if this would gain a slightly quicker improvement. Therefore, following a period of 15 minutes on 14 kg traction, two periods of rotation were given gently.

Sixth day

The patient reported feeling worse again and his flexion had lost some of what had been gained. It was then decided to give the traction and leave out any other treatment. The traction was gradually increased daily in poundage until 25 kg were being given for 15 minutes.

Fourteenth day

By this stage his symptoms were minimal, his forward flexion was 70 per cent recovered and he was able to reach two-thirds of the way down his shin. Straight leg raising on the left was 70 degrees and painless. On examining his muscle power, the extensor hallucis longus and toe extensors were normal and the tibialus anterior was almost fully recovered.

RESIDUAL INTERMITTENT NERVE-ROOT PAIN

Examination

History

Four months previously this woman aged 35 years had what she said had been diagnosed as a disc lesion with nerve-root compression. She had traction which relieved her symptoms considerably in the first month. Following this she did not have treatment but found that she still had intermittent symptoms in her left elbow. Physiotherapy was tried again but this time it did not help her symptoms. She complained of intermittent symptoms in the left elbow many times a day. They did not last long and were not severe but were unpleasant (*Figure 8.3*).

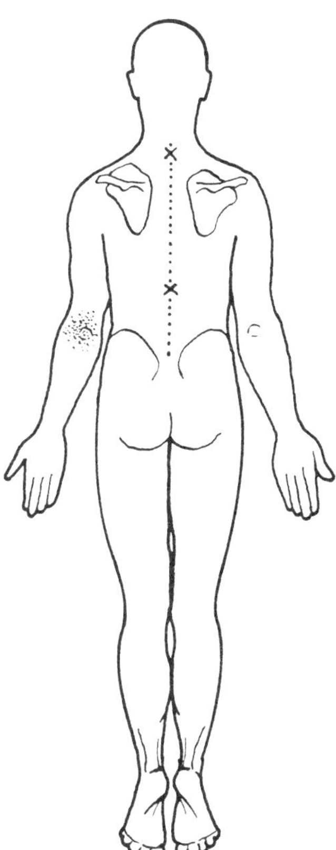

Figure 8.3. – Residual intermittent nerve-root pain

Physical findings

All cervical movements and arm movements were full range and painless. Even a sustained quadrant movement was pain free. There was marked weakness of her left triceps but the reflex activity appeared normal. On examination by palpation it was easily determined that there was a loss of at least 50 per cent movement at the left C6/7 intervertebral joint.

Treatment

Guiding factors

1. As the symptoms are unilateral the selection of techniques would be between postero-anterior unilateral vertebral pressure and rotation.
2. Traction would not be required not only because it has been attempted before without success but also because the symptoms are not severe.
3. Mobilization would be quicker in its effect than traction and therefore should be attempted first.
4. As the joint signs were found only with palpation it would be wise to use this sign as the first treatment movement.

First day

Postero-anterior unilateral vertebral pressure on the left side of C6/7 was given in three periods of 1 minute. The only assessment that could be made was that this movement appeared to improve slightly as treatment continued. The patient was warned of possible exacerbation as a result of the first treatment but was asked to note any change in the pattern of symptoms.

Second day

She reported that there had been a reduction of at least 50 per cent in the number of times she had had symptoms. On examination by palpation, the movements seemed to have retained the improvement which had been gained the previous day. The treatment was repeated.

Third day

She reported having had almost no symptoms but when they had come they were as uncomfortable as previously. The treatment was repeated and the movement was felt to be almost normal by the end of the third period. It was decided to leave treatment for a week to see whether further treatment was necessary. The patient was advised to come for treatment if the symptoms showed signs of returning.

One week later

As symptoms had gone the patient was pleased and treatment was discontinued.

CHRONIC LUMBAR NERVE-ROOT ACHE

Examination

History

This man aged 35 years had had recurrent back symptoms over a period of eight years. In the last 18 months he had had some symptoms in his left leg. Previous bouts had been successfully relieved by an osteopath. Two and a half months ago, while weeding in the garden, he noticed minor symptoms in his buttock and throughout his leg. These developed as the day progressed and over the next three days increased to a constant ache. This made sitting difficult and interfered with his work as a clerk. His osteopath had not been able to relieve the pain so he went to his doctor and thence for physiotherapy (*Figure 8.4*).

Physical findings

Flexion was to within 23 cm (9 inches) of the floor and straight leg raising was limited to 60 degrees. Other than these two signs his movements were painless. He had slight weakness of his calf and there was some tingling in the lateral border of the sole of his foot but no sensory change. His reflexes were normal.

Treatment

Guiding factors

1. As this is a probable discogenic nerve-root problem the choice of techniques lies between rotation and traction.

2. As his symptoms are not severe and mobilization is quicker in its effect it would be wiser to try rotation first.

3. As the nerve root is involved it may be necessary at a later stage to make use of straight leg raising as a technique.

First day

On determining that his symptoms were not irritable it was decided to use rotation quite strongly and in a sustained manner. The rotation was done, rotating the pelvis to the right, and this was sustained strongly. It was repeated four times. At the end of the treatment he said his symptoms felt a little easier and straight leg raising had improved by 5 cm (2 inches). Flexion had also improved.

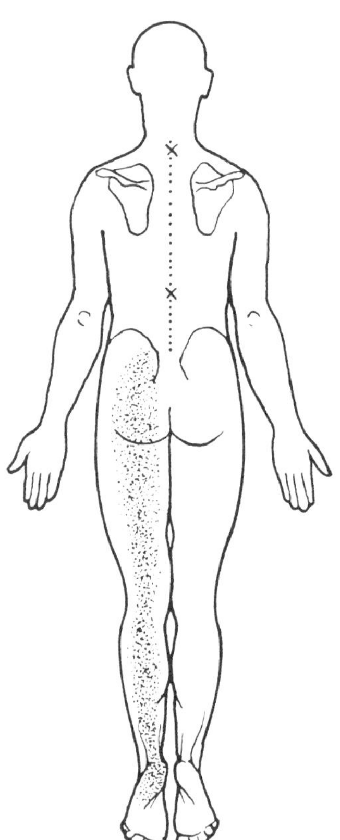

Figure 8.4. – Chronic lumbar nerve-root pain

Second day

He reported feeling much the same though his movements had maintained their slightly increased range. It was decided to repeat the rotation but also to add postero-anterior central vertebral pressure. This was done and movements improved a further 5 cm.

Third day

There was a slight lessening of pain, and the range of movements had been maintained. The treatment was repeated, after which the patient reported that his calf felt much more comfortable.

Fifth day

By the fifth day it was decided to add traction, following which the patient felt much better. His movements were improving, but more slowly, and it was thought that these should be progressing more quickly.

Seventh day

By this stage it was decided to give traction, followed by postero-anterior central vertebral pressure and rotation. To this was added straight leg raising as one strong stretch. Two days later the patient said he considered he was almost symptom free. His movements seemed almost normal for him and treatment was discontinued.

INSIDIOUS ONSET OF LEG PAIN

Examination

History

For 10 years a woman aged 35 years had had many bouts of back pain, each necessitating rest in bed. They had all begun suddenly from minor lifting incidents. Three months ago she noticed an ache superficially in the lateral aspect of the right thigh. Aching was intermittent at first, but became constant over a period of one week. A tingling feeling which also developed in the lateral aspect of the lower leg and foot later developed to an ache and a feeling of numbness on the dorsum of the foot (*Figure 8.5*). These symptoms developed over a period of three weeks. Her doctor put her into a plaster jacket for six weeks but the symptoms did not improve. Three weeks after the plaster was removed she was sent for a 'trial of manipulation and traction'.

Physical findings

With forward flexion she was able to reach to 40 cm (16 inches) from the floor. With this movement the leg pain increased, and a sciatic scoliosis, which caused a tilt of the trunk to the left, became evident. The scoliosis disappeared on resuming the upright position. Lateral

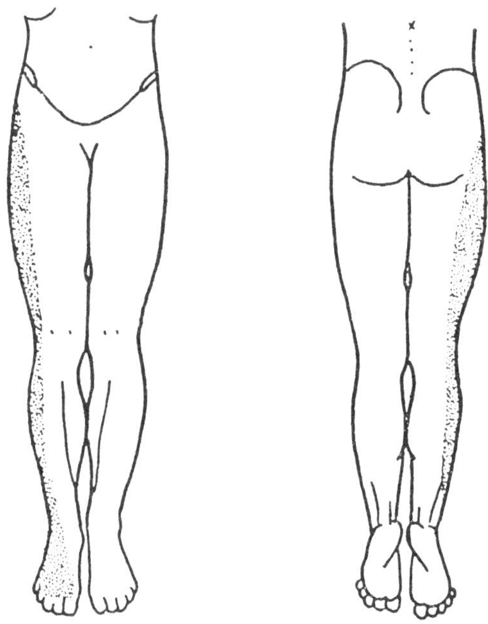

Figure 8.5. – Insidious onset of leg pain

flexion to the right performed in that range of forward flexion which caused the scoliosis was very limited and caused slight back pain. All other spinal movements were stiff but they were not noticeably painful. Firm pressure over the vertebral column did not cause any pain or muscle spasm, but there was a general feeling of intervertebral tightness in the lumbar spine. Right straight leg raising lacked 20 degrees of movement and was painful at the back of the whole leg. Reflexes, sensation and muscle power were all normal.

Treatment

Guiding factors

1. Slow onsets of this type are more likely to respond to traction than to manipulation.
2. A general limitation of intervertebral movement, if it is contributing to the symptoms, will be improved by mobilization rather than by traction.
3. This patient probably will be helped by a combination of traction and mobilization.
4. If mobilization were attempted, rotation should be the first choice.
5. As there are not neurological changes and straight leg raising is not markedly limited, the possibility of completely relieving symptoms is good.

First day

It was decided to institute traction first to assess its value before including mobilization.

Very gentle traction in supine was applied for 10 minutes. While the traction was on there was a lessening of pain in the leg, and on releasing the traction the symptoms remained eased. After a 5 minute rest the patient's straight leg raising had improved by 10 degrees. The patient went home and was asked to rest.

Second day

The patient felt that she had improved from the traction. She had not had any back discomfort. Forward flexion had improved by 5 cm (2 inches) and straight leg raising had maintained the improvement of 10 degrees.

Traction was repeated, but as there had been no trouble with back pain it was done in prone. A strong pull (35 kg) was given for 15 minutes and all leg pain disappeared. Some pain returned on releasing the traction. After a short rest, straight leg raising was found to have improved a little further.

Third day

Further slight improvement was felt by the patient. Forward flexion was 32 cm (13 inches) from the floor (an improvement of 2.5 cm (1 inch)), and straight leg raising still lacked 10 degrees.

The same strength of traction was used and similar relief of symptoms was experienced. Traction was maintained for 30 minutes.

Fourth day

In comparison with the first day there had been considerable improvement, but the rate of progress appeared to have been less over the last two days. Forward flexion now lacked 31 cm (12 inches) and straight leg raising lacked 5 degrees.

Stronger traction (70 kg) was given and the patient was then given a long rest.

Fifth day

Forward flexion lacked 25 cm (10 inches), straight leg raising was full and there was further symptomatic improvement.

As it was felt that progress should have been quicker mobilization was commenced. Rotation with the patient lying on her left side was given 4 times. Following each there was an improvement in forward flexion which consisted of a 5 cm (2 inches) improvement after the first and second times, 2 cm (0.8 inch) after the third and only 1 cm (0.4 inch) after the fourth. Strong traction followed the mobilization.

Sixth day

The patient felt much better. Her back felt freer and the leg ache was almost gone. Forward flexion had maintained its increased range and the finger tips were now 11 cm (3 inches) from the floor. Straight leg raising was normal.

A repetition of the rotation increased forward flexion to 2 cm (0.8 inch) from the floor. Traction was also repeated.

Seventh–ninth days

The routine of the fifth and sixth days was repeated, and by the tenth day the patient was free of all symptoms. Her straight leg raising was normal and forward flexion was full with all signs of the sciatic scoliosis gone. She had lost all tingling sensation by the seventh day. All active and passive movements were much freer than when examined the first day.

POORLY DEFINED LEG SYMPTOMS

Examination

History

For two years a man aged 45 years had noticed intermittent tingling which began over the dorsum of the left foot and gradually extended to the lateral aspect of the leg, thigh and buttock (*Figure 8.6*).

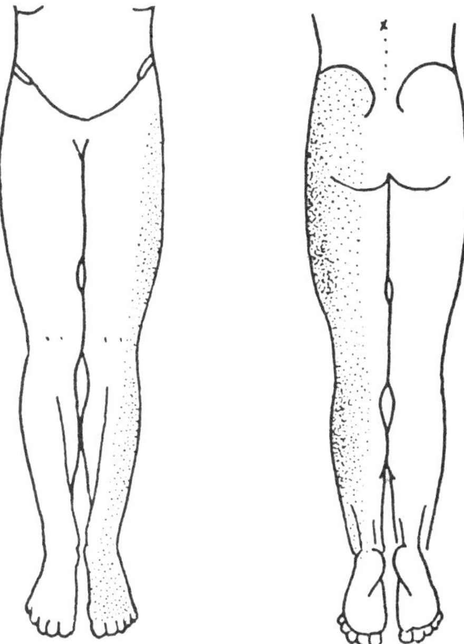

Figure 8.6. – Poorly defined leg symptoms with good movements

Two weeks ago he had been hospitalized for a heart condition and during this period the symptoms had worsened until at the time of treatment he had a constant dull ache in the left lateral buttock, thigh and leg and tingling over the dorsum of the foot.

Physical findings

Active movements of the spine were full and painless with the exception of forward flexion which caused a dragging feeling posteriorly in the left leg when his finger tips were 13 cm (5 inches) from the floor. Passive movements of the lumbar spine showed a marked limitation of the flexion-extension movement between the fourth and fifth lumbar vertebrae. Other tests of the spine, sacro-iliac joints and hips were normal.

The referring physician asked for two days of treatment as the patient was then returning to his home in the country.

Treatment

Guiding factors

1. The only objective sign is the L4/5 stiffness.
2. There is no muscle spasm protecting movement of the L4/5 intervertebral joint.
3. As only two days of treatment are possible and as the L4/5 stiffness, if this is the cause of the symptoms, has probably taken at least two years to reach its present stage, it could waste time to begin with mobilizing techniques.
4. From the above three points it would appear best to begin with manipulation of the intervertebral joint between L4 and L5.

First day

The rotary manipulation localized to the L4/5 joint was done twice to the right and twice to the left. The range of forward flexion improved each time until he was able to touch his toes without any dragging feeling in the left leg. The leg ache improved from the beginning and the foot tingling had gone after the four manipulations.

Second day

The patient was still able to touch his toes, and all limb and buttock pain had gone. Tingling had been intermittent and less severe since the manipulation. The L4/5 joint was sore from the manipulation.

The first day's treatment was repeated and this cleared the tingling in the foot.

On retesting, the L4/5 movement was greatly improved.

The patient wrote 10 days later to say that he had remained symptom free.

CERVICAL
PAIN SIMULATING CARDIAC DISEASE

Examination

History

A man aged 54 years was treated seven years ago for Ménière's disease and deafness. Three years later he had a very bad bout of left chest and arm pain which came on during the night. He later recalled that he had been waking with a feeling of slight neck stiffness for a few days before this onset. At that stage his doctor considered that a heart condition was the cause of the pain and he was treated for this.

Ten days ago he was again wakened by left chest and arm pain, and since then the pain had been unbearable at times (*Figure 8.7*).

His referring specialist said there was little evidence of cardiac disease, and as neck movements were restricted, manipulation and traction should be given as a diagnostic trial.

Physical findings

Neck movements were markedly restricted. Extension was impossible, forward flexion, left lateral flexion and left rotation lacked 60 degrees of their range, right lateral flexion and right rotation were limited by approximately 25 degrees. All of these movements caused pain in the arm.

Radiologically the body of C6 was narrowed vertically, and there was marked narrowing of the C6/7 interbody space with overriding of the apophyseal facets.

Treatment

Guiding factors

1. Pain in the left chest and arm which may simulate cardiac disease can arise from T4 or C7 levels.

2. With such severe symptoms and with all movements limited by a marked increase in arm pain, traction would be preferable to manipulation.
3. With marked limitation of movement and with a definite painful limitation of forward flexion the result can be expected to be slow.
4. As pain subsides with traction, and flexion becomes free, mobilization could be used to hasten the result.

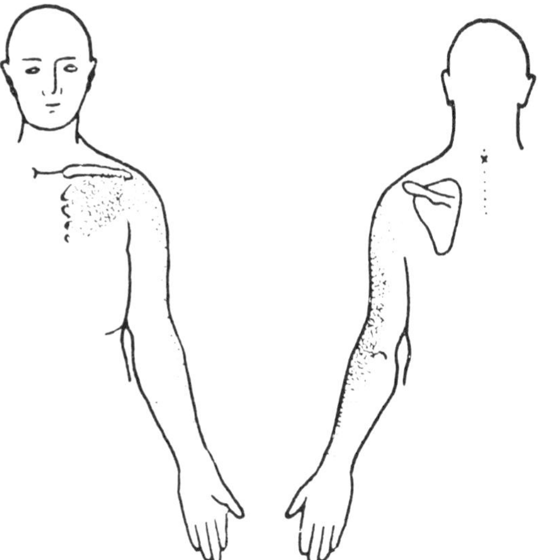

Figure 8.7. – Severe left chest and arm pain simulating cardiac disease

First day

As extension was so limited, cervical traction in flexion was given which almost completely relieved the pain (approximately 35 degrees). Treatment comprised two stretches, each of 10 minutes' duration. Pain returned on lowering the traction each time. The patient was warned of the possible flare-up of symptoms following the first treatment. He was attempting to continue his own clerical business throughout treatment.

Second day

Movements and pain were approximately the same as on the first day. Traction was repeated but it was given as a stretch of 15 minutes. Some degree of relief remained on releasing the traction.

Third day

Pain had eased a little and rotation showed a little improvement. Traction was repeated.

Fourth–seventh day

Marked progress continued with this daily traction.

Eighth day

By this stage pain had been reduced and all movements were less limited. Forward flexion was painless, and pain was in the same areas, namely the chest and the whole of the arm.

As symptoms were less severe and forward flexion was painless, it was decided to commence mobilization as well as continuing with the traction. Cervical rotation to the right carried out three times resulted in freedom from the forearm part of the pain and lessening of the upper arm pain, but the chest pain remained unchanged.

The thoracic spine between T1 and T5 was then mobilized three times pushing the spinous processes from right to left with transverse vertebral pressure. This relieved the chest pain but only slightly improved the forearm pain.

The usual traction was given and this completely relieved the forearm pain.

Ninth day

The pain had eased its usual amount, but movements had made more progress than previously. As thoracic soreness had increased from the mobilizing of T1–T5, only traction was given this day.

Tenth day

Local tenderness had improved, so the eighth day's treatment was repeated.

By the thirteenth day the alternate day mobilizing plus the daily traction resulted in freedom of movements, and only occasional sensations of ache in the arm.

PAIN SIMULATING SUPRASPINATUS TENDINITIS

Examination

Reference of pain from the vertebral column into joints is common and it is sometimes difficult to determine the origin of, say, shoulder pain, as demonstrated in the example which follows. When pain is referred, the joint signs consist of pain on movement without restriction. Sometimes there is pain in an associated area such as the scapula to guide the examiner but this is not necessarily so. Sometimes there are no vertebral column signs to indicate that the shoulder pain arises in the neck. The only way of finding out is to treat the neck and observe the shoulder pain. The response to treatment, when the neck is the cause, is always quick which makes assessment easier. This problem of vertebral cause of peripheral joint pain is common in the hip and shoulder and less common in the elbow or knee. The following case history is given as one example.

History

A young man aged 25 years was referred for physiotherapy treatment to his right shoulder which had been painful for two months.

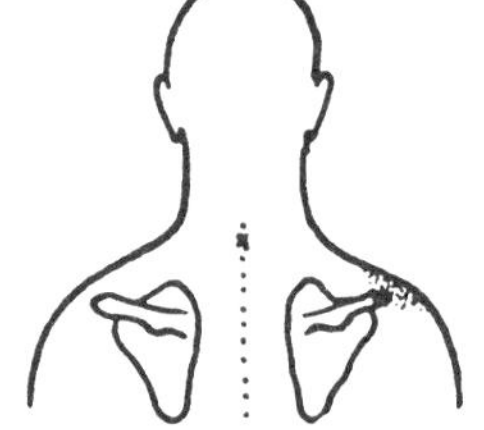

Figure 8.8. – Shoulder symptoms of cervical origin

Cortisone injections into the shoulder 18 days ago had caused a severe reaction.

The patient said the symptoms had come on gradually and he knew of no previous history of pain or injury. His symptoms consisted of an ache in the shoulder at night, and jabs of pain on top of the shoulder with movements of the arm during the day (*Figure 8.8*).

Physical findings

There was an arc of pain felt on top of the shoulder during mid-range abduction. A static contraction of supraspinatus muscle also caused pain on top of the shoulder. Passive movements of the acromioclavicular joint and glenohumeral joint were painless. All cervical movements were full range and painless. Except for slight tenderness in the region of the insertion of the right supraspinatus tendon, all tissues felt normal.

Treatment

Guiding factors

Shoulder treatment with emphasis on the supraspinatus tendon is to be given by short-wave diathermy and deep-friction massage to the tendon.

First–tenth days

During the first 10 days of treatment there were some nights when the shoulder did not ache. However, the arc of pain on abduction remained unchanged. On the eleventh day the site of the pain had changed to the middle of the supraspinous fossa.

Eleventh day

With the pain in a new position, cervical movements were rechecked and were found to be full, but rotation to the right and extension reproduced this right supraspinous fossa pain. With closer questioning the patient recalled pain in this area approximately two weeks before his shoulder pain developed. He also mentioned that in recent years he occasionally wakened with a slightly stiff neck which always disappeared within one or two hours of getting up. Mobilization of the cervical spine by left rotation was used as an oscillation for 1 minute and, upon favourable assessment of progress was repeated twice more. Abduction had then lost its painful arc and cervical movements were painless. The static test of the supraspinatus had also become painless. Local shoulder treatment was discontinued.

Twelfth day

The patient reported feeling much better, but this cervical rotation to the right still caused supraspinous fossa pain. Cervical extension and shoulder abduction were still painless. Rotation mobilization to the left was repeated three times and resulted in painless neck movements.

Thirteenth day

Pain had returned to the top of the shoulder and the painful arc of abduction had also returned. Cervical rotation to the right again caused pain in the right supraspinous fossa. Treatment mobilizing the cervical spine with a rotation to the left was repeated and resulted in freedom from all symptoms and signs, including the arc of pain with abduction.

Fourteenth day

Treatment was cancelled as the patient had no pain, and neck and shoulder movements were painless.

Treatment of further developments

There was a slight return of supraspinous fossa pain two weeks later which was cleared with mobilizing the cervical spine by rotation to the left on two consecutive days. He was later known to have remained symptom free for four months.

It should not be concluded from this case history that all shoulder conditions which have a painful arc of movement must be treated by mobilization of the cervical spine, but that such symptoms may have a cervical component.

PAIN SIMULATING MIGRAINE

Examination

History

A woman aged 40 years had a 21 year history of what the doctor had called migraine. During this time her longest period without pain had been two years. In each bout of pain the symptoms began at the back of the neck and then spread into the right occipital area and then over the head to the right ear and the right frontal area. The pain, which she described as a vicious throb, lasted from two to eight days, enforcing bed rest in the early stages. Symptoms of pain were accompanied by nausea and blurring vision. The only prodrome was a 'feeling of well-being' (*Figure 8.9*).

At the time of treatment the patient was having two attacks per week and was controlling them with drugs.

Physical findings (at the end of an attack)

Head and neck movements were quite full, but flexion and extension gave general discomfort in the right upper neck area. Right lateral

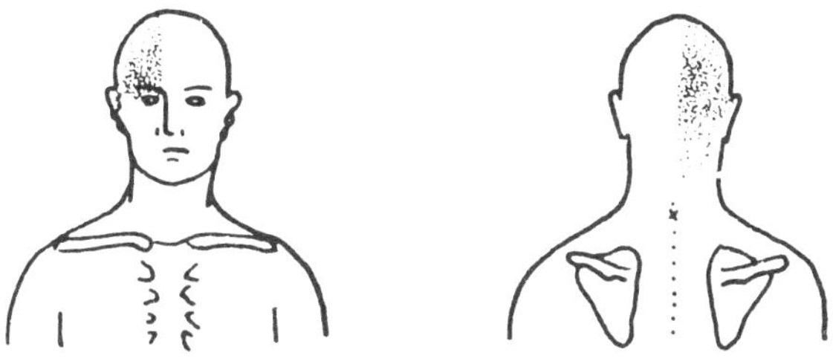

Figure 8.9. – Cervical headache

flexion gave moderate pain on both sides of the neck at the level of C1, whereas left lateral flexion hurt only to the right of C1. Rotation to the left was normal but to the right it caused pain to the right of C1.

Treatment

Guiding factors

1. While the patient's symptoms are severe, gentle and sustained traction in neutral would possibly ease the symptoms considerably.
2. Rotation is usually the best procedure for helping neck conditions, particularly when they are unilateral.
3. It needs to be explained to the patient that, once the pain to the right of C1 (which can be produced by testing movements) has been eliminated, treatment will only be given during attacks, and therefore the end-result may appear slow in coming.

4. The progress should consist of a lessening of the severity of the attacks and an extension of the pain-free period between the attacks.
5. Treatment should be instituted as soon as an attack begins, whatever the hour or day.
6. While treating during an attack, the treatment sessions can be expected to be long because extended rests should be given between techniques.
7. The changes which can be anticipated from the various procedures should be the same as would be expected with other vertebral syndromes.
8. The first aim is to make all cervical movements free of the pain at the right of C1 and to note how freedom from this alters the patient's pain cycle.

First–third day

Rotation mobilizations (done only to the left) were given as gentle but sustained procedures, twice the first day and four times on the second and third days. This produced a gradual clearing of the pain felt to the right of the first cervical vertebra.

Fourth day

The patient reported with all of the disturbances which accompany an attack but she did not have the usual throbbing head pain. The pain to the right of C1 had reappeared and had become more noticeable.

Gentle traction in neutral was given for 10 minutes and this eased the feeling of nausea and cleared her blurred vision. These symptoms did not return on releasing the traction. After a 5 minute rest the traction was repeated.

Fifth and sixth days

The nausea, although less, was still present, returning two and four hours respectively after the fourth and fifth day's treatments.

Traction was repeated in two periods, one of 20 minutes and the other of 10 minutes, on each day but this only produced a slight improvement.

Seventh day

Vision was normal and nausea was absent, but the pain to the right of C1 was still in evidence on rotation, especially if this was done to the right, and there was slight right frontal pain.

Rotation mobilization to the left was done four times as a much stronger oscillatory procedure. This resulted in a clearing of all symptoms and signs.

Eighth day

The patient reported feeling well, and the only remaining sign was pain to the right of C1 when the head was put into full extension and then laterally flexed and rotated to the right.

Rotation mobilization to the left was done twice as a strong full range procedure, allowing a 10 minute rest between. This made the patient free of pain on testing.

Treatment of further developments–1

The patient remained symptom free for 10 days (a much longer period of freedom then usual), and then returned with pain on the right side of the neck radiating over the right side of the head to the frontal area, with blurred vision and a feeling of nausea.

On examination, rotation to the right caused pain in the right side of the neck at the C1 level. This pain increased both in intensity and area to a right hemicranial pain if the rotation was combined with right lateral flexion and full extension (the upper cervical quadrant).

First day

The patient was given left rotation manipulation without traction three times during a 2 hour period which allowed for long periods of rest. rest. Symptoms were greatly eased and movements became less painful.

Second and third days

The patient felt pleased that she had not had to resort to drugs. There were fewer symptoms and by the third day she only had slight right frontal pain with testing rotation in the position of right lateral flexion and extension.

Left rotation manipulations were repeated with shorter rests between as they became unnecessary. By the end of the treatment on the third day she was both symptom free and sign free again.

Fourth and fifth days

There was a mild overnight recurrence of right hemicranial ache, not pain, which indicated that treatment should continue. There was no nausea or blurring of vision. During the treatment on the fourth and fifth days longitudinal movement, rotation to the right and postero-anterior central vertebral pressure were attempted in turn, but as each was used it caused an increase in symptoms, and rotation to the left had to be reinstituted in order to settle them. It was now known that rotation manipulation to the left was the effective treatment in this case.

Sixth and seventh days

Rotation manipulation to the left was the only technique used, and by the end of this period the patient was again symptom free and sign free.

Treatment of further developments–2

The patient remained symptom free for 13 days, indicating further improvement, and then developed moderate pain in the right occipital and adjacent neck area with slight right frontal pain. The feeling of nausea was minimal. The usual sign of pain with rotation to the right was present.

First day

At this stage rotation left manipulation without traction was the most effective treatment for this patient, and it was known that it could be done as a strong procedure with safety. As nausea was not excessive, long rests between manipulations were unnecessary. Rotation to the left was given four times as a very strong and sustained oscillating movement followed by a manipulative flick. The patient's neck on the left side was then too sore to allow further treatment. Active rotation to the right was almost painless, and all nausea and head pain had gone.

Second day

There was no nausea and only slight frontal pain. Rotation to the right still caused some pain to the right of C1.

Maximum-range forced rotation to the left was given three times with complete relief of symptoms and signs.

Treatment of further developments–3

The patient remained symptom free for a further three weeks; she then developed a mild right frontal pain. Active rotation to the right was painless even when done in conjunction with right lateral flexion and extension.

First day

Rotation manipulation to the left was given twice, followed by a 30 minute period of rest. As the symptom did not return further manipulation was considered unnecessary.

This treatment was given in 1957, and she is known to have remained free from attacks until she died in 1965.

SCAPULAR PAIN

Examination

History

One week ago while yawning and stretching a woman aged 40 years felt a sharp pain over the left scapula. During the next two hours the ache increased slightly in intensity and spread over a greater area to cover the left side of the lower neck and the left middle and upper scapular area (*Figure 8.10*). After that the symptoms remained unaltered.

The patient had had a similar episode a year ago which recovered without treatment in four days.

Physical findings

The symptoms consisted of a constant nagging scapular ache which was aggravated by movement and partially relieved by rest. Trunk and shoulder movements were full and painless, but the cervical movements, except for left lateral flexion and right rotation, were all very limited and caused scapular pain. Forward flexion lacked 50 per cent of its movement, and although it was possible to initiate extension, pain then prevented further movement. Rotation of the head to the left was limited by 50 per cent and pain prevented all but the first few degrees of right lateral flexion. (This combination of limited

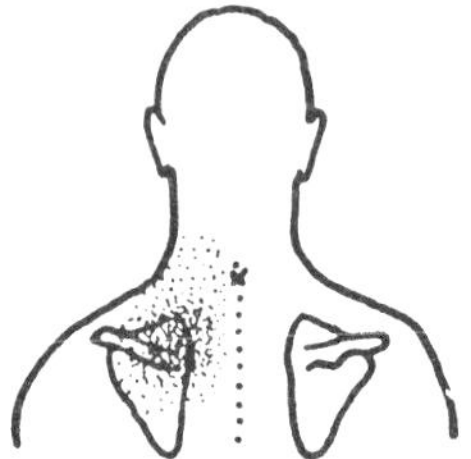

Figure 8.10. – Scapular pain

rotation to one side and lateral flexion to the opposite side is unusual.) With all of these movements pain in the left scapula was markedly increased. The only tenderness which could be found was over the spinous processes between T2 and T4.

Treatment

Guiding factors

1. Scapular pain can be caused by either a cervical or an upper thoracic condition; therefore both areas may need to be treated.
2. As the cervical movements are so limited, it would be wiser to treat this area first.
3. Conditions of sudden onset usually respond more rapidly to manipulation than to traction.
4. Rotation right would probably be the main technique here.

First Day

Mobilization of the cervical spine by rotation to the right was given very gently for 20 seconds. Following this, cervical extension and right lateral flexion had increased 20 degrees. The technique was repeated but as there was no pain or muscle spasm with the oscillation it was done with greater pressure. Following three applications of this rotation the patient had 50 per cent of her range of extension and right lateral flexion; full flexion and left rotation only lacked 20 degrees. All these movements still caused scapular pain. The patient was warned of the possibility of an increase in symptoms following treatment.

Second day

There had been no increase of symptoms and the patient felt much better. The range of movement had remained the same as had been obtained following the first treatment. The same mobilization was given but it was done seven times. There was no improvement with the last two applications of the rotation but overall the movements made further improvement. Flexion and right lateral flexion were full and painless. Rotation to the left increased by 10 degrees and now lacked the last 10 degrees of movement, while extension increased 10 degrees still lacking approximately 30 degrees of movement. Both these movements caused left scapular pain.

Third day

The improved movement was maintained and it was decided that, as progress had been slower on the second day, the upper thoracic spine should be included in the mobilization. As it was known how much improvement the rotation had produced on the second day, the thoracic mobilizing was done first to assess the comparative values of each. Transverse vertebral pressure was directed against the right side of the spinous processes of T2–T4. The technique was done firmly for 1 minute. The result was full left rotation and extension of the head, although both movements still caused pain. Following two further applications of transverse vertebral pressure, all pain had gone.

Fourth day

The patient could feel pain only in the left scapular area on full extension of the head or full rotation to the left. For the final treatment the patient was given transverse vertebral pressure against the spinous processes of T2–T4 followed by rotation to the right for the cervical spine. All movements were painless following the mobilization. No further treatment was required as the patient was free of symptoms and signs on the following day.

ACUTE TORTICOLLIS

Examination

History

A boy aged 16 years was wakened two nights ago at 3 a.m. by pain in the right side of his neck. He had never had any trouble with his neck previously and had not been carrying out any unusual work during the few days immediately prior to the incidence and had not been unwell (*Figure 8.11*).

Physical findings

The head and neck were held in a position of approximately 35 degrees of left lateral flexion and slight forward flexion. The patient said that there had been no improvement following one day of complete rest in bed.

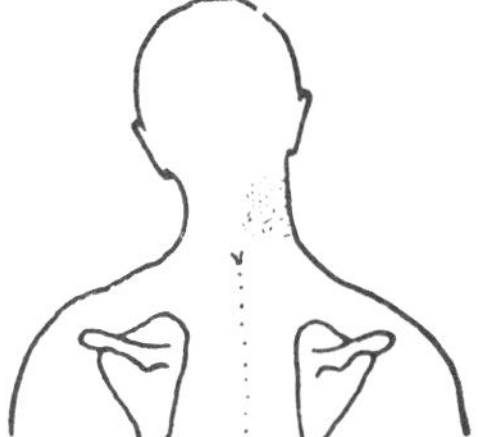

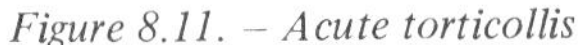

Figure 8.11. – Acute torticollis

His active range of flexion was full but gave some right middle neck pain. Both extension and right lateral flexion were grossly limited by the pain. Rotation to the left and right gave pain, but with rotation to the left the range was full, while to the right it was moderately restricted.

Treatment

Guiding factors

1. As there is some flexion deformity of the neck the result is likely to be slower than if only lateral flexion deformity were present.
2. If a day of rest has not made any difference, the patient is unlikely to respond to treatment as quickly or easily as would some patients with symptoms and signs of this type.
3. If manipulation is given it should be done gently, being guided by the patient's comfort.
4. The best result will possibly be obtained by doing a small amount of mobilizing to produce an increase in range of movement followed by gentle traction to maintain the improvement

while allowing soreness to subside. More mobilizing could then follow. This cycle should be repeated until the maximum progress has been gained. The last part of the treatment would need to be a period of traction.

5. As the patient is unable to extend his neck the traction will need to be given in flexion. This also applies to the mobilization used.
6. Following treatment the patient will need to rest with pillows supporting the neck.
7. If there is marked improvement during treatment on each of the first two days but with an overnight deterioration, a soft collar may be required to help maintain the progress. Under these circumstances the collar should not be needed for many days.
8. As symptoms are right sided the ideal technique will be rotation to the left but as there is deformity, care will be needed to ensure that a physiological rotary movement is produced.

First day

A rotation mobilization to the left was given first. This was done with the neck comfortably flexed. The rotation was taken gently to the limit of the range allowed by the pain and spasm. Once the limit was reached a gentle oscillation was carried out, attempting all the time to increase the spasm-free range. This was continued for approximately 1 minute. As there was quite a marked improvement from this one mobilization, it was decided to give traction in flexion while lying. This was done for 15 minutes. By doing this the following mobilizations would possibly be more effective and of less discomfort to the patient than if more mobilization was done at the beginning.

Following the 15 minutes' traction the angle of deformity was reduced but there was still marked limitation of right lateral flexion. Extension was greatly improved. Rotation mobilizing to the left was repeated three times, producing further improvement. During the mobilizing the rotation was easier to produce and the muscle spasm was much less. Traction was repeated.

The range of lateral flexion was then 50 per cent of normal and extension was 75 per cent of normal, but each movement still caused right neck pain. Some indication of the deformity was still present but the patient was able to adopt the normal head position without pain. Rotation was repeated three times. It was possible to do this much more strongly at this stage. Traction was repeated.

Following this, terminal extension caused pain, right lateral flexion was 75 per cent of full range and the deformity was almost gone. Rotation mobilization to the left was repeated twice more and traction reapplied. Movements were then full but were performed cautiously, and the deformity had gone.

The patient was asked to rest, using adequate neck support. As he had been using a rubber pillow, its disadvantage was explained; being rubber it has the tendency to maintain its shape, and during sleep this will result in a constant nudging against the relaxed neck. Although this may seem trivial, it is sufficient to irritate an easily disturbed neck. To give treatment every assistance, the patient was shown how to make an ordinary flock or feather pillow into a butterfly shape by shaking the stuffing to the ends and tying the centre isthmus lightly with ribbon. He was asked to lie with the isthmus under his neck for support, leaving the wings to stabilize the head. Then, whether he lies on his back or side, he has adequate support for the neck and the head. If necessary, a second small pillow can be used temporarily under the 'butterfly' pillow to give the amount of flexion needed to relieve the pain.

Second day

The deformity was almost gone, extension was full but caused slight right neck pain at the limit of its movement. Right lateral flexion was limited by approximately 25 per cent of its movement. Rotation to the left was full and painless, but to the right there was pain at the limit of the range. There had been more progress than was anticipated (*see* Treatment, (1) and (2)). Therefore more could be done without causing the patient discomfort.

Rotation left was repeated as a strong oscillating procedure. This made right lateral flexion almost full range after three mobilizations, but further repetition of the rotation did not produce much further increase. Extension was now full and painless, as was rotation left. Both lateral flexion right and rotation right caused terminal pain. Treatment was changed to mobilizing with left lateral flexion, and after being carried out twice it produced slight improvement. As the patient's neck was sore from the stronger procedures, he was given supine traction in flexion.

Following this there was no deformity and only pain with rotation to the right. One strong rotation was then given but this time to the right. Assessment was made difficult by soreness from the mobilization, but the patient was told that he need not rest at home.

Third day

There was no deformity and only right neck pain with full right lateral flexion and full right rotation.

The patient was manipulated twice with rotation without traction to the left, after which the movements were painless.

CERVICAL JOINT LOCKING

Examination

History

A girl aged 15 years while playing basketball had suddenly turned her head to the left and it had become stuck in this position. She felt pain on the right side of her neck. She had had no previous neck injury or symptoms and was not otherwise unhealthy (*Figure 8.11*).

Physical findings

She was unable to extend her head, or laterally flex or rotate it to the right. Examination by passive intervertebral movement showed the C2/3 joint to be fixed.

Treatment

Guiding factors

1. As it occurred easily it may clear easily.
2. Gentle longitudinal movement and rotation should be tried first.
3. If mobilization does not help a localized manipulation should be used to open the C2/3 joint on the right.
4. Complete restoration of range should be achieved on the first day though the movement may still be sore.

First day

Longitudinal movement was tried without success. Rotation to the left was tried next and this produced slight improvement. Repeating the movement did not help further. A localized diagonal thrust was used next tipping the patient's head to the left, patiently coaxing the position to relieve spasm first. One manipulation completely restored movement. The test for range by passive intervertebral movement was made following the manipulation to ensure that range was restored. Heat and massage were then given to relieve soreness.

Second day

Movement was normal but soreness was still present. Palliative treatment was given but further manipulation was considered unnecessary.

SHOOTING OCCIPITAL PAIN

Examination

History

A man aged 38 years bent over a handbasin five weeks ago, and sustained a sharp pain across the neck at the level of C1. Following this he was unable to move his head without pain.

He complained of 'shooting' pains across his upper neck at the level of C1 when turning his head, and an ache which spread downwards in the midline from C1 to T1 (*Figure 8.12*).

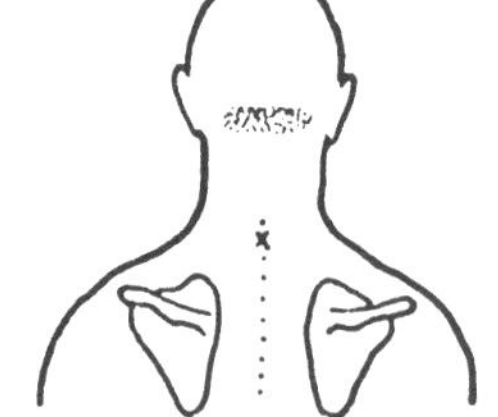

Figure 8.12. – Shooting occipital pain with movements

Physical findings

Neck flexion caused a pulling feeling in the area of the upper cervical spine but was full range if carried out cautiously. Extension and lateral flexion were painless. Rotation to each side was full range and caused moderate pain in the suboccipital area, but all movements had to be done slowly. Quick movements in flexion or rotation produced sharp suboccipital pain.

The referring doctor asked for treatment by traction and manipulation, to be attempted in that order.

Treatment

Guiding factors

1. As the symptoms are predominantly sharp pains with movements, an ineffective procedure should be changed quickly for another.
2. Sudden onsets with immediate limitations which do not become progressively worse over the following two or three days, are more likely to be helped by mobilization than by traction.
3. Upper cervical conditions are usually more difficult to help than mid-cervical conditions.
4. Rotation is usually the most effective procedure for the cervical spine, although postero-anterior central vertebral pressure is usually best for evenly distributed symptoms.
5. If traction is to be used, traction in neutral would be preferred to traction in flexion, as the condition is probably arising from the upper cervical spine.
6. As the patient can only attend for treatment for two consecutive days in nine it will be reasonable to give a long treatment on the second day despite soreness if progress is being achieved, as the patient will have a week before further treatment can be given.

First day

Traction in neutral was applied gently at first, but as this produced no improvement in the pain felt with movements while it was on, it was gradually increased until a firm traction was applied for 10 minutes. After the traction there was a feeling of burning suboccipitally and a feeling of general loosening of the neck, but there was no improvement in the sharp pains. It seemed pointless continuing with traction as there had been no quick progress.

With the patient lying, longitudinal movement as an oscillatory procedure was applied. After 20 seconds of this, rotation to the left was improved but other movements remained unchanged. This was repeated twice more without further change.

As right rotation now caused more pain than left rotation, it was decided to use left rotation as the next mobilization. This was done firstly as an oscillating procedure, then as a manipulation without traction. As this did not produce any improvement the same order was tried with rotation to the right, but this also did not produce any improvement. No further treatment was given that day, and the patient was warned of a possible exacerbation of symptoms following the treatment.

Second day

The patient reported a bad night with a lot of shooting pains, but these symptoms had subsided to their usual level today.

As traction and rotation had failed, postero-anterior central vertebral pressure was used next, localizing it to C1 and C2, commencing gently for approximately 15 seconds. There was an immediate improvement in the freedom of rotationary movements following this technique.

This mobilization was continued as it was producing a steady improvement in the freedom from pain with movements. Because the patient could not come in again for a week, the technique was carried out 12 times with gradually increasing pressure. The patient was again warned of the possibility of temporary flare up of his symptoms.

Third day (one week later)

Thirty minutes after the last treatment the patient had vomited and had a lot of shooting suboccipital pain, but by the following day he felt markedly improved, and had been almost free of pain ever since. Currently his symptoms were ‘a feeling of limitation to turning the head but no real jabs of pain’.

The same postero-anterior central vertebral pressure was used for a further five times. This made rotation painless and unrestricted.

Fourth day (following day)

Except for a slight pain on full quick active rotation the patient felt normal. There was no recurrence of vomiting. The treatment given on the third day was repeated, resulting in full free rotation.

The patient wrote one week later stating that he had lost all his symptoms.

LUMBAR

LOW BACK PAIN

Examination

History

A woman aged 43 years was limited in the amount of housework she could do because of backache and pain with movement of the back. Since the age of 20 she had had bouts of back pain usually following heavy work.

She had had her present bout for two weeks, during which time it had not improved (*Figure 8.13*).

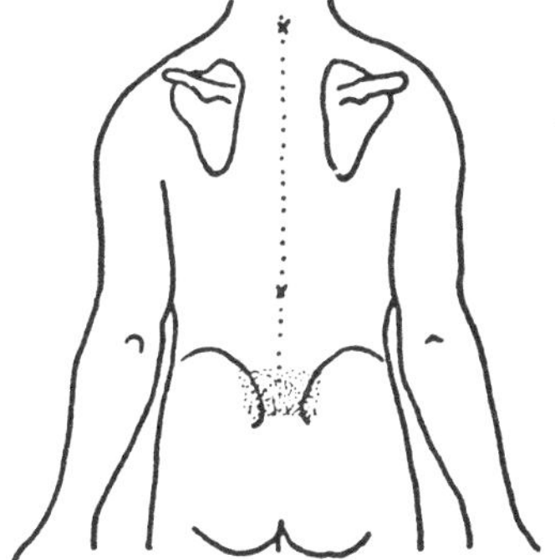

Figure 8.13. – Low back pain with marked radiological degenerative changes

The ache was relieved by short rests, but a full night's rest in bed caused stiffness of the lower back. This stiffness readily disappeared on moving about but the backache became much worse by the end of the day. Sitting increased her backache and she always experienced difficulty rising from a chair. Sneezing caused considerable back pain.

Physical findings

With forward flexion the patient's lower lumbar spine was lordosed and she was only able to reach her knees before pain prevented further movement. Backward bending was limited and lateral flexion to the right was more limited and more painful than to the left. Rotation and straight leg raising were normal. The lumbar spine was generally tender in the area of pain (L4–S1). Radiologically the body of L4 was almost sitting on L5 and they were fused on the left. The lumbosacral disc space was extremely narrow, and this was narrower on the left. This created a scoliosis convex to the right from L4 to S1 and there was a compensating scoliosis above L4 convex to the left together with a slight amount of rotation. Passive intervertebral movements of the lower spine could not be adequately tested for range, because of pain.

Treatment

Guiding factors

1. Painful movements when associated with marked radiological degenerative changes are often helped by gentle oscillating mobilization, particularly postero-anterior central vertebral pressure.
2. Even though the symptoms are bilateral, the pain felt with lateral flexion is worse when done to the right. It may therefore be better to use a rotation mobilization using the right side as the dominantly painful side.
3. Symptoms which have a gradual onset usually respond better to traction than to manipulation.

First day

Postero-anterior central vertebral pressure was chosen and was done for a period of 20 seconds as a very gentle oscillating procedure over L4 and L5. Forward flexion became more limited and the patient was only able to reach to 50 cm (20 inches) from the floor.

Mobilization was then changed to a gentle oscillating rotation with the patient lying on her left side. As this produced improvement in the range of forward flexion it was repeated three times. Forward flexion improved to 30 cm (13 inches) from the floor. Warning of a possible exacerbation was given.

Second day

The patient reported feeling easier for a while after treatment, but by the time she reached home the symptoms were very bad and she had a bad night. On examination forward flexion was still 30 cm (12 inches) from the floor. The amount of treatment was possibly the cause of the exacerbation, and not the technique used, so rotation was repeated three times with the patient lying on her left side. To reduce the possibility of a further exacerbation it was decided to stop at three times. Forward flexion improved by only 5 cm (2 inches).

Third day

The patient reported another bad night. Forward flexion remained 25 cm (10 inches) from the floor. Traction was considered to be the next step. Because movement was required, it was decided to use intermittent variable traction. Twelve kilograms were given for 10 minutes with a 5 second 'hold' period and no 'rest' period. At this low poundage she felt relieved of pain but said that if it had been any stronger it would have given her back pain.

On releasing the traction there was moderate back soreness. After a short rest the patient reported feeling better than before the traction. Forward flexion was not tested because this movement is often stiffer for a short period immediately following traction.

Fourth day

The patient felt greatly improved and forward flexion was now 20 cm (8 inches) from the floor. Traction was repeated.

Fifth–ninth days

There was steady and marked progress from day to day and traction was able to be slightly increased in pressure each day, until on the ninth day she felt no back discomfort with 30 kg of traction. The duration of traction did not exceed 15 minutes.

After the fifth traction (on the ninth day) all movements were full and painless actively, and she had been able to do housework without discomfort.

ACUTE BACK PAIN

Examination

History

During the last five years a heavy man aged 62 years had had three comparatively minor bouts of back pain, each of sudden onset from trifling incidents. His present bout commenced with a slight backache following weeding in the garden one week ago. The pain improved but was aggravated by an eight-hour drive in his car three days ago. Gradually the symptoms became more severe and changed in nature from the ache to a sharp pain with movement which eventually prevented walking. After two days in bed without any improvement in his symptoms, his doctor requested manipulation. At the time of treatment the patient was in bed unable to move because of jabs of pain in the centre of the lower back (*Figure 8.14*).

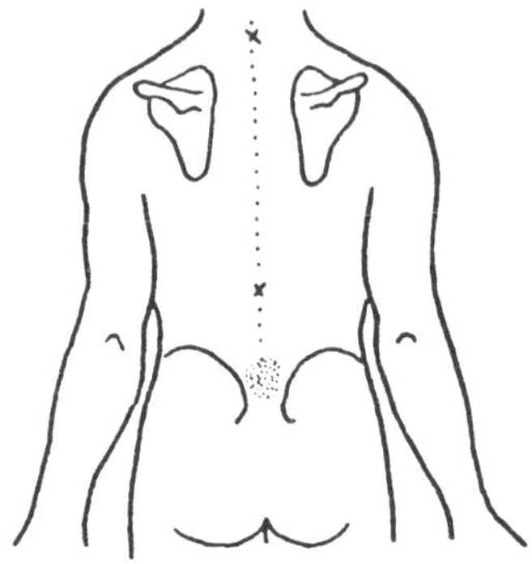

Figure 8.14. – Acute back pain confining patient to bed

Physical findings

It was impossible to examine more than straight leg raising, spreading and compressing the ilia, and neck flexion, as the patient was unable to move. Straight leg raising was almost full on both sides but more back pain was produced with raising the right leg than with raising the left. Flexion of the neck with the chin on the chest produced slight back pain and the sacro-iliac joint test was negative.

Treatment

Guiding factors

1. Examination is too limited to be conclusive but at least the symptoms are localized to the back and straight leg raising is good.

2. The fact that the response to straight leg raising varies slightly when comparing the left leg with the right leg may call for a unilateral technique when the patient is more mobile.

First day

The only technique possible with such an immobile patient, and possibly the best choice in view of the nature of the patient's symptoms, is longitudinal movement. The movement was done gently but sharply as three tugs using both legs. It caused marked pain each time at the site of his symptoms. Following this the pain with neck flexion was less. The tugs were repeated and neck flexion then became painless. Straight leg raising was then normal on the left, and although full range on the right, it still produced some back pain. The patient was still unwilling to try to move in bed. It was then decided to give the longitudinal movement using the right leg only. This was done in the same way as the two-leg technique, as it was obvious that the patient would not be able to kick. This procedure was done twice with two tugs each time. Right straight leg raising was then normal. The patient was given adequate warning that some exacerbation might occur during the next few hours.

Second day

There was only a slight flare-up of symptoms, and the patient was able to walk about but he was unable to bend. He had lost most of his 'catching' pain. On examination he had a slight protective scoliosis with the displacement of his shoulders being to his left side. Forward flexion was very limited and this caused central pain at the level of L5. Right lateral flexion was very limited and painful, but to the left it was full and painless. Backward bending, straight leg raising and neck flexion were normal.

The protective scoliosis resulting in a tilt to the left and the unilateral straight leg raising of the previous day suggested a unilateral problem (predominantly right sided) even though symptoms were central.

Rotation mobilizing was given with the patient lying on his left side. After two rotations the protective scoliosis had gone and lateral flexion right was full and painless. Forward flexion had improved but was still limited and painful. Rotation was repeated twice more without any further improvement. It was suggested that the patient should rest for an hour, after which he should walk about as much as possible, provided that the symptoms were not aggravated.

Third day

There was no exacerbation and the patient had been up most of the day. Also there were fewer symptoms. The scoliosis had returned but right lateral flexion was full and painless. Forward flexion was still limited.

Rotation, which was repeated twice, eliminated the scoliosis and partly improved the range of forward flexion. This technique was repeated twice more but did not produce any change.

Longitudinal movement using the kicking action of the patient's right leg was used four times. With each of the first three, there was an increase in the range of forward flexion until it became almost full, but the fourth did not produce any further improvement.

The patient was asked to move about normally.

Fourth day

There was no scoliosis and only slight limitation of forward flexion. The patient said he felt almost normal.

Rotation was repeated twice and followed by two applications of longitudinal movement using the patient's right leg. Forward flexion was then full range and painless.

Forward flexion remained normal and treatment was discontinued.

L1 BUTTOCK PAIN

Examination

History

A man aged 55 years gradually developed right buttock pain over a period of five days while engaged on heavy shovel work six months ago. He was able to continue work, and although the aching did not become any worse it did not improve. After a long period of unsuccessful treatment involving what he called 'adjustments', he went to his local doctor. After a week of bed rest failed to help him, his doctor suggested a further trial of manipulation (*Figure 8.15*).

Physical findings

His symptoms consisted of a constant ache felt superficially in the right upper gluteal area. The ache did not seem to vary much with moderate activity or rest. With the exception of extension which reproduced the buttock pain, his spinal movements were painless although all movements were stiff. His thoracolumbar area was kyphosed but the patient said that it had always been so. There was no tenderness in the buttock or spine, but with firm pressure over the spinous processes of L1 and L2, a deeply situated protective muscle spasm could be felt. With the application of this pressure it was possible to feel a limitation of movement in this postero-anterior direction when compared with the areas above and below this level. By questioning the patient it was noted that his treatment by adjustments had consisted of rotation of the lumbar spine, pressure over the lower lumbar spine, and a whip-cracking action of the back produced by using the patient's leg as the handle of the whip while the patient was lying prone.

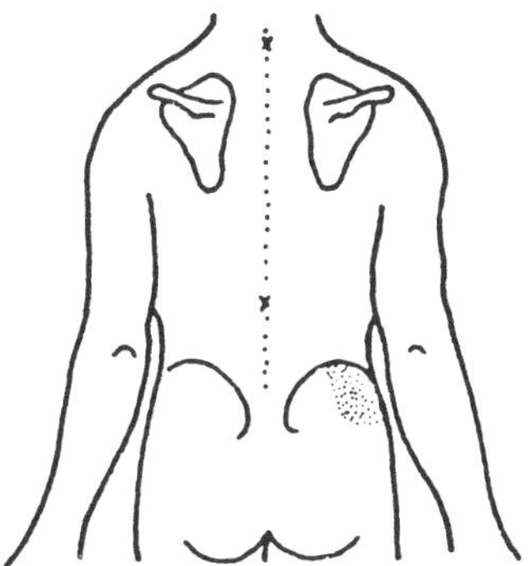

Figure 8.15. – L1 buttock pain

Treatment

Guiding factors

1. When a patient has been unsuccessfully treated elsewhere by manipulation one expects more difficulty in alleviating the symptoms.
2. The whip-cracking and pressure of the previous treatment would have been effective only on the lower lumbar spine. Rotation is more valuable for treating the lower lumbar spine than the upper lumbar spine.
3. In view of the deep spasm in the upper lumbar area and the limitation of postero-anterior movement, it would be better to direct mobilization at this level using postero-anterior central vertebral pressure.

4. It is possible for buttock pain to arise from the upper lumbar spine.
5. As rotation did not help in the patient's earlier treatment, it would be better to begin with postero-anterior central vertebral pressure or transverse vertebral pressure.
6. Because the symptoms developed slowly, and did not respond to adjustments it may be better to begin treatment with traction.

First day

With the presence of muscle spasm and the likelihood of the symptoms having an upper lumbar origin, it was decided to begin by mobilizing between T12 and L2. Postero-anterior central vertebral pressure was given firmly, attempting to give the maximum pressure possible without causing muscle spasm. One minute was spent mobilizing the area at this pressure. The procedure caused no change in the patient's symptoms or signs. This technique was repeated twice more because it was felt that the muscle spasm was lessening. By the end of the treatment the ache in the buttock had eased by 50 per cent.

Second day

Although there was little change, the patient considered he could feel some improvement for the first time in six months. This indicated that treatment was probably being directed at the right level. Postero-anterior central vertebral pressure was repeated but this technique was interspersed with transverse vertebral pressure pushing the spinous processes from left to right. The result following four applications of each technique was a further noticeable improvement in symptoms.

Third–sixth days

The second day's treatment was repeated during these four days. Symptoms gradually lessened day by day until, by the sixth day postero-anterior movement felt normal and it was free of muscle spasm.

It may be that if traction had been incorporated into the treatment routine on the third day, the total treatment time might have been shortened by one or perhaps two days. However, it seemed unwise to change from measures which were obviously proving successful.

SPONDYLITIC SPINE WITH
SUPERIMPOSED LOCALIZED LESION

Examination

History

An elderly man developed sharp pain in his left groin and quadriceps area following rest in bed for a kidney infection. He complained of a constant dull ache with intermittent sharp pains (*Figure 8.16*).

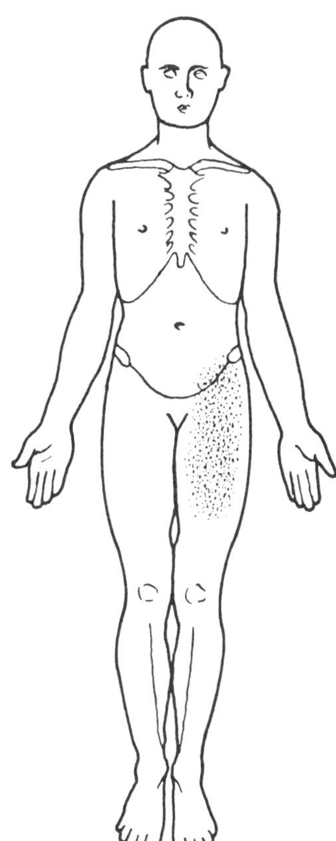

Figure 8.16. – Superimposed localized lesion

Physical findings

Radiologically he had marked spondylitic changes throughout his lumbar spine. Examination of his lumbar movements revealed that extension and left lateral flexion were both markedly limiting, causing pain in the left thigh. All other movements were pain free. Palpation in the L2/3 area revealed that transverse pressure at this joint, pushing towards the right, reproduced his right quadriceps pain.

Treatment

Guiding factors

1. An elderly patient with a lot of spondylitic change, having a superimposed localized joint lesion, is likely to be very difficult to help.
2. The localized mobilizing techniques are more likely to be helpful than the general techniques.
3. Traction, if it is to be used, will need to be of the intermittent variable type rather than the constant type.
4. It is likely that all suitable techniques will need to be used in concert.

First day

Transverse pressure towards the left at the L2/3 level and above and below this joint was performed three times. There was an improvement in extension and left lateral flexion but the movement was still very painful.

Second day

There was no unfavourable reaction from the first treatment so intermittent variable traction was added after the transverse pressures. The traction used was gentle and for a short time; 12 kg was given for 10 minutes with 3 second hold periods and no rest period.

Fourth day

There appeared to be a gradual but slow improvement in the range of extension and left lateral flexion so the treatment was continued and postero-anterior central vertebral pressure was added.

Sixth day

A further technique, that of lumbar rotation, pelvis to the right, was added.

Subsequent days

This treatment was continued daily for three weeks, at the end of which time he said he had had no pain in his leg for the previous three days and had been able to play 18 holes of golf without trouble. Treatment was discontinued.

COCCYGODYNIA

Examination

History

Six months ago, after an unusually long ride on a bicycle which had a wide seat, a woman aged 34 years developed pain in the region of the coccyx. This pain gradually increased until it reached a stage when she was unable to sit through a full cinema programme. The area ached for at least an hour after prolonged sitting, but provided she did not sit again she would remain symptom free.

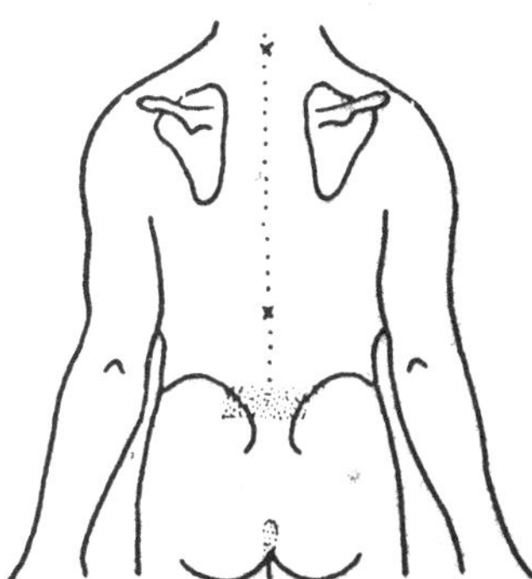

Figure 8.17. – Coccygodynia

Since the age of 16 she had had minor low back ache following gardening or heavy housework but this symptom had not altered during the last six months (*Figure 8.17*).

Her referring doctor felt that her symptoms might be from her lower back rather than of local coccygeal origin, and requested a trial of manipulative treatment directed to the back, to aid in assessing the source of the symptoms.

Physical findings

All movements of the lumbar spine were full and painless, but the patient was able to elicit pain in the coccyx by sitting on a hard seat and leaning back 10 degrees. Both the coccyx and lumbosacral joint were tender on pressure.

Treatment

Guiding factors

1. During each treatment period the only guides to progress are tenderness to pressure and the patient's ability to lean backwards while sitting on a hard seat.
2. As the symptoms are not unilaterally distributed the first choice for mobilizing should be postero-anterior central vertebral pressure.
3. As tenderness is one of the guides, it might be better to begin treatment with rotation to avoid the possibility of causing back soreness which could make it difficult for the patient to assess coccygeal soreness.
4. If rotation is used as the first mobilization it may be necessary to perform it to one side only at one treatment, and then assess the patient's ability to sit during the following 24 hours.

First day

Treatment by mobilizing with postero-anterior central vertebral pressure was given first as a gentle oscillating procedure from L3 to L5. Although there was some tenderness over L5, there was no muscle spasm. On reassessing the patient's ability to sit and lean backwards, the pain was still produced after 10 degrees of movement. The procedure was repeated twice more, after which the degree of leaning backwards had increased to 20 degrees. A further mobilization was given but this did not produce any further increase, so treatment was stopped.

Second day

The patient had not noticed any improvement but it now required 20 degrees of leaning backwards to produce the coccygeal pain while sitting. As this improvement had been maintained, it was decided to repeat the postero-anterior central vertebral pressure. After the first three times there was an improvement of 5 degrees with the sitting test but there was no further progress after the fourth.

Third day

There was a marked increase in lower back discomfort but no improvement in the ability to sit for prolonged periods. Coccygeal pain was caused by 15 degrees of leaning backwards in sitting. This was almost back to the original range. Rotation with the patient lying on her left side was the next mobilization chosen. This side was chosen merely because only one side should be used on one day. Four applications produced an improvement of 10 degrees (to 25 degrees) in the sitting test.

Fourth day

As no improvement could be reported and the sitting test had maintained its range of 25 degrees from the previous day, the rotation was applied with the patient lying on her right side. After three applications of this technique there was a further increase of 10 degrees (to 35 degrees) in the sitting test, but a fourth use of the rotation did not produce any further improvement.

Fifth day

All low back discomfort had gone and the patient noticed that the coccygeal ache had taken longer than usual to come on with sitting. On examination, the tenderness over the coccyx was approximately the same but the sitting and leaning back test had maintained its range of 35 degrees. Rotation with the patient lying on her right side was repeated three times, after which the patient could sit and lean backwards without feeling any discomfort. Also there was noticeably less coccygeal tenderness.

Sixth day

The patient considered that her ability to sit without pain had improved to 80 per cent of normal. There was very little tenderness on palpation but at the limit of leaning backwards in sitting the patient could feel coccygeal discomfort. The rotation was repeated four times, after which the sitting test was normal and tenderness had gone. It was decided to discontinue treatment for one week to assess progress, and suggested that the patient should return earlier if the symptoms became worse.

One week later

There were only odd times when pain was present, and she had been to the cinema twice during this time. On examination the sitting test was normal and palpation was painless. The rotation mobilization was repeated four times and treatment discontinued.

JUVENILE DISC LESION

Examination

History

Following a boating accident, a boy aged 19 years developed pain in his right buttock extending into the hamstring area. He had no previous history of back injury. Although symptoms were not severe they were preventing him from his normal work and he could not rest properly at night (*Figure 8.18*).

Physical findings

On standing he had a contralateral tilt which increased with the limited range of forward flexion he had. He was unable to reach beyond his knees but the limitation was due more to tightness than a feeling of pain in his buttock or leg. Right straight leg raising was also limited to 40 degrees but all other movements were full range and painless. There were no neurological changes.

Treatment

Guiding factors

1. Being young, this patient will be slow in his response to treatment.
2. Because the diagnosis is a disc lesion, rotation and traction are probably the two most important techniques.
3. Probably the techniques will need to be used quite firmly.
4. It is probable that treatment will effect an improvement in symptoms without making as much improvement in the signs.

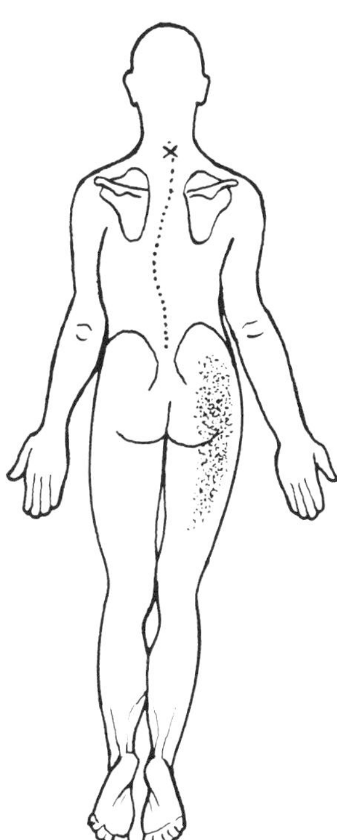

Figure 8.18. – Juvenile disc lesion

First day

Rotation of the pelvis to the left was performed four times and although this did not seem to make much difference to his movements, the patient was able to say that his leg felt freer.

Second day

He had retained the free feeling in his leg for four hours but it then returned to the previous state. The treatment was repeated and postero-anterior central vertebral pressure was added. The treatment again produced a freeing of his leg.

Third day

He retained the free feeling in his leg for longer though by the third day his symptoms were much as they had been. Treatment was repeated and traction was also added. This again produced freedom which was maintained for a similar period.

Subsequent days

The same treatment of rotation, central pressures and traction were repeated for the next five days during which time the symptoms became much easier. The freedom was retained from treatment to treatment and the scoliosis was reduced by 50 per cent. Straight leg raising and forward flexion were essentially the same, except that the pain felt at the limit of the ranges was decidedly less. Treatment was discontinued and the patient was reviewed one month later. At this stage his symptoms had remained relieved and his movements were approximately the same. On review 12 months later his scoliosis had gone, his straight leg raising and forward flexion had both improved by 30 per cent but were not normal. However, at this range they were pain free.

BILATERAL LEG PAIN

It is perfectly obvious that not all patients will respond to treatment by mobilization or manipulation. However, even when treatment is unsuccessful, if it is administered in a methodical and constructive manner the result can be so conclusive as to be of advantage in itself to the referring doctor. Frequently it is obvious that a patient requires surgery and would not respond to conservative measures. Although this is so, the unexpected occurs sufficiently often to justify a trial of manipulation because the number of treatments required to reach a conclusive result is usually few.

Examination

History

A girl aged 27 years had a five year history of trouble with her lower back and intermittent symptoms radiating into the buttocks and ham-string area. The onset had been insidious with periods of back pain during the first 18 months before pain spread into her leg. She had

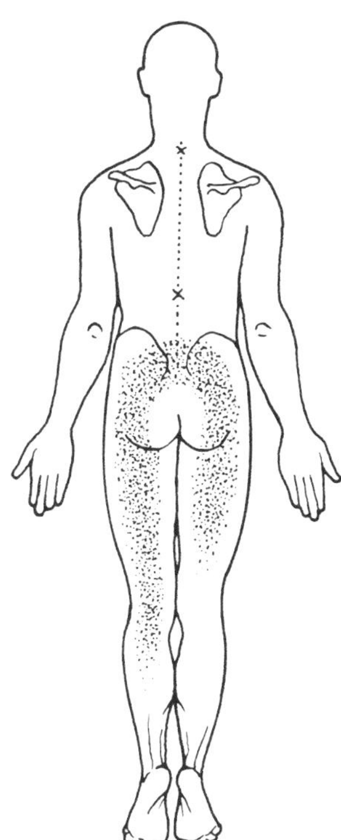

Figure 8.19. – Bilateral leg pain

been able to continue with her domestic work throughout this time. Two weeks prior to admission to hospital she had been cleaning floor-level cupboards and after working in the bent position for half an hour was unable to straighten. She was admitted to hospital and put on constant lumbar traction. After 11 days there had been no improvement in her symptoms or her signs (*Figure 8.19*).

Physical findings

On examination she was only able to reach her knees in flexion and she was unable to laterally flex to the left at all. Right lateral flexion was approximately 50 per cent of full range and she only had 10 degrees of extension. Straight leg raising on the left was 30 degrees and on the right was 45 degrees. Movement produced by pressure over the fourth and fifth lumbar spinous processes was limited by 50 per cent in all directions and at this point was strongly protected by muscle spasm. There were no neurological changes.

Treatment

Guiding factors

1. Symptoms are likely to be discogenic in origin; therefore the treatment techniques most likely to succeed are rotation and traction.
2. She has had traction administered on a constant basis without success; therefore further traction is unlikely to succeed.
3. The techniques which can be used in quick succession to give clear-cut information for the lumbar spine are rotation, central pressure, traction, and possibly straight leg raising.
4. Patients with bilateral leg symptoms are always slow to respond to treatment and difficult to help.
5. As this patient has a lot of pain as well as marked limitation of movement care will be necessary with techniques to avoid exacerbation.
6. Very careful assessment will need to be made to be sure of the effect of treatment as quickly as possible.
7. If rotation is to be used then the left side is the dominant side both from the point of view of signs and symptoms.

First day

Rotation to the right was administered firstly as a Grade I movement. However this irritated the symptoms while it was being done and produced no improvement in straight leg raising or other signs. The same movement was then attempted as a very gentle Grade IV. Less pain was provoked during this technique. On examination her forward flexion had improved 5 cm (2 inches) and her left lateral flexion showed signs of the first part of movement. The technique was repeated but did not produce any further improvement. The patient commented that the symptoms in her back were much worse.

Second day

Symptomatically she had been much worse. However it was her back which was worse and not her leg symptoms. On examination, her flexion and left lateral flexion had maintained their progress. The same rotation was attempted again but muscle spasm was present, preventing as good movement as could be achieved previously. On re-examination her movements had not improved further. It was decided to discontinue with that rotation and to attempt rotation on the other side. This could be done a little less easily than to the right and the technique did not produce any improvement in movements. The patient then lay prone and postero-anterior central vertebral pressure was attempted but this movement was found to be worse than on the day of the initial examination. Following its use as a very gentle Grade I technique movements were reassessed and found to be unchanged.

Third day

The patient reported again feeling worse in her back. Movements had not changed from that achieved following the first day's treatment. Attempted rotation and postero-anterior central vertebral pressure were both more difficult to achieve this day than on the second day. It seemed fairly obvious that there was no point in continuing treatment further.

A myelogram revealed a massive lumbosacral central protrusion and decompression surgery produced relief of symptoms.

THORACIC

'GLOVE' DISTRIBUTION OF SYMPTOMS

The T4 syndrome is commonly referred to. This does not mean that T4/5 is the joint always involved. It may refer to T3–T7, but it does imply symptoms of an ill-defined nature probably having their reference via the autonomic nervous system. It can be applied to symptoms in the arm or head. Symptoms are dull in nature and cover the whole of the head or hand or arm. The following example is one where symptoms were felt locally at the T4 level. However this is not essential though signs at the appropriate thoracic joint can always be found when symptoms arise from it.

Examination

History

A woman aged 42 years complained of intermittent 'pins and needles' involving the whole of the right hand. The symptoms appeared at least five times during a day lasting for as long as an hour each time. There were no symptoms at night. She had had these symptoms to a lesser degree during the last two years but they had recently increased in intensity and duration. As far as she knew there was no injury or strain which could have caused the onset two years ago or the more recent increase of symptoms.

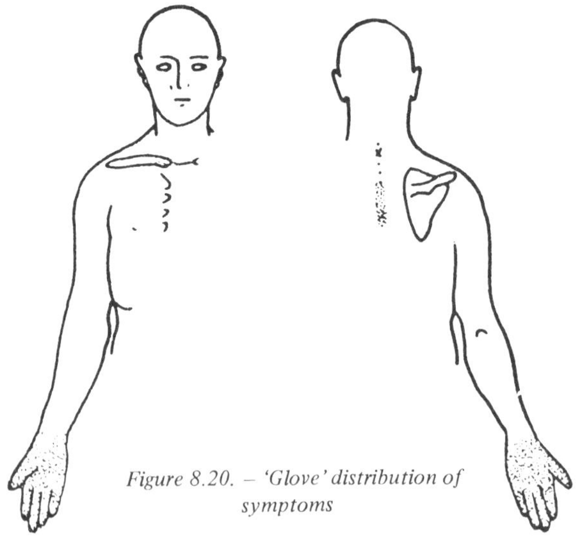

Figure 8.20. – 'Glove' distribution of symptoms

There was an area of extreme sensitivity in the mid-thoracic area which she had had for many years without change. Although hard rubbing of this area eased the sensitivity, she could not tolerate soft rubbing (*Figure 8.20*).

Treatment by traction and mobilization was requested.

Physical findings

Forward flexion was the only cervical movement which was painful. This movement lacked 40 per cent of its range and caused sharp pain along the anterior aspect of the right arm from the shoulder to the wrist. Trunk and upper limb movements were full and painless. There was no tenderness in the cervical spine but T5 was extremely tender and pressure here caused pain in the region of the right elbow. The patient was able to produce tingling in the hand by going through the actions of combing her hair, and these symptoms could be relieved by shaking her hand vigorously.

Treatment

Guiding factors

1. As there has not been a sudden or traumatic origin to account for these symptoms, traction may be the technique to try first.

2. Traction in flexion should be used before traction in neutral as the symptoms could hardly be of upper cervical origin.

3. Of the mobilizing techniques, rotation of the cervical spine should be used before postero-anterior central vertebral pressure as the symptoms are distributed unilaterally.

4. If none of the above techniques relieve the symptoms mobilization of the T5 area should be included. It must be remembered that the autonomic nerve supply for the arm arises from as low as T8.

First day

Traction in flexion was applied with firm pressure (approximately 15 kg) for 10 minutes. As there were no symptoms present in the hand at the time of treatment the pressure of the traction could not be gauged to suit the symptoms. On releasing the traction, neck flexion had improved a little, but hand tingling could still be produced by the patient combing her hair. After applying traction in flexion for a further 15 minutes, neck movements and hand tingling were unchanged.

Second day

The patient felt that there may have been a slight lessening of the intensity of the hand symptoms but the discomfort felt with combing her hair was unchanged. Neck flexion had maintained the slight improvement from the previous day. Traction in flexion was repeated, but this time it was carried out much more strongly (25 kg) as there had been little change, favourable or otherwise, from the previous traction. It was given for periods of 20 minutes and 15 minutes. Following the treatment, neck flexion had increased a further 5 degrees (making a total improvement of approximately 10 degrees) but the hair-combing test was still unchanged.

Third day

Neck flexion had maintained its slight improvement but there had been no further improvement in the hand symptoms. To enable the traction to be given more strongly, it was changed to traction in neutral and it was applied at a pressure which almost lifted the patient from the chair. While in this position she attempted the hair-combing test and found that although she could still bring about a tingling it was less intense. The patient was only able to tolerate 3 minutes of this traction the first time and 2 minutes the second, because of pain in the mid-thoracic area. Following the second traction her neck flexion was 5 degrees less than previously and the hair-combing test was unchanged.

Fourth day

The patient reported feeling about the same as she was before treatment, and on examination there seemed to have been no progress. Treatment was changed from traction to mobilization, and the first technique used was cervical rotation to the left. Remembering that the patient had been given strong traction without any ill effects, the mobilizing was done firmly from the beginning and the movement was sustained for 1 minute. Following this the hair-combing test was unchanged and neck flexion had improved 10 degrees. The rotation was repeated even more strongly but this did not produce any change in symptoms or signs. As no headway was being made the next mobilization given was a strongly applied postero-anterior central vertebral pressure alternating three times with transverse vertebral pressure directed against the left side of the spinous processes between C4 and T1. However, these techniques did not produce enough change to warrant continuing with them. It was decided therefore to mobilize the mid-thoracic spine before attempting cervical lateral flexion. Postero-anterior central vertebral pressure was applied from T3 to T7 at a pressure which did not cause pain in the patient's elbow. The oscillating was continued for 1.5 minutes. Following this treatment, neck flexion was full and painless and the hair-combing test had improved by approximately 50 per cent. While the mobilizing was being repeated it was found that the pressure could be markedly increased without causing local pain or referred pain. By the third application of the mobilization the patient was unable to induce the hand tingling by combing her hair.

Fifth–seventh days

There was a marked reduction in severity and duration of symptoms following the fourth day's treatment and neck flexion had remained full in its range although it still caused anterior arm pain. The postero-anterior central vertebral pressure was repeated between T3 and T7 without producing any elbow pain and again made the patient free of symptoms and signs. After treatment on the sixth day the patient remained symptom-free, but as T5 was still tender the mobilizing was repeated on the seventh day.

Treatment of further developments

One month later there was a mild recurrence of symptoms which was eliminated by two days of mobilizing the mid-thoracic area.

This case history has been included to show that the therapist must be aware that atypical symptoms can and do occur, and that one must be ready to treat the less obvious areas sometimes.

THORACIC BACKACHE

Examination

History

A woman aged 31 years first noticed thoracic backache four years ago. It came on following heavy work of an unusual nature and took two weeks to subside. After this attack she had similar aches following any particularly heavy work even though there was never any incident of sudden pain with this work. The ache would subside in two weeks. More recently the ache had become continuous, but it was always further aggravated by heavy work. On waking each morning there was a marked feeling of stiffness in this area of the thoracic spine (*Figure 8.21*), but the stiffness would disappear after she had been up and about for 30 minutes.

Physical findings

Symptoms were evenly distributed to each side of the spine. There were few positive signs. Trunk rotation to each side was limited by 20–25 degrees, and each movement caused pain 2.5 cm (1 inch) to the left of the T8/9 area. When the intervertebral joints were tested passively, there was a limitation of rotation between T4 and T5 and between T5 and T6. There was very marked tenderness to pressure over the spinous processes of T4, T5 and T6, and to a lesser extent over T3 and T7. When firm pressure was applied over this area of the spine, strong muscular contraction came into play to prevent intervertebral movement.

Treatment

Guiding factors

1. Mobilization will need to be kept within the limits of the spasm.
2. Symptoms are evenly distributed but there is left-sided pain with rotation to left or right which may therefore require a unilateral technique.
3. The thoracic spine responds best to postero-anterior central vertebral pressure first and transverse vertebral pressure towards the painful side (left side in this case) next.
4. With this patient there are three things to eliminate, namely the ache, the stiffness on rising, and the tenderness with limitation of movement between T4 and T6. The tenderness and movement will be helped by mobilization, but the ache and stiffness may require traction.
5. As mobilization is quicker in its effect, it should be used first.

First day

Postero-anterior central vertebral pressure was given first over the spinous processes from T3 down to T8. There was marked tenderness between T4 and T6 necessitating a gentler pressure. The oscillating was done steadily, taking it approximately 1.5 minutes to cover the area. The spasm did not prove to be any obstacle as localized tenderness prevented the depth of oscillation which would have caused the muscle spasm. There was an increase of 10 degrees in the rotation to each side following this procedure and pain was still left sided.

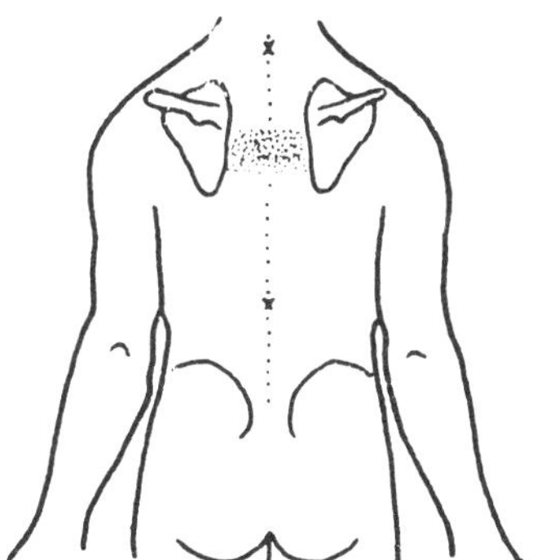

Figure 8.21. – Thoracic backache

This gently oscillating mobilization was repeated another three times. Rotation, which improved but was not yet full range, caused a feeling of general thoracic soreness rather than a left-sided pain. After a short rest the patient thought the ache was less than before the treatment.

Adequate warning of a possible increase of symptoms was given and she was asked to refrain from any work which she knew would aggravate her symptoms.

Second day

The ache and the stiffness on rising were unchanged. The centre of the patient's back was sore (presumably from the mobilizing) and rotation to the left produced left-sided pain, but now lacked only 15 degrees of its full range.

The same postero-anterior central vertebral pressure was given but it was done more firmly. Even though the area was sore it was possible to increase the pressure to the level of the muscle spasm. This was repeated four times, still maintaining the oscillating and taking 1.5 minutes to complete each time. The range of movement was then full and painless, but the spine felt very sore.

It was decided to leave treatment for 48 hours to allow the soreness to subside and thus make assessment more informative.

Third day

During the day following treatment the patient's back was sore, but she reported that the ache was less severe. Stiffness on rising had remained unchanged. Rotation was now only slightly limited, but still caused left-sided pain. There was less tenderness than at the beginning of treatment, and there was now no muscle spasm.

Postero-anterior central vertebral pressure was repeated gently as a continuous oscillation four times, and was interspersed with transverse vertebral pressure pushing against the right side of the spinous processes from T3 to T7, pushing them towards the painful left side. This was done three times. Rotation became full and painless, being the best result obtained with treatment of this patient so far.

It was decided to leave assessment for three days to allow all soreness to subside again.

Fourth day

All soreness had gone and backache was almost nil. However, the patient still had stiffness on rising, and although rotation was full, it gave a general feeling of soreness in the thoracic area.

The movements appeared normal but some backache and stiffness remained, so it was decided to give the patient traction.

The passive range of intervertebral rotation was found to have improved and to be almost normal. As some limitation remained it was decided that the mobilizations should be repeated. Had this movement not improved it would have been necessary to manipulate these intervertebral joints.

The oscillating techniques of the third day's treatment were repeated. There was no muscle spasm and very little soreness. Following this, the patient was given traction in two periods lasting 15 minutes and 10 minutes. The angle of pull on the cervical halter was approximately 30 degrees with the horizontal, and although the patient had not had any low back pain, the flexed hip and knee position was adopted.

Fifth day

In the morning she reported feeling very much better. There was no ache and almost no stiffness on rising. Rotation was normal both actively and on passively testing the movement at the intervertebral joint.

No mobilization was given, but traction was repeated for another two periods of 15 minutes and 10 minutes.

She reported one week later having had no backache or stiffness since the last treatment.

TRAUMATIC GIRDLE PAIN

Examination

History

Following a vehicular accident one week ago, a man aged 33 years suffered a collapse of the left upper lobe of the lung and girdle pain (left side greater than right side) at the fifth thoracic level. Because of chest pain breathing was difficult, coughing was impossible, and the man was unable to lift his left arm above his head. He had two nerve blocks but these gave only temporary relief (*Figure 8.22*).

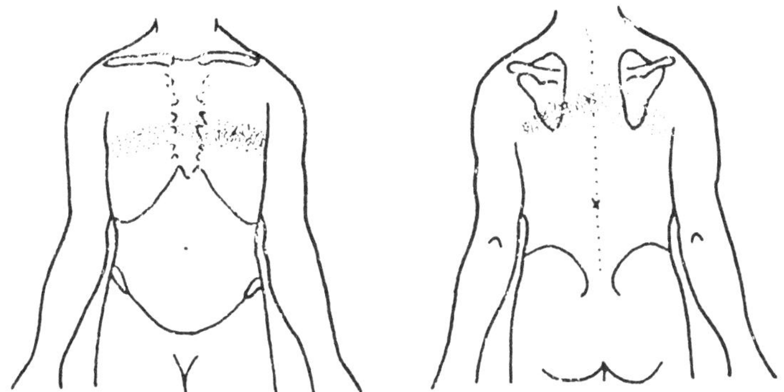

Figure 8.22. – Traumatic girdle pain

Physical findings

The trunk was held rigid as if to avoid all movement, as movements of the head caused chest pain. On the left side of the trunk the constant pain radiated throughout the fifth thoracic level from the vertebra around the thoracic cage to the sternum. The right-sided pain which was mild and intermittent would subside with rest. Trunk rotation to the left caused pain throughout the area but particularly posteriorly on the left after 10 degrees of movement. Rotation to the right caused pain after 40 degrees. With lateral flexion of the trunk, pain was produced at the beginning of the movement to the left and after 20 degrees of the movement to the right. Trunk flexion could be performed more readily than other movements but it still had to be done slowly. Without any obvious movements of the trunk, 50 degrees of head and neck extension caused the thoracic pain. Cervical rotation to the left, which lacked 20 degrees movement, also caused thoracic pain. Tenderness was most marked over the spinous processes of the third to the sixth thoracic vertebrae.

Treatment

Guiding factors

1. As symptoms are severe and movements are grossly limited, mobilizing will need to be done extremely gently.
2. Traction may be made difficult by the patient's inability to lie on his back without pain but perhaps it could be done sitting.
3. Although symptoms and signs have a unilateral dominance, postero-anterior central vertebral pressure will probably be the best procedure as it is the main technique for the thoracic area and as symptoms spread to both sides.

First day

Postero-anterior central vertebral pressure was given very gently over the spinous processes from the second to the seventh thoracic vertebrae. The mobilizing, which was done so softly that spasm and pain were avoided, was continued over a period of two minutes. Trunk rotation to the left improved from 10 to 25 degrees movement. The procedure was repeated twice more, after which rotation to the left was 45 degrees. All other movements improved including raising the arm. The patient said that the pain had had the 'sting' taken out of it. To avoid joint soreness it was decided to stop treatment for that day. Warning was given of the possibility of an increase in symptoms later in the day.

Second day

The patient reported having felt wonderful for five hours, but that in the morning he had felt worse. On examination, the arm movement had remained improved and trunk rotation to the left was possible through 30 degrees. This is an example of a patient feeling worse possibly due to treatment soreness but whose signs show improvement. Patients may complain of severe pain and may continue to feel that their pain is worse, despite improvement in signs, for as long as five days. However, the improvement in signs guides the therapist in the choice of techniques. Postero-anterior central vertebral pressure, repeated as a firmer procedure, was more uncomfortable than on the first day, but it still was not done firmly enough to cause muscle spasm. The procedure was repeated three times and the result was an increase in trunk rotation to the left to 60 degrees.

Third day

The patient felt much better and left trunk rotation was possibly through 45 degrees. Transverse vertebral pressure was used against the right side of the spinous processes of the second–seventh thoracic vertebrae, moving them towards the more painful left side. After two applications of this technique rotation of the trunk to the left was possible through 65 degrees. This technique did not appear to be superior to the previous procedure in the results it produced. Postero-anterior central vertebral pressure was then carried out twice, resulting in a range of painless rotation to the left of 75 degrees. The overall rate of progress was considered to be satisfactory.

Fourth–sixth days

Treatment was continued as a combination of postero-anterior central vertebral pressure and transverse vertebral pressure, alternating from one to the other four times. These mobilizations were gradually increased in pressure day by day as symptomatic progress was made. Traction was not given for two reasons: the rate of progress was satisfactory, and the patient could afford only the minimum of time necessary for treatment now that he was able to resume the full responsibilities of his job. By the sixth day his pain was only of nuisance value and movements were full although left trunk rotation and extension still caused slight left thoracic pain. Arm movements were normal and there was no discomfort with breathing or coughing.

Further treatment

Treatment was then continued on alternate days for the next three visits, this break being caused by the pressure of his work. The same routine as had been used previously was repeated strongly, and by the last visit movements were normal and painless and the ache had gone.

ABDOMINAL PAINS AND VAGUE SIGNS

The following case history is an example of uncertain diagnosis where manipulation was used as a diagnostic trial. It is included in this chapter to show how manipulation, although an empirical form of treatment, can be used methodically and constructively as an active yet safe eliminative treatment.

Examination

History

This patient was a girl aged 12 years training for competitive swimming. While swimming 18 months ago she had a severe bout of left-sided abdominal pain, and had to be lifted out of the water. She was able to return to swimming three weeks later, and then had only occasional twinges. Two months ago vague left-sided abdominal symptoms began to return, and gradually became more persistent, preventing full swimming training. On questioning she mentioned mild soreness across the back between the levels of T12 and L2 (*Figure 8.23*) during 'out of pool training' six months ago.

Her only symptom at the time of treatment was a predominantly left-sided abdominal pain brought on by swimming and to a lesser extent by prolonged walking.

Her referring doctor suggested that she should discontinue swimming temporarily but that after a trial of manipulation she should go back into the water to assess progress.

Physical findings

On examination, all active movements were painless but active lateral flexion to the left appeared to be limited between the T12 and L2 spinous processes when compared with the same movements to the right. Passively testing the range of intervertebral movement revealed a limitation between T12 and L1 and between L1 and L2.

With the patient prone, strong pressure against the left side of the spinous process of T12 pushing it towards the right sometimes caused a pain in the left side of the abdomen.

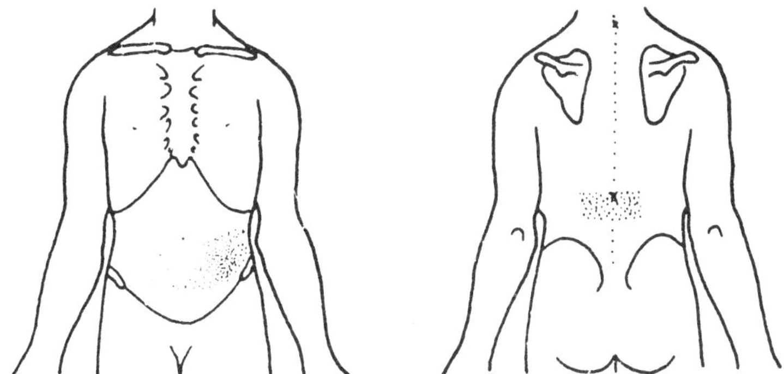

Figure 8.23. – Abdominal pains and vague signs in a young patient

Treatment

Guiding factors

1. Young people with persistent symptoms of a severity necessitating treatment are often more difficult to help than middle-aged people with similar symptoms.
2. If the symptoms arise from the thoracolumbar junction, the three main mobilizations are postero-anterior central vertebral pressure, transverse vertebral pressure and rotation as used for the lumbar spine, and the order of preference would be as listed.
3. With a limitation in the active range of movement between T12 and L2 as it exists in this patient, the transverse vertebral pressure mobilization could be done either to restore the movement, or could follow the general principle of pushing the spinous processes towards the painful side. Each of these principles would result in transverse vertebral pressures but from opposite sides.
4. The intervertebral joints T12–L1 and L1/2 can be manipulated if symptoms do not improve with mobilization.
5. Her only two true guides to progress are pain with walking and pain with swimming. If walking can be regulated, and thereby used as a guide, the swimming test can justifiably be tried when walking becomes painless.

First day

Postero-anterior central vertebral pressure was chosen to be used in conjunction with transverse vertebral pressure directed against the left side of the spinous process from T11 down to L2, aiming at reducing the active limitation of left lateral flexion (contrary to the principle 'push towards the pain'). These two mobilizations were carried out three times in each direction. The girl was asked to walk two miles before breakfast to assess the timing and the severity of pain.

Second day

The patient reported left abdominal pains of short duration after 500 yards and again after 900 yards. Active left lateral flexion looked unchanged and there was some local vertebral soreness from the previous day's treatment. As no reason could be seen for assuming that the patient was either worse or better the previous day's treatment was repeated. She was asked to repeat her walking test before breakfast.

Third day

Pain was less severe with walking on this morning. Left-sided twinges were experienced once at 600 yards and once at 800 yards. As this indicated possible progress, the same mobilizing procedure was repeated.

Fourth day

Twinges of pain experienced with the walking test were approximately the same as the previous day.

Lateral flexion appeared unaltered. It was felt that this should have improved and also that the walking test should have shown further progress after the third day's treatment. Treatment was therefore altered to transverse vertebral pressure only, but directed against the right side of the spinous processes of T11 and T12, pushing towards the painful side. This was carried out four times, each time lasting approximately a minute with an assessment of her active left lateral flexion between. This movement did not appear to change.

Fifth day

There was no pain with walking this morning, and on examination left lateral flexion showed slight improvement. The fourth day's treatment was repeated and it was suggested that a half-a-mile swim should be attempted.

Sixth day

Only two momentary twinges were felt with the swim. Lateral flexion had improved a little more. Very strong pressure against the left side of T12 no longer produced abdominal pain. The treatment of the fourth and fifth days was repeated, and a two mile swim was suggested.

Seventh day

No symptoms resulted from further swimming. Lateral flexion appeared to be unchanged from the sixth day. It was decided to discontinue treatment as normal swimming training the preceding day did not produce any symptoms.

At the end of her full summer training programme four months later she reported that there had been no further trouble.

Appendix 1

Movement Diagram: A Teaching Aid and a Means of Communication

It is emphasized that the movement diagram should be used solely as a teaching aid or means of communication. When examining, say, postero-anterior movement of the C3/4 intervertebral joint produced by pressure on the spinous processes (*see Figure 2.11,* page 35) newcomers to this method of examination will find it difficult to know what they are feeling. However the Movement Diagram makes them analyse the movement in terms of range, pain and muscle spasm. Also it makes them analyse the manner in which these factors affect the movement.

The components considered in the diagram are *pain, spasm-free resistance* (stiffness) and *muscle spasm* found on joint examination, their relative strength and behaviour in all parts of the available range and in relation to each other. Thus the response of the joint to movement is shown in a very detailed way. The theory of the movement diagram is described in this appendix by discussing its components separately. The practical compilation of a diagram for one direction of movement of one joint on a particular patient is given in Appendix 2.

Each of the above components is an extensive subject in itself and it should be realized that discussion in this appendix is deliberately limited in the following ways. Discussion of pain is confined to pain felt at the site of the joint examined; referred pain is not dealt with, although if the essence of the exercise is grasped, it will be seen how the diagram can be extended to include referred pain. The spasm referred to is protective muscle spasm secondary to joint disorder; spasticity caused by upper motor neurone disease and the voluntary contraction of muscles is excluded. Frequently this voluntary contraction is out of all proportion to the pain being experienced yet in very direct proportion to the patient's apprehension about the examiner's handling of the joint. Careless handling will provoke such a reaction and thereby obscure the real clinical findings. Resistance (stiffness) free of muscle spasm is discussed only from the clinical point of view; that is, discussion about the pathology causing the stiffness is excluded.

A movement diagram is compiled by drawing graphs for the behaviour of pain, physical resistance and muscle spasm, depicting the position in the range at which each is felt (this is shown on the horizontal line AB) and the intensity of each (which is shown on the vertical line AC) (*Figure A1.1*).

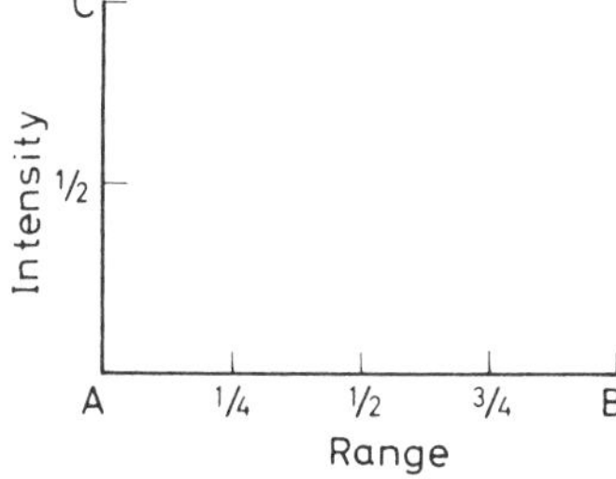

Figure A1.1. – Beginning of movement diagram

The base line AB represents any range of movement from the starting position at A to the limit of the normal range at B. It makes no difference whether the movement depicted is small or large, whether it involves one joint or a group of joints working together, or whether it represents the whole range or part of the range. For example, AB might represent 2 mm of postero-anterior movement on the spinous process of C4 or 90 degrees of cervical rotation to the left.

Point B is *always constant*, and *always* at the extreme of normal average range of passive movement. On the other hand, point A, the starting position of the movement, is variable: its position may be the extreme of range opposite B or somewhere in mid-range, whichever is most suitable for the diagram. For example, if cervical rotation is the movement being represented and the pain or limitation occurs only in the last 10 degrees of the range, the diagram will more clearly demonstrate the behaviour of the three factors if the base line represents 20 degrees rather than 90 degrees of cervical rotation. For the purpose of clarity position A is defined by stating the angle or amplitude represented by the base line AB. In the above example, if the base line represents 90 degrees, A must be at the position with the head facing straight forwards and similarly, if the base line represents 20 degrees, position A is with the head turned 70 degrees to the left (assuming of course that the normal average range of rotation is 90 degrees to each side).

As the movement diagram is used to depict what can be felt when examining passive movement, it must be clearly understood that point B represents the extreme of passive movement, and that this lies variably, but very importantly, beyond the extreme of active movement.

The vertical axis AC represents the intensity of the factors being plotted; point A represents complete absence of the factor and point C represents the factor's maximum intensity. The meaning of 'maximum' in relation to each factor is discussed later for further clarification.

The basic diagram is completed by vertical and horizontal lines drawn from B and C to meet at D (*Figure A1.2*).

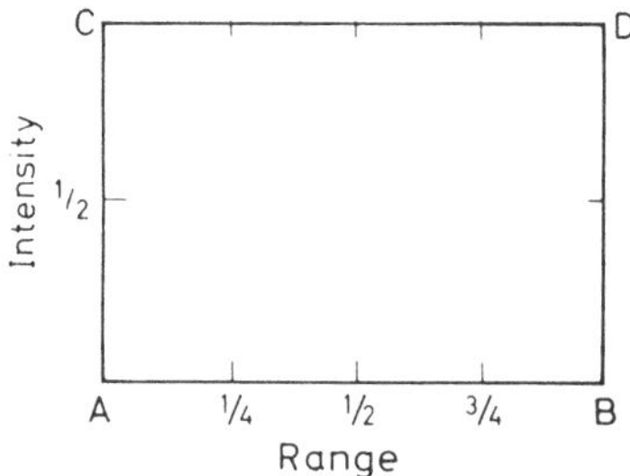

Figure A1.2. – Completion of movement diagram

PAIN

The initial fact to be established is whether or not the patient has any pain while the joint is at rest.

The first step is to move the joint slowly and carefully into the range being tested, asking the patient to report immediately when any discomfort is felt. The position at which this is first felt is noted.

The second step consists of several small oscillatory movements in different parts of the pain-free range, gradually moving further into the range up to the point where pain is first felt, thus establishing the exact position of the onset of the pain. There is no danger of exacerbation if sufficient care is used and if the examiner bears in mind that it is the very first provocation of pain which is being sought. The point at which this occurs is called P_1 and is marked on the base line of the diagram (*Figure A1.3*).

Thus there are two steps to establishing P_1:

1. a single slow movement first, and then
2. small oscillatory movements.

If the pain is reasonably severe then the point found with the single slow movement will be deeper in the range than that found with oscillatory movements. Having thus found where the pain is first felt, the oscillatory test movements will be carried out in a part of the range which will not provoke exacerbation.

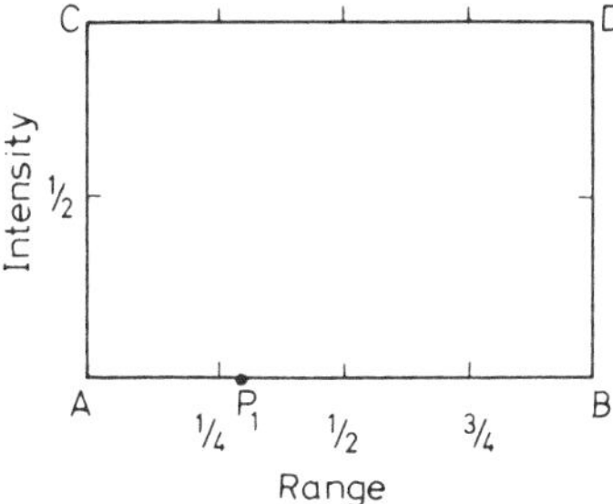

Figure A1.3. – Onset of pain

The next step is to determine the available range of movement. This is done by slowly moving the joint through pain until the limit of the range is reached. This point is marked on the base line as L (*Figure A1.4*).

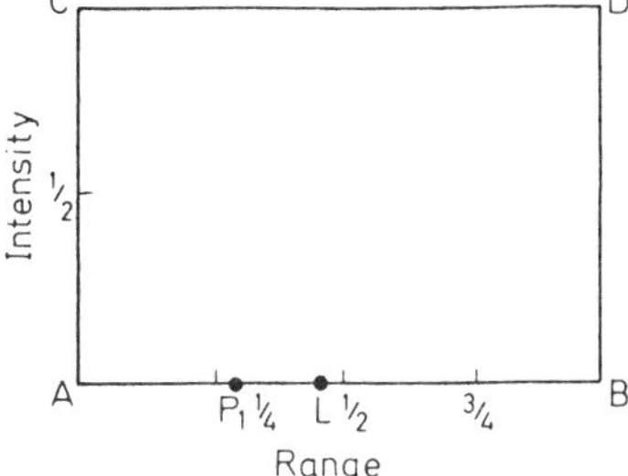

Figure A1.4. – Limit of the range

As we are only discussing pain at this stage P_2 is then marked vertically above L at maximum intensity (*Figure A1.5*).

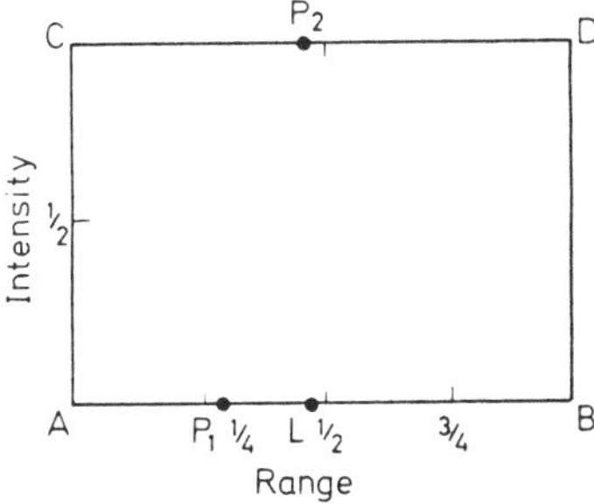

Figure A1.5. – Maximum intensity of pain

To represent on the graph the behaviour of the pain between P_1 and P_2, the intensity of pain in any one position is assessed as lying somewhere on the vertical axis of the graph (i.e. between A and C) between no pain at all (i.e. A) and the maximum (i.e. C). It is important to realize that maximum intensity of pain in the diagram represents the maximum amount of pain the physiotherapist is prepared to provoke. This point is well within, and quite different from, a level representing intolerable pain for the patient. Estimation of 'maximum' in this way is, of course, entirely subjective, and varies from person to person.

If pain increases evenly with movement into the painful range the line joining P_1 and P_2 is a straight line (*Figure A1.6*).

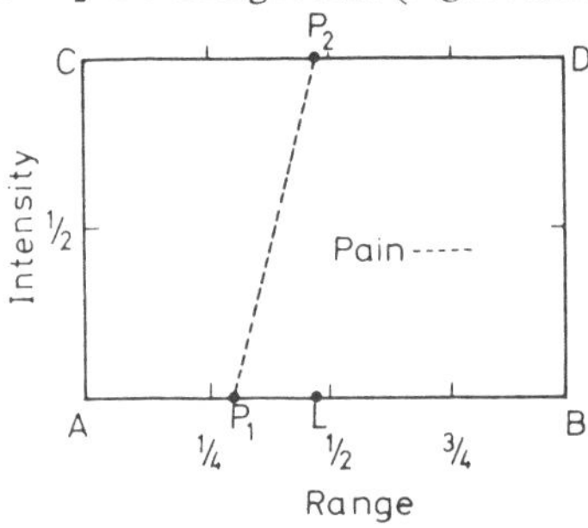

Figure A1.6. – Pain increasing evenly with movement

However, pain may not increase evenly in this way, its build-up may be irregular, calling for a graph which is curved or angular. Pain may be first felt at about quarter range and may initially increase quickly to near maximum; then the movement can be taken further until a limiting intensity at three-quarter range is reached (*Figure A1.7*).

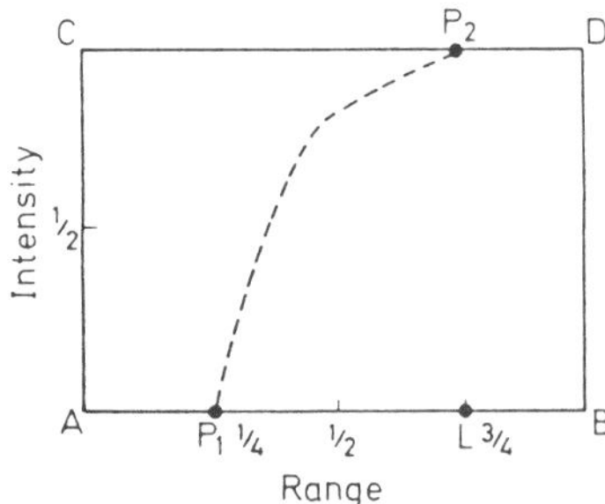

Figure A1.7. – Irregular increase of pain

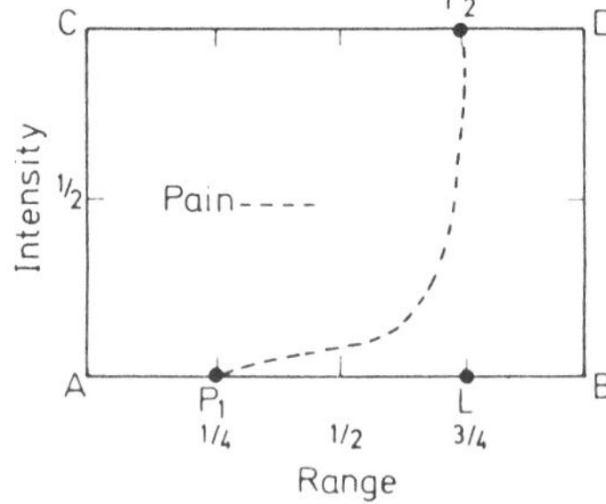

Figure A1.8. – Pain reaching a maximum at three-quarter range

In another example pain may be first felt at quarter range and remain at a low level until suddenly its intensity increases, reaching a maximum at three-quarter range (*Figure A1.8*).

The examples given demonstrate pain which limits movement of the joint, but there are instances where pain may never reach a limiting intensity. *Figure A1.9* is an example where a little pain may be felt at

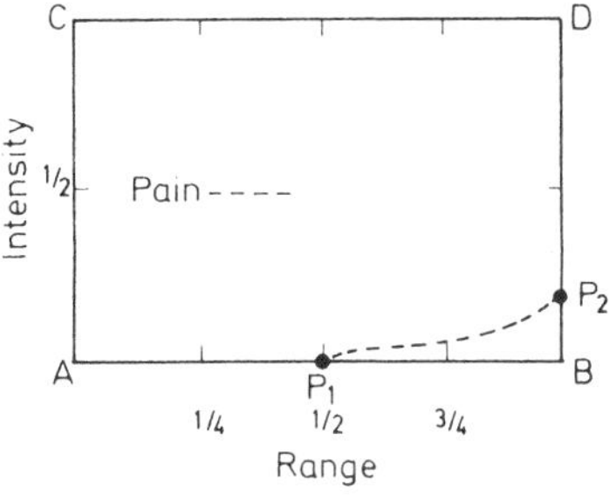

Figure A1.9. – Pain with no limiting intensity

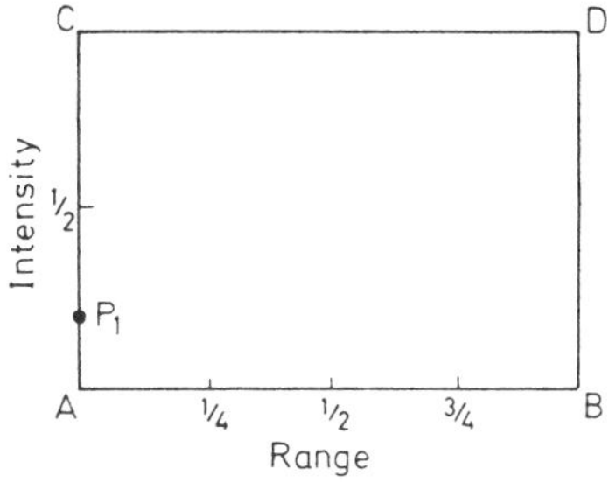

Figure A1.10. – Pain in joint at rest

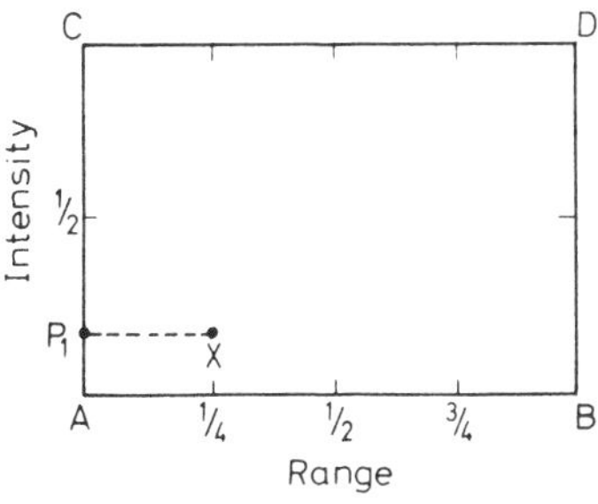

Figure A1.11. – Level where pain begins to increase

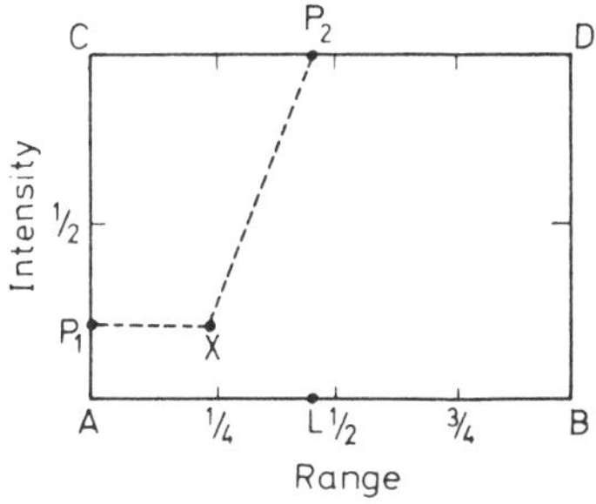

Figure A1.12. – Pain due to subsequent movement

half range but the pain scarcely increases beyond this point in the range and the end of normal range may be reached without provoking anything approaching such intensity as would forbid further movement. There is thus no point L, and P_2 appears on the vertical line BD to indicate the intensity of the pain at that point.

If we now return to an example where the joint is painful at rest, mentioned at the beginning of this appendix, an estimate must be made of the amount of pain present at rest and this appears as P_1 on the vertical axis AC (*Figure A1.10*). Movement is then begun slowly and carefully until the original level of pain begins to increase (X in *Figure A1.11*). The behaviour of pain beyond this point is plotted in the manner already described and an example of such a graph is given in *Figure A1.12*.

When the joint is painful at rest the symptoms are easily exacerbated by poor handling. However, if examination is carried out with care and skill no difficulty is encountered.

Again it must be emphasized that this evaluation of pain is purely subjective. Nevertheless it presents an invaluable method whereby students can learn to perceive different behaviours of pain, and their appreciation of these variations of pain patterns will mature as this type of assessment is practised from patient to patient and checked against the judgement of a more experienced physiotherapist.

RESISTANCE (FREE OF MUSCLE SPASM)

A normal joint, when completely relaxed and moved passively, has the feel of being well oiled and friction free. It can be likened to wet soap sliding on wet glass. It is important for a physiotherapist using passive movement as a form of treatment to appreciate the difference between a free-running, friction-free movement and one which, although being full range, has minor resistance within the range of movement.

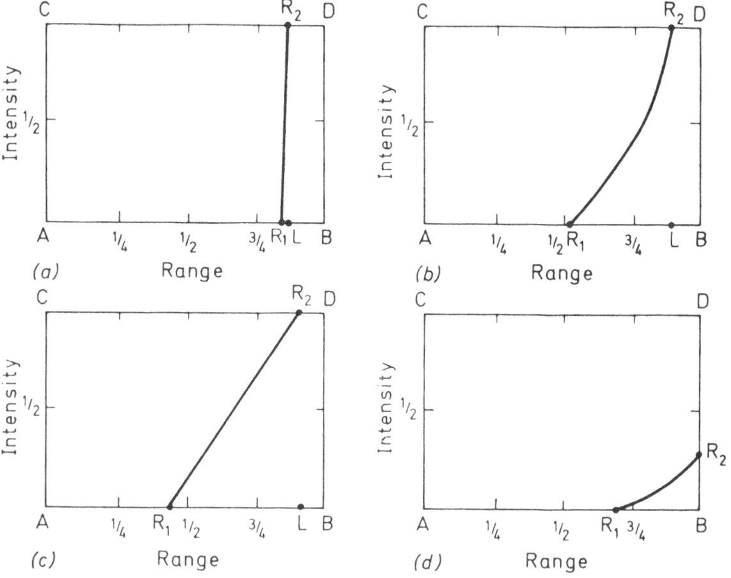

Figure A1.13. – Spasm-free resistance

The best way to appreciate the free running of a joint is to support and hold around the joint with one hand while, with the other hand, producing an oscillatory movement back and forth through a chosen path of the range. If this movement is felt to be friction free then the oscillatory movement can be moved more deeply into the range. In this way the total available range can be assessed. With experience, by comparing patients and also comparing a patient's right side with his left side, the physiotherapist will quickly learn to appreciate minor resistance to movement. Point R_1 is then established and marked on the base line AB. The joint movement is then taken to the limit of the range. If resistance limits movement, the range is assessed and marked by L on the base line.

Vertically above L, R_2 is drawn on CD to indicate that it is resistance which limited the range. Following this the behaviour of the resistance between R_1 and R_2 is assessed by movements back and forth in the range between R_1 and L and the line depicting the behaviour of the resistance is drawn on the diagram (*Figure A1.13*). As with pain, resistance can vary in its behaviour and examples are shown in *Figure A1.13a, b, c* and *d*.

MUSCLE SPASM

There are two kinds of muscle spasm to consider: one which always limits range and occupies a small part of it, and another which occurs as a quick contraction to prevent a painful movement.

Frequently, whether it is spasm or stiffness which is limiting the range can only be accurately assessed by repeated movement, taken somewhat beyond the point at which resistance is first encountered and performed at different speeds. Muscle spasm can be shown to have the power of recoil. In contrast, resistance which is free of muscle activity does not have this quality; rather it is constant in strength at any given point in the range. Also, any increase in strength will be directly in proportion to the depth in range, regardless of the speed with which movement is carried out; that is, the resistance felt at one point in movement will always be less than that felt at a point deeper in the range. (If pain is severe, or irritability high, it may be impossible to carry out this method of assessment, and full examination of physical resistance is then, quite correctly, not completed. As always, a balance must be sought between gaining sufficient information to guide treatment and avoiding exacerbation of the symptoms by over-examination).

The first kind of muscle spasm will feel like spring steel and will push back against the testing movement, particularly if the test movement is varied in speed and in position in the range.

Testing this kind of spasm is done by moving the joint to the point at which spasm is first elicited, and this point is noted on the base line at S_1. Further movement is then attempted. If maximum intensity is reached before the end of range, spasm thus becomes a limiting factor.

This limit is noted by L on the base line and S_2 is marked vertically above L on the upper horizontal. The graph for the behaviour of spasm is plotted between S_1 and S_2 (*Figure A1.14*). It will be found that when muscle spasm limits range it always reaches its maximum quickly, and thus occupies only a small part of the range. Therefore it will always be depicted as a near-vertical line (*Figure A1.14a* and *b*). In some cases when the joint condition is less severe, a little spasm which increases slightly but never prohibits full movement may be felt just before the end of range (*Figure A1.14c*).

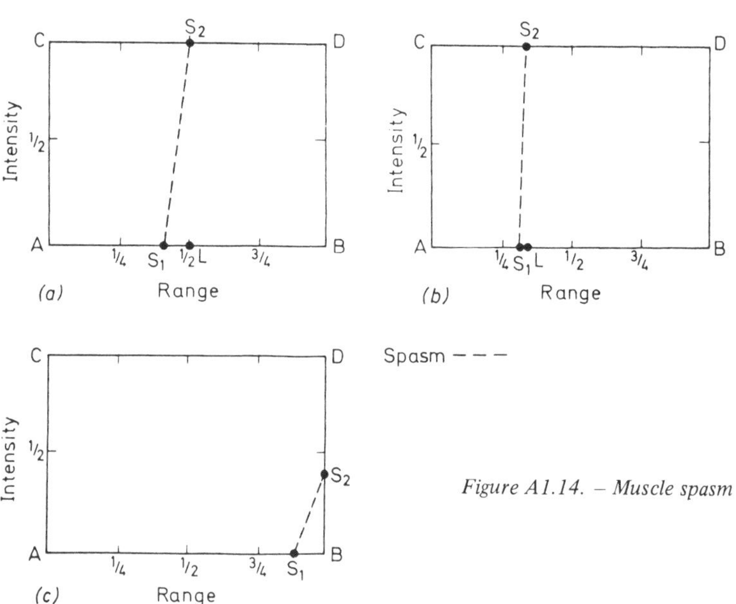

Figure A1.14. – Muscle spasm

The second kind of muscle spasm is directly proportional to the severity of the patient's pain: movement of the joint in varying parts of the range causes sharply limiting quick muscular contraction. This usually occurs when a very painful joint is moved without adequate care and can be completely avoided if the joint is well supported and moved gently. This spasm is reflex in type, coming into action very rapidly during the test movement. A very similar kind of muscular contraction can occur as a voluntary action by the patient, indicating a sharp increase in pain. If the physiotherapist varies the speed of her test movements she will be able to distinguish quickly between the reflex spasm and the voluntary spasm because of the speed with which

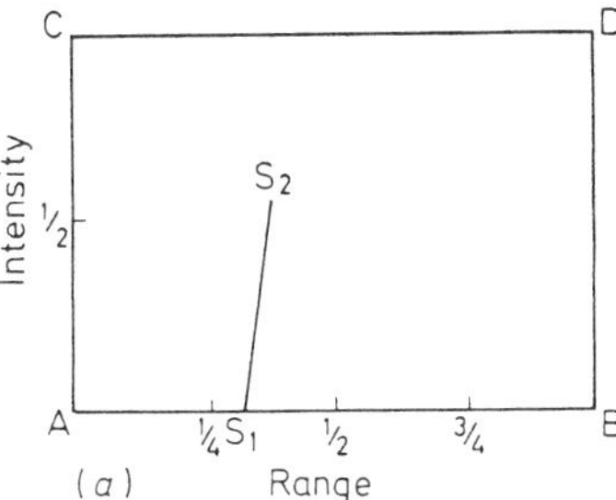

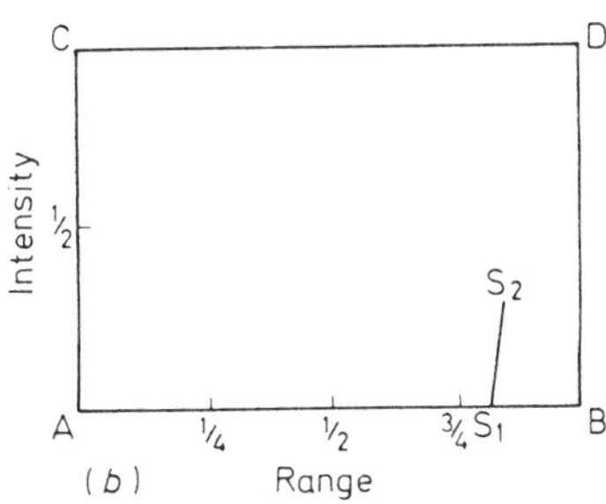

Figure A1.15. – Spasm which does not limit range of movement

the spasm occurs–reflex spasm occurs more quickly in response to a provoking movement than does voluntary spasm. This second kind of spasm, which does not limit a range of movement, can usually be avoided by careful handling during the test.

To represent this kind of spasm, a near-vertical line is drawn from the base line; its height and position on the base line will signify whether or not the spasm is easy to provoke and will also give some indication of its strength. Two examples are drawn of the extremes which may be found (*Figure A1.15a* and *b*).

Appendix 2

Compiling a Movement Diagram

This book places great emphasis on the behaviour of pain with the different movements of disordered joints. Pain is of major importance to the patient and therefore takes priority in the examination of joint movement. The following is the practicality of the diagram. When testing (say) the C3/4 joint by postero-anterior pressure on the spinous process of C3 (or any other palpation test on pages 34–42) the routine is as follows:

1. Gentle, increasing pressure is applied very slowly to the spinous process of C3 in a postero-anterior direction and the patient is asked to report when he first feels pain. This point in the range is noted and the physiotherapist should then release some of the pressure from the spinous process and perform small oscillatory movements. Again she asks the patient if he feels any pain. If he does not, the oscillation should then be carried out slightly deeper into the range and conversely if he does, the oscillatory movement should be withdrawn in the range. By these oscillatory movements in different parts of the range the point at which pain is first felt with movement can be identified and is then recorded on the base line of the movement diagram as P_1 (*Figure A2.1*). The estimation of P_1 is best achieved by performing the oscillations at what the physiotherapist feels is $^1/_4$ range, then at $^1/_3$ range and then $^1/_2$ range. By this means P_1 can be very accurately assessed. Therefore there are two steps to establishing P_1:

   (*a*) a single slow movement, and
   (*b*) small oscillatory movements.

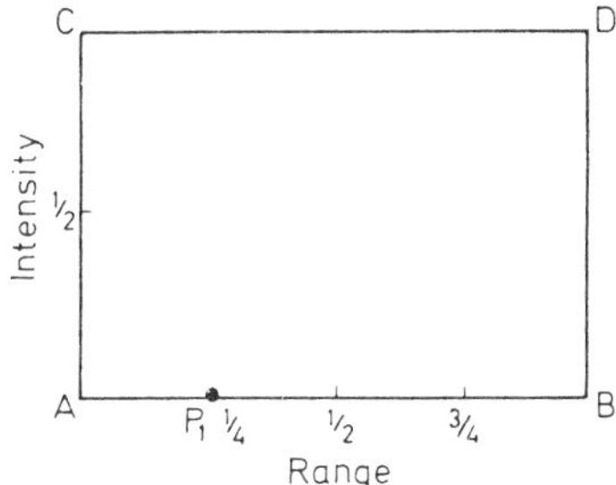

Figure A2.1. – Point at which pain is first felt

2. Having found P_1 the physiotherapist should continue with the postero-anterior movements until she reaches the limit of the range. She identifies that position of the range and records it on the base line of the movement diagram as point L (*Figure A2.2*). If the movement being tested were hypermobile the point L would be shown as being beyond B (*Figure A2.3*).

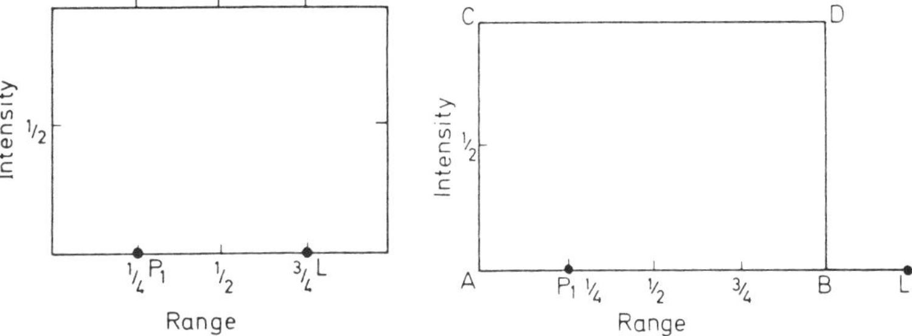

Figure A2.2. – Limit of the range

Figure A2.3. – Hypermobile movement

3. For the hypermobile or hypomobile joint the next step is to decide *why* the movement was stopped at point L. If we assume for the purpose of the example the movement was hypomobile and that it was physical resistance, free of muscle spasm, which prevented the movement, then vertically above L on the horizontal projection CD, the point where these two lines meet is marked as R_2 (*Figure A2.4a*). If the joint were hypermobile the diagram would be as in *Figure A2.4b*.

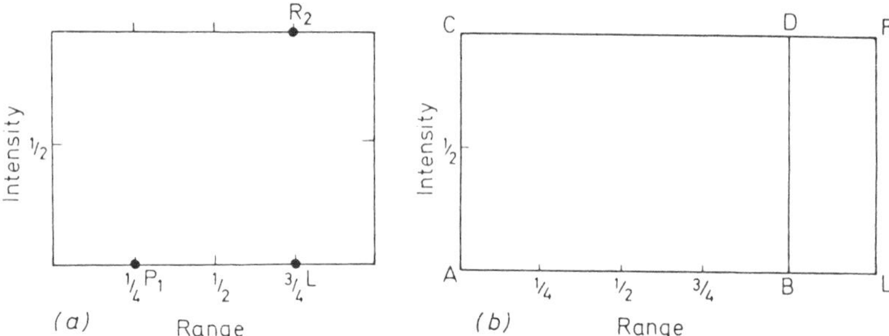

Figure A2.4. – Spasm-free resistance limiting movement in (a) hypomobile joint and (b) hypermobile joint

4. The physiotherapist then decides the intensity of the pain at the limit of the range. This can be estimated in relation to what maximum would feel like and also what 50 per cent of maximum would feel like. By this means the intensity of the pain is fairly easily decided thus enabling the physiotherapist to put P_2 on the vertical above L in its accurately estimated position (*Figure A2.5*).

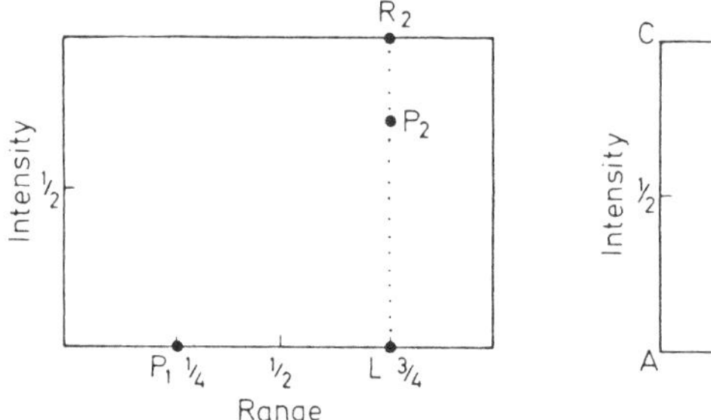

Figure A2.5. – Intensity of pain

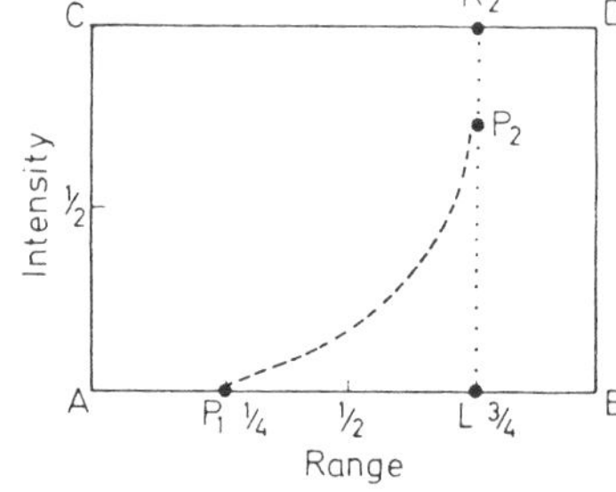

Figure A2.6. – Behaviour of the pain

5. The C3/4 joint is then moved in a postero-anterior direction between P_1 and L to determine, by watching the patient's hands and face and also by questioning him, how the pain behaves between P_1 and P_2. The line representing the behaviour of pain is then drawn on the movement diagram, that is, the line P_1 P_2 is completed (*Figure A2.6*).

6. Having completed the representation of pain, resistance must be considered. This is achieved by receding further back in the range than the point P_1 where, with carefully applied and carefully felt oscillatory movements, the presence or not of any resistance is ascertained. Where it commences is noted and marked on the base line AB as R_1 (*Figure A2.7*).

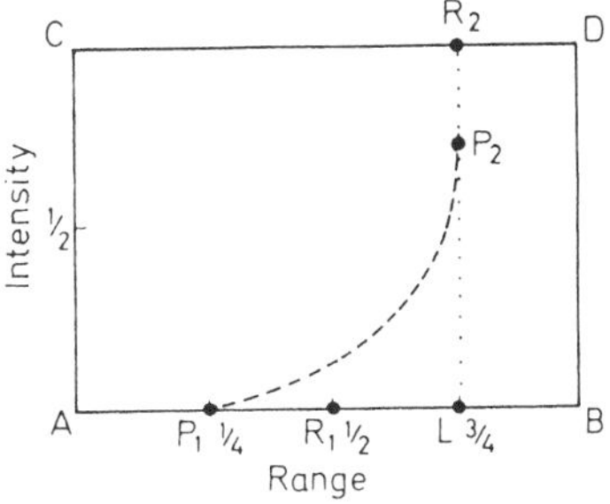

Figure A2.7. – Commencement of resistance

7. By moving the joint between R_1 and L the behaviour of the resistance can be determined and plotted on the graph between the points R_1 and R_2 (*Figure A2.8*).

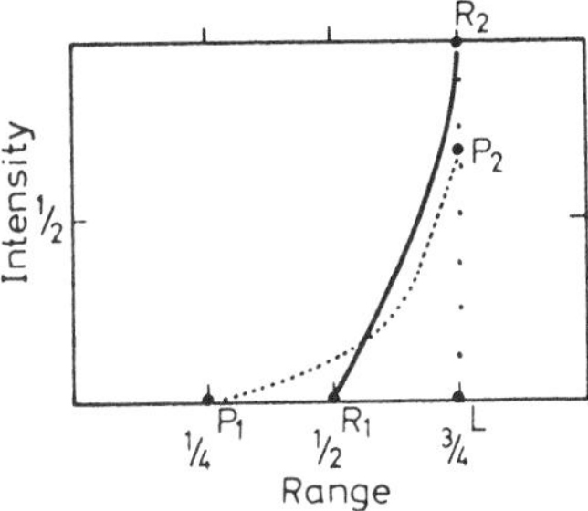

Figure A2.8 – Behaviour of resistance

8. If no muscle spasm has been felt during this examination and if the patient's pain is not excessive, the physiotherapist should continue the oscillatory postero-anterior movements on C3 but perform them more sharply and quicker to determine whether any spasm can be provoked. If no spasm can be provoked, then there is nothing to record on the movement diagram. However, if with quick sharper movements a reflex type of muscle spasm is elicited to protect the movement this should be

drawn on the movement diagram in a manner which will indicate how easy or difficult it is to provoke (i.e. by placing the spasm line towards A if it is easy to provoke, and towards B if it is difficult to provoke). The strength of the spasm so provoked is indicated by the height of the spasm line (*Figure A2.9*).

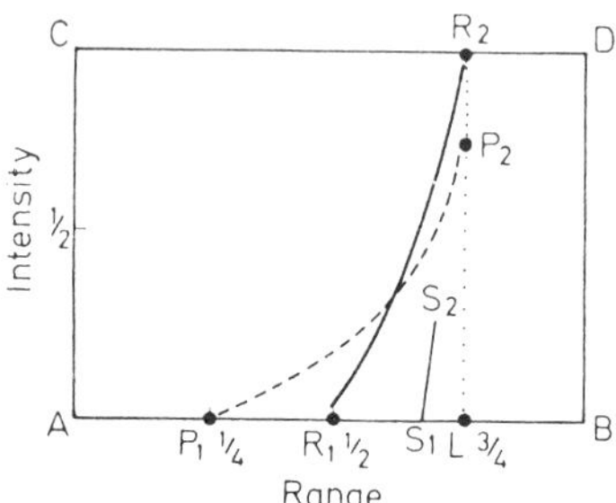

Figure A2.9. – Strength of spasm

Thus the diagram for that movement is compiled showing the behaviour of all elements. It is then possible to assess any relationships between the factors found on the examination. The relationships give a distinct guide as to the treatment which should be given particularly in relation to the 'grade' of the treatment movements.

Index